Medical School for Everyone: Grand Rounds Cases

Roy Benaroch, M.D.

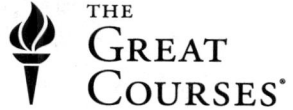

PUBLISHED BY:

THE GREAT COURSES
Corporate Headquarters
4840 Westfields Boulevard, Suite 500
Chantilly, Virginia 20151-2299
Phone: 1-800-832-2412
Fax: 703-378-3819
www.thegreatcourses.com

Copyright © The Teaching Company, 2014

Printed in the United States of America

This book is in copyright. All rights reserved.

Without limiting the rights under copyright reserved above,
no part of this publication may be reproduced, stored in
or introduced into a retrieval system, or transmitted,
in any form, or by any means
(electronic, mechanical, photocopying, recording, or otherwise),
without the prior written permission of
The Teaching Company.

Roy Benaroch, M.D.
Adjunct Assistant Professor of Pediatrics
Emory University School of Medicine

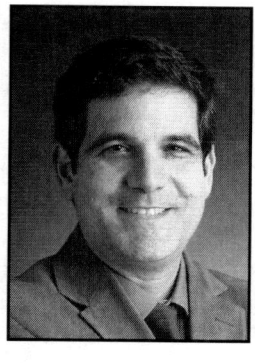

Dr. Roy Benaroch is a general pediatrician, an author, and an educator. He earned his B.S. in Engineering at Tulane University, followed by his M.D. at Emory University. He completed his residency through Emory University's affiliated hospitals in 1997, serving as chief resident and instructor of pediatrics in 1998. He has continued his involvement on the Emory faculty as an Adjunct Assistant Professor of Pediatrics. Dr. Benaroch was board certified in general pediatrics in 1997 and practices full time at Pediatric Physicians, PC, located near Atlanta, Georgia.

In addition to his clinical responsibilities as a pediatrician, Dr. Benaroch teaches medical students and residents at his practice and gives regular lectures to physician's assistants at Emory University.

Dr. Benaroch has published two books on parenting and pediatric health topics: *Solving Health and Behavioral Problems from Birth through Preschool: A Parent's Guide* and *A Guide to Getting the Best Health Care for Your Child*. He also has a blog for parents and health professionals at pediatricinsider.com. His essays on pediatric health have been widely published on the Internet, and he has served as a featured expert on WebMD.com.

In addition to his work in private practice and as a teacher and writer, Dr. Benaroch also serves on the board of directors of the Cobb Health Futures Foundation, Inc., a nonprofit group dedicated to public health for people of all backgrounds. ∎

Table of Contents

INTRODUCTION

Professor Biography i
Course Scope 1

LECTURE GUIDES

LECTURE 1
I Never Feel Good 3

LECTURE 2
A Persistent Fever 22

LECTURE 3
Puzzling Pain 41

LECTURE 4
Just Look at Me 60

LECTURE 5
Headaches in Wonderland 78

LECTURE 6
The Tennis Player 97

LECTURE 7
Sudden Collapse 116

LECTURE 8
School Failure 135

LECTURE 9
Dizzy Attacks 154

LECTURE 10
Weight Loss 174

Table of Contents

LECTURE 11
I Can't Walk 193

LECTURE 12
Learning from Failure 212

LECTURE 13
The Children Who Come and Go 231

LECTURE 14
Guardians' Day 250

LECTURE 15
Dickens's Diagnosis 269

LECTURE 16
Shaking Sammi 288

LECTURE 17
Hickam's Dictum 306

LECTURE 18
Forgetting Jerusalem 326

LECTURE 19
Sherlock's Investigation 344

LECTURE 20
The Boy Who Doesn't Speak 363

LECTURE 21
Antarctic Adventure 382

LECTURE 22
A Sunday Drive 400

LECTURE 23
Cough, Cough, Cough 419

Table of Contents

LECTURE 24
A Confused Father..438

SUPPLEMENTAL MATERIAL

Glossary 458
Bibliography...469

Disclaimer

This series of lectures is intended to increase your understanding of how doctors diagnose and treat diseases and how you can improve your own health by being an active and informed patient. However, these lectures are not designed for use as medical references to diagnose, treat, or prevent medical illnesses or trauma, and neither The Teaching Company nor the lecturer is responsible for your use of this educational material or its consequences. Furthermore, participating in this course does not create a doctor-patient relationship. The information contained in these lectures is neither intended to dictate what constitutes reasonable, appropriate, or best care for any given health issue and does not take into account the unique circumstances that define the health issues of the patient. If you have questions about the diagnosis, treatment, or prevention of a medical condition or illness, you should consult your personal physician. The opinions and positions provided in these lectures reflect the opinions and positions of the relevant lecturer and do not necessarily reflect the opinions or positions of The Teaching Company or its affiliates.

The Teaching Company expressly DISCLAIMS LIABILITY for any DIRECT, INDIRECT, INCIDENTAL, SPECIAL, OR CONSEQUENTIAL DAMAGES OR LOST PROFITS that result directly or indirectly from the use of these lectures. In states which do not allow some or all of the above limitations of liability, liability shall be limited to the greatest extent allowed by law.

Medical School for Everyone: Grand Rounds Cases

Scope:

We're all fascinated by medical knowledge. From popular television shows to our own visits to the doctor to reports of medical breakthroughs, the culture of medical knowledge has become commonplace in our everyday world. Understanding medicine isn't just enlightening—it can improve your own health and help you cultivate a more beneficial relationship with your doctors.

This course offers a miniature medical school curriculum for nondoctors, structured into a "grand rounds" format similar to how medical students and experienced physicians are taught at hospitals and universities. Each lecture concentrates on a single clinical case. A real patient will be presented, from the initial complaint through the diagnostic process to the treatment decisions, discussing the details of each step. You will follow along as each diagnostic clue is uncovered, with the goal of taking the next best step toward helping the patient. Every lecture is, in a way, a medical mystery—and by the end of each lecture, you will not only understand more about the diagnosis, but also gain insight into how doctors work and think. You will get an insider's view of the art of medical decision making that's rarely revealed to patients.

Topics covered include an overview of many common diseases, including their symptoms and evaluation and treatment; the diagnostic tools of the physician, including the medical history and physical exam along with lab tests, radiology, and other modalities used to diagnose and treat disease; and how patients can best help their own doctors get the information they need. Along the way, you will pick up diagnostic pearls about disease, along with information that is typically only known to medical professionals: their lingo, their style of thinking, and how they go about evaluating patients.

The case histories cover a wide range of patient ages and concerns. You will meet a young man with a chronic fever and a woman with abdominal pain. There's a preteen with a mysterious rash, a woman with dizzy spells, and a woman with an itchy rash that keeps coming back. You will meet patients who are fatigued and patients who are coughing; patients with chest pain and trouble talking; patients with blurry vision; and a surgeon who had to diagnose and treat himself. Some problems may seem simple at first; some unfold quickly into catastrophe. Some illustrate that there's always hope, and others reveal the limits of what modern medicine can and cannot do. What brings these cases together is a common thread: that medical doctors and patients alike can learn from patient experiences. In fact, doctors' best teachers are their patients.

Patients—and medical professionals, and those considering or pursuing a career in medicine—will enjoy solving the mysteries in each case and learning solid medical information about diagnosis and treatment. But the lasting lessons of this course will be the ones best remembered: how to communicate with physicians, how to help coordinate care when seeing multiple specialists, and how to get the most out of every medical encounter. There are plenty of immediately practical lessons, too: what to do when someone nearby collapses and what kinds of symptoms warrant immediate evaluation. You will also learn about how to talk with people facing serious illnesses—how to share bad news and how to help steer people toward wellness and recovery.

This course reveals how doctors think and how, as a patient, you can improve your own medical experiences through a better understanding of their education and training. By the end of the course, you will not just understand the field of medicine better, but you will also become a better—and healthier—patient. ■

I Never Feel Good
Lecture 1

In this course, you'll be exposed to a wide variety of symptoms and diseases, and you'll get a good appreciation for how the body works in health and disease. More importantly, though, by the end of this course, you'll have a much better understanding of how doctors think. By learning this, you will also learn how to be a better patient yourself. Understanding what doctors do—and how and why they do it—will make you a better patient and improve your health.

From Chief Complaint to Diagnosis
- Imagine that you are working in an **internal medicine** clinic. A 55-year-old woman comes to the clinic with a **chief complaint** of "I never feel good." A patient's chief complaint is a quote, in the patient's own words, of what his or her main concern is. Why did this person come to see the doctor? It's a very important bit of information, because it focuses the evaluation on what the patient is worried about.

- Sometimes chief complaints don't end up being the main thing that the doctor is worried about and don't directly point to the final diagnosis. But the chief complaint is still something crucial to know when you're getting started.

- In this case, the chief complaint is vague: "I never feel good." It doesn't really help us narrow down anything, but it does tell us that the patient is really suffering and always feels bad in some way—and maybe has felt bad for a long time.

- After the chief complaint, we take a **history of present illness (HPI)**, which is the patient's story of what's going on, when it started, and what sort of factors influence the symptoms. When we take an HPI, it's important to let the patient do most of the talking. We'll give a bit of a lead or push now and then, with questions to clarify the story, but this is the time for the patient to tell us what's going on—not the other way around.

- The 55-year-old woman presented a constellation of symptoms, with a history of several seemingly unrelated problems. She had broken a bone and was noted to be deficient in vitamin D; she was also **anemic**, or deficient in iron. She had very low energy. She had a number of different gastrointestinal (GI) complaints spanning several years, some of which seemed to come and go, perhaps at times related to the ingestion of milk.

- The history, our most important diagnostic tool, is followed by a physical exam—to clarify our suspicions and to drive some considerations higher or lower on our list of possibilities.

- After the physical exam, it's time to see if we can make a list of possible diagnoses and then narrow and refine the list based on all of the information we have. When there are many symptoms, as in this case, it may not be possible to fit all of them into one diagnosis, and that's okay. After all, not everyone with disease X has every single symptom that's typical of disease X, and sometimes people with disease X also have a little bit of disease Y.

- To confirm a diagnosis from a list, or to strike off other diagnoses as being not possible, the next step in our evaluation is to order tests. These can include blood work, X-rays, or other sorts of investigations. Labs and X-rays aren't done to fish around and find a diagnosis, but to confirm or refute what we already suspect. That is how doctors think.

- For this patient, her gallbladder ultrasound came back normal, and a chest X-ray was normal, including normal heart size. An electrocardiogram was normal, further confirming that there was no heart disease. Blood tests revealed normal thyroid functioning, low vitamin D levels, and mild anemia. In addition, there was no evidence of ongoing **inflammation** or infection.

- A test confirmed the diagnosis that best fits what we know so far: A blood test was **positive** for **antibodies** seen in celiac disease. The diagnosis of celiac was then confirmed by a gut wall biopsy.

- The key to making the diagnosis is to get all of the information together and to think broadly about what could account for everything. Listening to the patient tell her story is the source of our best clues.

Celiac Disease
- Celiac disease is a chronic disorder that causes malabsorption of nutrients from the gut, leading to a myriad of symptoms that can include fatigue, anemia, and almost any GI symptom. In celiac disease, malabsorption of nutrients can also affect the bones—decreased absorption of dietary Vitamin D, phosphorus, and calcium can cause decreased bone density.

- With celiac disease, the lining of the gut—the small, fingerlike projections where absorption of food nutrients occurs—is damaged, and the net effect is that nutrients are not absorbed across the gut wall into the blood for use by the body.

- The **primary** symptoms of celiac disease are caused by inadequate nutrient availability and also by the GI effects of having, essentially, food staying in the gut instead of moving into your body. This includes diarrhea, bloating, and abdominal pain.

- Sometimes, constipation can be more of a problem than diarrhea, or—as in the case of the 55-year-old patient—there can be periods of time when these seemingly opposite symptoms go back and forth. Many celiac symptoms also occur outside of the gut.

- Celiac disease was known to the ancient Greeks, who referred to a condition called *koiliakos*, meaning "suffering of the bowels." A patient case written in the second century described a man with stomach pain who was underweight, pale, weak, and incapable of working—which is still a pretty good description of a severe case in modern times. The Greek term was translated to the term "celiac" in 1856.

- Around that time, it was recognized that this was a disease that could be managed by diet. In 1954, Dutch pediatrician Willem Dicke linked the disease to the ingestion of wheat protein. It's speculated that his experience seeing patients improve during the famine of 1944, when wheat was scarce, may have helped him recognize the critical role of wheat in this illness.

- Though the symptoms of celiac disease are varied and affect many organ systems, it only has one cause: ingesting certain proteins found in wheat, barley, and rye. These are natural proteins from a family called gluten proteins. Celiac disease is sometimes called "gluten enteropathy" or "celiac sprue."

- When gluten-containing foods are eaten by people with celiac disease, these proteins are modified or processed so that they

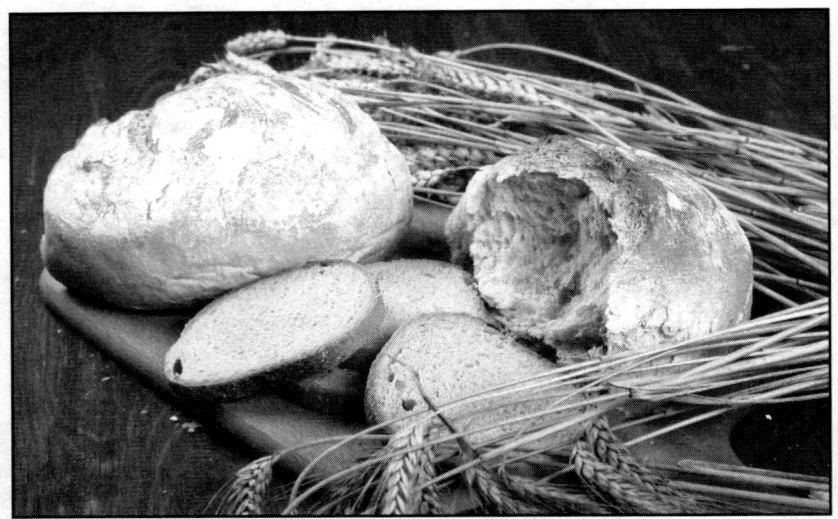

People with celiac disease cannot tolerate gluten, which is a substance that is found in wheat and flour.

trigger a cross reaction with gut tissue. Basically, the body's own immune system is tricked into attacking healthy cells in the gut (and probably elsewhere, too).

- Celiac disease is in a sense an autoimmune disease—the body attacks itself—but it's an autoimmune disease that has specific and avoidable trigger. It's the gluten proteins that trigger the reaction, and once gluten is no longer part of the diet, the disease itself can almost always be reversed.

Treatment and Diagnosis of Celiac Disease

- The treatment of celiac disease is, simply enough, a gluten-free diet. However, because wheat-based products are very common in a typical Western diet, a gluten-free diet might not be so simple in practice. Though wheat is the main food to avoid, people with celiac should also not eat barley or rye, and it's often suggested that oat products be avoided, too, because typically harvested oats are often contaminated with wheat grains that presumably blow across the crops.

- At this time, there are no medications to prevent or treat the autoimmune damage that occurs when wheat is ingested, and people with celiac need to avoid eating gluten-containing products for the rest of their lives. Avoiding wheat not only helps relieve the immediate symptoms of celiac disease but also reduces the risk of long-term complications of untreated celiac disease, including osteoporosis and an increased risk of cancer.

- For many years, the only way to diagnose celiac disease was by small intestinal biopsy. Dr. Dicke, who made the link with wheat after World War II, also first described the "villous atrophy" characteristic of celiac disease when biopsies are examined under the microscope. Biopsies are still used to definitively diagnose celiac and to monitor patient's progress.

- However, the availability of reliable, relatively inexpensive blood tests to diagnose celiac has changed our approach to this disease.

In the past, only people with persistent and severe symptoms would undergo the procedure necessary to get the biopsies, so celiac was viewed as a disease that was relatively uncommon and always presented with severe gut symptoms.

- The availability of these blood tests has made it easy to test children and adults, and it's become clear that many (if not most) celiac patients have mild symptoms. There are probably many people who have no symptoms whatsoever, though they may be at risk for long-term complications.

- Though current, state-of-the-art blood tests have very good correlation with biopsies, older tests were not as reliable. Patients need to be careful that their physicians are ordering the best tests, and they need to beware that some providers may give a misleading diagnosis based on the wrong tests.

- There are also **genetic** tests available, but it's important that patients understand what these mean. Almost all patients with celiac disease have one of two genetic markers that can be demonstrated in blood or mouth swab samples. If you don't have either of these markers, your lifetime risk of celiac is zero, or at least very close to zero. However, many people do have these markers and do not go on to develop celiac disease. These genetic tests are not affected by a patient's diet.

- While there are no medical downsides to a gluten-free diet, it can be difficult to maintain this diet, as required, for the rest of someone's life. That's why we usually confirm positive celiac antibody tests by biopsy. This may be especially important in children, who tend to be picky eaters and may not take well to a gluten-free diet.

Important Terms

anemia: Low red blood cell count.

antibodies: Serum immunoglobulins that are part of the immune system.

chief complaint (often abbreviated "CC"; "chief concern" is also used): A traditional part of a medical encounter that is typically recorded in the patient's own words, expressing the main reason that the patient sought care.

genetic: Relating to the genes, or the sequences of DNA encoded in cells that direct their functioning.

history of present illness (HPI): A chronologic account of a patient's symptoms.

inflammation: A physiologic reaction to infection or stress that can include redness, swelling, pain, and warmth.

internal medicine: A medical specialty that concentrates on the diagnosis and management of nonsurgical problems in adults.

positive: In medical lingo, "positive" is used to denote a finding that is present. It does not imply whether this finding is good or bad.

primary: A problem or finding that isn't caused by something else. For example, a primary headache isn't caused by some other medical condition.

Suggested Reading

Green and Jones, *Celiac Disease*.

Groopman, *How Doctors Think*.

Questions to Consider

1. Other than lack of sleep, what could make a person feel fatigued?

2. In a medical encounter, should the doctor or the patient do most of the talking? Why?

I Never Feel Good
Lecture 1—Transcript

Welcome, everyone, to Medical School! An essential part of learning to think like a doctor is the grand rounds experience. In each lecture, we'll meet and examine a patient with a medical problem. Keep your eyes and ears open and see if you can figure out the solution to each mystery. Today, we're in the general medicine clinic, and our first patient is a 55 year old woman. She's made an appointment to see you. You're her physician. You start by introducing yourself, then you say, "What can I do for you today?" Your patient answers, "I never feel good."

These Grand Round sessions are a traditional part of every medical education. Each one is an in-depth discussion of a patient case from initial presentation, to diagnosis, to treatment. We'll gather our history—that's the story, the reason the patient came in. Then we'll perform a physical exam and develop what's called a differential diagnosis of what might be going on. If needed, we'll order tests to confirm our suspicions; then we'll come up with a plan to help our patient.

So, what should you expect to learn from these cases? You'll certainly see a wide variety of symptoms and diseases, and you'll get a good appreciation for how the body works in health and in disease. More importantly, though, by the end of this series, you'll have a much better understanding of how doctors think. How doctors figure out what's wrong with a patient, how we use our skills to rule in or rule out certain diagnoses, how we come up with a diagnosis and a treatment plan, and how we work with patients to improve health and prevent and treat disease. Obviously, I'm not your physician, and I can't give you personal medical advice—that's what your own doctor is for. But by listening to these lectures, you will learn how to communicate more effectively with your doctor. Understanding what doctors do, and how and why they do it, will make you a better patient, and will improve your own health.

Our grand rounds case today is the 55-year old woman we've just met, who says she never feels good. In medical encounters, doctors start every case with a patient's age and gender, followed by the so-called "chief complaint."

This is a quote, usually in the patient's own words, of what the main concern is. Why did this person come to see the doctor? It's a very important piece of information, because it focuses the evaluation on what the patient is worried about.

Sometimes chief complaints don't end up being the main thing that the doctor is worried about and don't directly point to the final diagnosis, but it's still something crucial to know when you're getting started. In this case, our chief complaint is vague. "I never feel good." It doesn't really help us narrow down anything. But it does tell us that our patient is suffering and always feels bad in some way, and maybe, has been for a long time. There could be a clue there.

After the chief complaint, we'll take a history of the present illness, often abbreviated as an HPI. This is a story, the patient's story, of what's going on, when it started, what sort of factors influence the symptoms. When we take an HPI, it's important to let the patient do most of the talking. We'll give a bit of a lead or push now and then with questions to clarify the story, but this is the time for the patient to tell us what's going on, not the other way around.

Our patient says that she used to be healthy and vigorous and used to enjoy playing tennis. About five years ago she began to find that her energy wasn't as good. At about the same time, she broke her wrist and had to stop playing. She wonders now if maybe stopping tennis was a mistake. At the time, the doctor who treated her broken wrist thought that her bones didn't look strong on an x-ray, so she was referred to a specialist and eventually started on calcium supplements and hormone pills, often used in post-menopausal women to increase bone density. She recalls that those medicines—there were a series of different medicines, actually—they caused a lot of stomach symptoms, and she ended up stopping them after a year.

She was also supposed to take iron, because she was told she was anemic but ended up thinking that the iron made her stomach feel worse, so she's stopped that too. Still, even after stopping these medications, she's continued to have intermittent belly aches and constipation and sometimes diarrhea at times, and she often feels bloated and nauseous. She recalls that she wanted to stop drinking milk; she had read that lactose intolerance could cause some of her symptoms, but her doctors didn't want her to stop, because she needed calcium for her bones. Eventually, she ignored her doctors and did stop all dairy products, and she thinks that this has maybe helped a little. In the meantime, though, she had to retire from her job as a teacher because she found that she just didn't have the energy to stay on her feet all day. She sleeps well, wakes up feeling rested, and seems to eat a healthy diet.

That's our HPI, the patient's story. It's sometimes helpful to ask questions to clarify some of these symptoms—the onset and the nature of those symptoms, and the factors that make them better or make them worse. But for now, we're going to move on to the next step past this initial history.

The next thing to review is usually the patient's family and social history to see if any of this background information gives us useful clues. We already know our patient is a retired teacher. We learn that she lives with her husband and has two children who have moved away from home. Her family health history reveals that her mother died at age 50 of breast cancer and her father had a stroke at age 81. She doesn't smoke or drink alcohol and says she doesn't take any prescription medicines, herbs, or street drugs. She does take a vitamin every day and also takes over-the-counter Pepto-Bismol regularly, which at least, sometimes, seems to help her stomach.

Our next step will be a physical exam, but before we get into that, let's pause and look over the case and organize our thoughts. We're planning to do a comprehensive physical exam, but it's good to think about what we're going to look for even before doing the exam. On any exam, we ought to keep our eyes wide open for clues, but we're more likely to see those clues if we at least know what we're looking for.

To help stay on track, let's come up with a problem list. What are the things are wrong here? We have a woman who's been ill for about five years. She had a fracture and is said to have had decreased bone density. She has very low energy. We're told she has had anemia—that's a low count of red blood cells. She also has a number of abdominal complaints, including pain, nausea, sometimes diarrhea, and sometimes constipation. That is quite a problem list!

Well, have you got it figured out yet? Actually, you shouldn't have. If at this point the doctor is thinking of a single likely diagnosis, the doctor himself is likely to get it wrong. Our job as doctors isn't to lunge at the first diagnosis that seems to fit, but to keep an open mind, and think about broad categories of problems that we can narrow down as we get more information. Thinking of a diagnosis too early ends up anchoring your mind, so you're more likely to overlook clues that don't fit your expectations.

On to the physical exam. Our patient is a thin woman, and she looks a little anxious. She's seen a lot of doctors over the last several years and may be becoming, understandably, a bit distrustful. Today, we're going to focus only on the most pertinent positives and negatives from the exam. Specifically, her vital signs, that is, her pulse, blood pressure, respiratory rate, and temperature are normal. Her lungs sound clear, and her breathing is easy. Her heart exam and circulation are normal, and her abdominal exam reveals kind of a diffuse, mild tenderness wherever you press. A rectal examination was unrevealing, and afterwards, a quick test for blood in stool was negative.

OK, we have our chief complaint: "I never feel good." We have our HPI, some additional history, and a physical exam. It's time to see if we can make a list of possible diagnoses and then narrow and refine the list based on all of the information we have. When there are many symptoms, as there are in this case, it may not be possible to fit all of them into one diagnosis, and that's OK. After all, not everyone with disease X has every single symptom that's typical of disease X, and sometimes people with disease X also have a little bit of disease Y. Patients do not routinely read medical textbooks, and sometimes they don't present with the exact symptoms they're "supposed to have."

OK, let's start with one symptom, make a broad list of diagnoses, and then add symptoms to her story to see what goes up, goes down, or falls off of our list. Let's start with chronic fatigue. The most common cause of fatigue is, of course, inadequate sleep. That can mean not enough hours of sleep or inadequate quality of sleep. Even if there are enough hours of sleep, if sleep is frequently interrupted, it will not be restful. Sometimes, sleep is interrupted by severe snoring by the patient or the spouse, or frequent trips to the bathroom, or frequent wakenings from a baby. Another common cause of poor sleep quality is restless legs syndrome, again, either of the patient or the spouse. In our case, none of this sounds likely, so we can leave sleep problems off of our list.

Fatigue can also be caused by depression. Now, you may be surprised that I'd bring up a psychiatric diagnosis so early, but keep in mind that depression is very common and causes a lot of genuine, serious symptoms and impairment. People with depression also complain of a lot of aches and pains—belly aches or headaches. So this diagnosis, in some ways, fits here. We'll keep it in mind.

Another potential cause to add to our fatigue list would be heart disease. If the heart can't pump enough blood, a kind of fatigue called exercise intolerance can occur; that's basically when a person can't keep up with a certain level of exercise as expected. Our patient's fatigue doesn't really seem related to exercise, and her normal physical exam really doesn't fit with a person who has had significant heart disease for five years. So, let's leave heart disease at the bottom of our list of possibilities. A number of endocrine problems can also cause fatigue, including diabetes and thyroid disease. We'll make sure to test for these.

Further expanding our list, anything that causes anemia or low blood iron can cause low energy or fatigue. We were told that our patient was diagnosed with anemia in the past. Could that be the main problem here? If the anemia is caused by blood loss, say, in the gut, from some chronic inflammation or infection, that could, perhaps, explain some her GI symptoms too.

Many infections can cause fatigue, including a mononucleosis, for example, but our patient's fatigue has lasted too long for that to fit well. Many cancers can also make a patient feel fatigued, but again, with a five year history, that seems unlikely. I don't think you could have symptoms from cancer for this long without the diagnosis becoming much more obvious. We'll move cancer lower down on our list. Many medications, including both prescription and non-prescription drugs, cause fatigue, as do many drugs of abuse. Our patient tells us she doesn't use any of these products, but we'll keep in mind that our patients are not always forthcoming about drug or alcohol habits. This next idea doesn't fit our patient, but it's always worth considering for a woman with fatigue and nausea. Could she be pregnant? Our patient is past menopause, so we'll leave that off the list.

OK, that's a good start. Now, let's look at the data we've got and see how we might adjust our list. Our physical exam didn't reveal a whole lot, but it did focus our concern on the belly. She had some tenderness there, and a lot of her symptoms seem to be belly related. Have we thought enough about problems with the gut that might also cause fatigue? What sorts of diagnoses can cause nausea, pain, diarrhea, and constipation, and are some of those same "gut" diagnoses ones that perhaps have already appeared on our list of likely "fatigue" diagnoses?

We'll go through this list quicker. There are a lot of causes of acute, sudden abdominal symptoms, including many viral infections and food poisoning, but we can focus here, instead, on causes of chronic problems. Irritable bowel syndrome is very common and presents with abdominal discomfort, bloating, and either diarrhea or constipation, or sometimes both. But it doesn't really cause anemia and shouldn't cause fatigue, unless, of course, the gut symptoms interfere with sleep.

Abdominal ulcers can cause pain, though not so much those lower-down symptoms of diarrhea and constipation. Gall bladder disease could cause pain and nausea, and sometimes diarrhea, though it wouldn't particularly cause fatigue. How about inflammatory bowel disease, like Crohn's Disease; that can certainly cause at least most of the GI symptoms our patient reported, as well as causing GI blood loss, anemia, and fatigue. We mentioned depression, which could be related to chronic abdominal pain. But we wouldn't expect anemia with depression, unless the patient had stopped eating well. Lactose intolerance is a common cause of diarrhea and pain, though not constipation, and not fatigue.

How about celiac disease? That's a chronic disorder that causes malabsorption of nutrients from the gut, leading to a myriad of symptoms that can include fatigue, anemia, and almost any GI symptom. In celiac disease, malabsorption of nutrients can also affect the bones—decreased absorption of dietary Vitamin D, phosphorus, and calcium can cause decreased bone density. Do you recall the beginning of our patient's story? It started with a fracture, and the suggestion from some doctor that she needed more calcium in her diet.

We have some good candidates here, several possibilities that can cause her central symptoms of both fatigue and GI problems. To confirm a diagnosis from a list, or to strike off other diagnoses as not being possible, the next step in our evaluation is to order tests. These can include blood work, or x-rays, or other kinds of investigations.

As we go through our grand rounds series, we'll learn more about the ways medical imaging and blood tests are used, but for today, let me just summarize the tests that were done on our patient. A gall bladder ultrasound came back normal, and a chest x-ray was normal, including normal heart size. An EKG was normal, further confirming that there was no heart disease. Blood tests revealed normal blood sugar, meaning, she does not have diabetes; normal thyroid functioning; low vitamin D levels; and mild anemia. Her sed rate and CRP were normal—these normal blood tests mean that there was no ongoing inflammation or serious infection. One last blood test was done, a test for antibodies that are usually present in people with celiac disease, and that test was positive. Our patient then had a gut wall biopsy, and celiac disease was confirmed.

Celiac disease is a chronic illness, primarily of the gut, characterized by malabsorption. The lining of the gut—the small, finger-like projections where absorption of food nutrients occurs—is damaged, and the net effect is that nutrients are not absorbed across the gut wall into the blood for use by the body. The primary symptoms of celiac disease are caused by inadequate nutrient availability and also by the GI effects of having, essentially, food staying in the gut instead of moving into your body. This includes diarrhea, and bloating, and abdominal pain. Sometimes, constipation can be more of a problem than diarrhea, or, as in our patient, there can be periods of time when these seemingly opposite symptoms go back and forth. Many celiac symptoms also occur outside of the gut; we'll talk more about those later.

Celiac disease was known to the ancient Greeks, who referred to a condition called koiliakos, meaning "suffering of the bowels." A patient case written in the second century described a man with stomach pain who was underweight, pale, weak, and incapable of working. That's a pretty good description, still, of a severe case. The Greek term was translated to the term celiac in 1856.

Around that time, it was recognized that this was a disease that could be managed by diet. In 1954, Dutch pediatrician Willem Dicke linked the disease to the ingestion of wheat protein. It's speculated that his experience seeing patients improve during the famine of 1944, when wheat was scarce, that may have helped him recognize the critical role of wheat in this illness.

Though the symptoms of celiac disease are varied and affect many organ systems, it only has one cause: ingesting certain proteins found in wheat, barley, and rye. These are natural proteins from a family called gluten proteins; you may also see the term gliadin, which refers to a more specific type of gluten. Celiac disease is sometimes called gluten enteropathy, or celiac sprue.

When gluten-containing foods are eaten by people with celiac disease, these proteins are modified, or processed, so that they trigger a cross reaction with gut tissue. Basically, the body's own immune system is tricked into attacking healthy cells in the gut, and probably elsewhere too. So, celiac disease is, in a sense, an autoimmune disease—the body is attacking itself. But it's an autoimmune disease that has a specific and avoidable trigger. It's the gluten proteins that trigger the reaction, and once gluten is no longer part of the diet, the disease itself can almost always be reversed.

As we've seen, the malabsorption that occurs with celiac disease causes gut symptoms like bloating, pain, and diarrhea. It also causes specific nutritional deficiencies, including iron deficiency, with resulting anemia; vitamin D deficiency, resulting in poor calcium absorption and less calcium in the bones; sometimes weight loss; and poor growth in children.

Our patient also reported that she thought some of her symptoms could have been made worse with the ingestion of diary products. This could have been a secondary phenomenon. Though celiac disease doesn't directly affect the digestion of milk, the damage to the gut tissue can reduce the availability of the enzyme lactase, which is necessary to process the milk sugar lactose. So, some people with celiac disease seem to also have what we'll call a secondary lactose intolerance. Secondary here means caused by something else. So our patient, she was right; her symptoms do get worse with dairy, even though a dairy allergy or lactose intolerance were not her main diagnoses.

In addition to these malabsorption symptoms, celiac disease can include many possible symptoms outside of the gut. These arise maybe because of the nutritional deficiencies, or sometimes because gluten can trigger autoimmune tissue destruction in other parts of the body. These so called extra intestinal manifestations, as with the other symptoms of celiac, are reversible once the patient is placed on a gluten-free diet.

The most common extra intestinal symptoms are easy fatigue and skin rashes, especially a characteristic itchy rash called dermatitis herpetiformis, which may occur with or without other manifestations of celiac disease. There are also a number of neurologic symptoms, including neuropathy, that's a form of nerve damage that can result in pain or tingling in the extremities, as well as a loss of control of body movements, which can make walking difficult.

The treatment of celiac disease is, simply enough, a gluten-free diet. That's simple to say, but may not be so simple to do; wheat-based products are very common in a typical Western diet. Though wheat is the main food to avoid, people with celiac should also not eat barley or rye, and it's often suggested that oat products also have to be avoided because typically harvested oats are often contaminated with wheat grains that presumably blow across the crops.

At this time, there are no medications to prevent or treat the autoimmune damage that occurs when wheat is ingested, and people with celiac disease need to avoid eating gluten-containing products for the rest of their lives. Avoiding wheat not only helps relieve the immediate symptoms of celiac, but also reduces the risk of long-term complications of untreated celiac disease, including osteoporosis and an increased risk of cancer.

With treatment, our patient's prognosis is excellent. She was very relieved to learn about celiac disease and became a bit of a gluten crusader in her household, making sure that there was no way her own food could even inadvertently be contaminated with wheat. Within two months of her dietary changes, all of her symptoms completely resolved, and she was able to resume playing tennis. She was also treated with extra iron and vitamin D for her anemia and low bone-mineral content. Unfortunately, there is no way to quickly replace years of lost bone calcium, so she will remain at a somewhat increased risk of fractures for some time.

There's an important distinction to be made between people who have different kinds of problems when they eat wheat products. Celiac disease, as we've discussed, is a specific autoimmune disorder that causes malabsorption, gut symptoms, and other problems, as we saw in our patient. It's not the same as wheat allergy. Allergy refers to a different kind of immune-mediated reaction and typically causes things like hives, vomiting, or sometimes difficulty breathing. People with wheat allergy do not have celiac disease, and people with celiac do not have wheat allergy. Another confusing term is gluten sensitivity. This is a somewhat controversial entity, where people have troublesome symptoms when they eat wheat, but they test negative for celiac disease and allergy. There's no good test to confirm gluten sensitivity, but there are many people who test negative for celiac and still seem to feel better when they avoid wheat-containing products.

For many years, the only way to confirm the diagnosis of celiac disease was by intestinal biopsy. Dr. Dicke, the Dutch physician who made the link with wheat after World War II, he also first described the "villous atrophy" characteristic of celiac disease when biopsies are examined under a microscope. Biopsies are still used to definitively diagnose celiac disease and to monitor patient progress.

However, the availability of reliable, relatively inexpensive blood tests to diagnose celiac has changed our approach to this disease. In the past, only people with persistent and severe symptoms would undergo the procedure necessary to get the biopsy, so, celiac disease was viewed as something relatively uncommon and something that always presented with severe gut symptoms. The availability of these blood tests has made it easy to test children and adults, and it's become clear that many, if not most, celiac patients have mild symptoms. Some patients have just unexplained anemia or mild elevations of their blood markers for liver disease. Some only have rashes or constipation, or GI complaints that may have been labeled irritable bowel syndrome.

There are probably many people who have no symptoms whatsoever, though they may be at risk for long-term complications. The prevalence of the actual diagnosis of celiac disease is about 1 in 1700 people, however, when blood donated to blood banks is tested, the rate of positive celiac tests may be about 1 in 100. So many people may have celiac disease without symptoms, and may not know it.

The current, state-of-the-art blood tests have very good correlation with biopsies, but older tests were not as reliable. Keeping up with the advantages and disadvantages of specific tests, and especially, newer tests as they're released, that the physicians responsibility, but patients should be able to ask, "How reliable is this test?" before the blood is drawn.

There are also genetic tests available, but it's important that patients understand what these mean. Almost all patients with celiac disease have genetic markers that can be demonstrated in blood or mouth swab samples. If you don't have the genetic markers, your lifetime risk of celiac is zero, or at least very close to zero. However, most people who do have these markers do not go on to develop celiac disease. Even among people who are genetically predisposed to celiac disease, with a positive genetic test, the lifetime risk of developing celiac disease is probably from 3 to 10 percent. So with genetic tests for celiac, a negative test means you have close to zero risk, and a positive result means you are at some risk, but will probably go the rest of your life without developing celiac disease.

While there are no medical down sides to a gluten-free diet—there are plenty of other nutritious foods to choose from—it can be difficult to maintain this diet, as required, for the rest of someone's life. That's why we usually confirm positive celiac antibody tests by biopsy. This may be especially important in children, who tend to be picky eaters and may not take well to a gluten-free diet.

Our patient today presented with a constellation of symptoms, with a history of several seemingly unrelated problems. She had had a broken bone and was noted to be deficient in vitamin D; she was also anemic, or deficient in iron; she had very low energy; she had a number of different GI complaints spanning several years, some of which seemed to come and go, perhaps at times related to the ingestion of milk. The key here, to making the diagnosis, was to get all of the information together and to think broadly about what could account for everything.

Listening to the patient tell her story was the source of our best clues, and that's something we're going to see again and again. The history, our most important diagnostic tool, is followed by a physical exam to clarify our suspicions and to drive some considerations higher or lower on our list of possibilities. Labs and x-rays are never done to fish around and find a diagnosis, but to confirm or refute what we already suspect. That is how doctors think.

Today, we've explored the first of our series of grand rounds, and you've gotten a flavor for the organization of these medical mysteries. Some of the upcoming cases will be diseases you've heard of, or perhaps you're very familiar with. Others might be a bit more arcane. All of them will illustrate how doctors and patients should think about diagnosing and treating disease.

Next up, a much newer disease, one not known by the ancient Greeks. We'll learn more about that next time.

A Persistent Fever
Lecture 2

In this lecture, you will learn about some of the basic tools of medical diagnosis—the history, the physical, some of the common tests, and X-rays. As a doctor, you'll see that your most important tools are your senses and your brain—listening to your patient, observing, and thinking about data you've collected. Listening can not only help you glean the clues you need, but can also help develop a trusting, two-way relationship with your patient.

Prolonged Fever

- Imagine that you are in an outpatient clinic—general internal medicine. The patient is a 33-year-old man with a chief complaint of "I can't get rid of this **fever**." He had been in excellent health until two months ago. Since then, he has run fevers almost every day, usually in the range of 101 to 102 degrees Fahrenheit. He has also developed a cough that is getting increasingly worse and uncomfortable ulcers or sores in his mouth.

- This is his history of present illness (HPI). The next part of a standard medical history is called a **review of systems (ROS)**. In contrast to the HPI, the ROS is a series of questions driven by the doctor. It's usually organized by organ system.

- A previously healthy man has had a prolonged fever, plus coughing and mouth sores, GI problems, rashes, fatigue, weight loss, achiness—it seems like just about everything is going wrong with this patient.

- Almost all fevers are caused by one of four broad categories of illness: infection, cancer, autoimmune disease, and miscellaneous. Of these, infections are by far the most common, especially for relatively brief fevers. But the longer the fever persists, the less likely it's going to be an infection—at least not a straightforward infection.

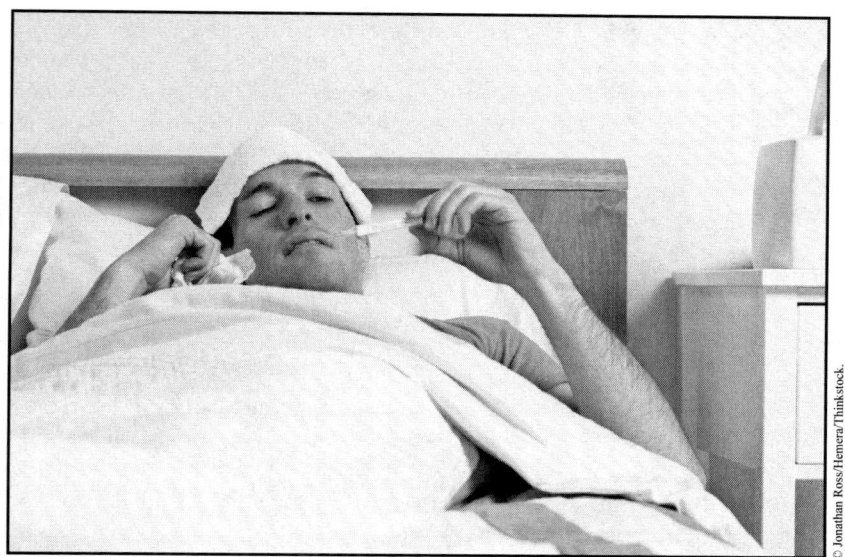

If you think you have a fever, a good way to measure your body temperature is by using a thermometer.

- A physical exam confirms that the patient is quite ill. He has what sounds like pneumonia. He also has white material in his mouth, which is thrush, an overgrowth of a yeast called **candida**. Thrush is commonly seen in newborns and young babies, but really should not occur in healthy, young men. The appearance of thrush suggests that something has gone wrong with his immune system. He also has some swollen lymph nodes, which are most commonly seen during infections.

- One of the most common blood tests done is a **complete blood count (CBC)**, which counts the quantities of the three basic types of blood cells: the red cells, which carry oxygen; the white cells, which fight disease; and the **platelets**, which help blood clot when it needs to. In addition, a CBC usually includes a differential (or "diff"), which breaks down the white cells into subtypes.

- Our patient's CBC with diff shows that all three cell lines are low: He is anemic, with low red cells, plus he has low white cells and low platelets. The diff shows a striking lack of a certain kind of white cell called a lymphocyte, which typically accounts for about 50 percent of the total white cells. Our patient has zero. Maybe that's related to what we're suspecting is some kind of immune disorder—one that's led to a serious infection, or infections, that our patient is not shaking off.

- A chest X-ray is a very important test that is used in a variety of circumstances, both as a screening and as a confirmatory test. Essentially, it's a photograph of the chest, but one taken using X-rays—which can pass through body tissues but are blocked by denser things—rather than visible light.

- When a chest X-ray is done, we can assess the health of the bones of the chest, the condition of the lung fields, and the size and shape of the shadow made by the fluid-filled heart. Our patient's chest X-ray shows fluffy white areas superimposed across both lung fields, where instead of air there is excess fluid. That fluid blocks some of the X-rays, so you get areas that look more dense than air ought to look. There is some kind of widespread problem in the lungs.

HIV/AIDS

- Acquired immunodeficiency syndrome (AIDS) is caused by the human immunodeficiency virus (HIV). HIV is a roughly spherical **virus** that is about 60 times smaller than a human **red blood cell** (which is actually rather large for a virus). It's one of a kind of viruses called retroviruses, which have their own unique enzymes and proteins that can insert their own genetic material into that of the infected host cells.

- Viruses are, in a way, not really living organisms. They don't have any way to extract energy from their environment and can't reproduce on their own. What they do is infect the cells of living organisms and use their own genetic instructions to take over the cell's machinery.

- The HIV virus takes the idea of controlling a cell one step further. As a retrovirus, HIV contains a special enzyme called reverse transcriptase that turns the virus RNA into DNA that is directly inserted into the DNA of the host cell.

- Furthermore, the HIV virus preferentially infects our own immune cells—the cells that are supposed to be fighting off infections. The host's own immune-fighting apparatus, instead of defending the body against HIV, is tricked into damaging our own cells and making more HIV virus to infect more of our cells.

- HIV doesn't necessarily make the host immediately ill. It can replicate and spread in a relatively small number of cells, leaving plenty of normal immune cells to do their job. It can take years for people with HIV infection to develop signs of serious illness.

- The diagnosis of AIDS is made when a person with HIV infection has clinical manifestations of disease, either caused by the virus itself or by an opportunistic infection. Without treatment, about 50 percent of people infected with HIV will develop AIDS within 10 years (though a small number of people seem to remain healthy indefinitely).

- In addition to destroying the host immune system, HIV infects cells in the brain (causing, eventually, a form of **dementia**) and perhaps cells in the gut and other tissues.

- Without a functioning immune system, serious illness can occur from out-of-control, ordinary infections. A fairly ordinary, innocuous infection can be much harder to clear and can have severe or prolonged symptoms. There are also less-ordinary infections, sometimes called opportunistic infections—which are caused by organisms that couldn't cause any problems for a healthy individual at all.

- Though we can still use antibiotics, antivirals, antiparasitics, and antifungal drugs to some benefit in AIDS patients, none of these drugs works as well as they would in a person with a normal immune system. Drugs help our immune system fight infections; they don't knock out infections very well on their own.

- There are several different ways that HIV infections can present. There is an acute phase, occurring two to four weeks after initial infection. The symptoms are usually fever, aches, sore throat, swollen lymph nodes, and sometimes a rash or GI symptoms. The symptoms are not very specific, and many of these acute infections are not diagnosed as HIV. (One common misdiagnosis, at this point, is infectious mononucleosis.) Many people have no symptoms at all during this earliest phase.

- Then, there's a prolonged period of latency, where the virus slowly spreads without symptoms. Depending on the "viral load" (that is, how many virus particles there are in the blood), a person at this stage can be more or less contagious—in some cases, very high viral loads and infectivity can be associated with minimal if any symptoms, at least for a while.

- During this stage, patients can be found by routine screening of sexually active adults or others with risk factors. If symptoms are present, they might include chronic enlarged lymph nodes, fever fatigue, weight loss, diarrhea, or cough—all of these can come and go and may not overlap at the same time, which may make the diagnosis easy to overlook. Catching people early, in the latent stage, before obvious symptoms of AIDS develop, leads to a better long-term prognosis.

- Full-blown AIDS, which usually occurs within 10 years of exposure, includes more severe symptoms, including fevers with soaking night sweats, cough and shortness of breath, chronic diarrhea, plaques in the mouth, rashes, distorted vision, and persistent fatigue. Which symptoms predominate depends on which opportunistic infections are present.

Testing and Treatment

- The most commonly used test for HIV is a blood test for antibodies to the virus, which usually becomes positive 3 to 12 weeks after infection during **seroconversion** (which is when the serological tests—the serum tests for antibodies—become positive). This delay in positivity means that someone with acute HIV, a new infection with symptoms, may still have a **negative** HIV test.

- In cases of suspected acute HIV, before seroconversion, a test for HIV genetic material in the blood using the polymerase chain reaction (PCR) technique can show infection. This same test, sometimes called the viral load, can also be used to see how heavily the blood is infected and, thus, how contagious a person might be.

- Another test commonly used in the evaluation and follow-up of an HIV patient is a CD4 count, a count of the T helper lymphocytes that are destroyed by HIV infection. A normal CD4 count is around 800 to 1,200; in advanced HIV and AIDS, this trends into the 100s or eventually down to zero.

- The most effective treatment of HIV starts early. There are medicines that can prevent the initial transmission of HIV—this can be used during the birth of a baby to an HIV-positive mom, after an inadvertent needlestick blood exposure for a health-care worker, or after an unsafe sexual encounter.

- When an HIV infection is diagnosed, there are about 30 different anti-HIV medications to stop the spread of the virus. These are used in a variety of combinations to make them more effective and also to prevent the virus from developing resistance. Current HIV medications need to be taken every day for the rest of a patient's life.

- We also have a number of medications to prevent and treat the opportunistic infections that cause a lot of the suffering in AIDS patients. Again, these need to be taken long term. Medication regimens for AIDS and HIV patients can be complex and expensive and may lead to significant side effects. It's also crucial to help people with HIV infections maintain good overall health and nutrition and to take steps to prevent transmission to other people.

Important Terms

candida: A common species of yeast.

complete blood count (CBC): A common laboratory test that quantifies the different types of cells in the blood.

dementia: A chronic disorder of brain functioning, most typically marked by memory problems in addition to other manifestations.

fever: An elevated body temperature.

negative: In medical use, "negative" means that the inquired symptom or finding is absent. It does not imply that this is good or bad.

platelets: A kind of blood cell involved in clotting.

red blood cells: The cells in the blood that carry oxygen.

review of systems (ROS): Part of the medical interview, with a series of questions organized by organ system to see if specific symptoms have been present.

seroconversion: When blood tests show that a person has been exposed to an infectious agent by demonstrating the presence of specific antibodies against that infection.

virus: A small infectious agent that does not contain its own cells or organelles.

Suggested Reading

Garrett, *The Coming Plague.*

Shilts, *And the Band Played On.*

AIDS.gov, http://aids.gov/.

Questions to Consider

1. What are some of the "new diseases" that first arose in the twentieth century?

2. What kinds of illnesses cause fever?

A Persistent Fever
Lecture 2—Transcript

Welcome back to grand rounds. Each grand rounds will focus on a single case—one sick child or adult. You'll see that every case follows a path, from the initial presentation, to the diagnosis, to the treatment. But that path can be twisty and windy, and often has multiple forks and decision points. It will be difficult at first to know what to expect around the next curve. As we go through these sessions, you'll get better at knowing where each case is likely to lead.

The key to accurate diagnosis and treatment will always be to pay attention to details and keep an open mind. It is never a good idea to latch onto your first assumptions. When the path seems to be leading to a dead end or seems to be straying far from what you expected, you may need to step back, retrace, and reconfirm the original story and the data. In other words, as with any mystery, there will be surprises.

We're in the outpatient clinic again today, general internal medicine. Our patient is a 33-year-old man with a chief complaint of "I can't get rid of this fever." He had been in excellent health until about two months ago. Since then, he's run fevers almost every day, usually in the 101°F to 102°F range. He's also developed a worsening cough and uncomfortable ulcers, or sores, in his mouth.

What we've presented so far is the HPI, or history of present illness. The next part of a standard medical history is called a review of systems. In contrast to the HPI, the ROS is a series of questions driven by the doctor. While the HPI is a statement from the patient about what's been going on—in a way, it's the story of the illness—the review of systems is the doctor's turn to find out, basically, what else has been going on. It's usually organized by organ system. You've probably completed an ROS yourself at a doctor visit. It's often presented as a checklist of possible symptoms for you to go through, one by one, and you mark off which ones you've been experiencing. In a way, it's a kind of fishing expedition: Which, of this long list of problems, has the patient had?

I don't want to belabor all of the possible questions on a detailed review of systems, but in this case, our patient had many other things wrong, even beyond the prolonged fever and cough. We'll go through the most pertinent parts of his ROS by system. Let's start with a general category and find out that our patient has lost weight and has had easy fatigue.

Next we ask about skin problems. He reports a number of different rashes, though the one that bothers him the most are these sores on the inside of his mouth. From questions about the GI system, we learn that there has been low appetite, and trouble swallowing, and frequent diarrhea. We ask about joints and muscles, and our patient reports a sort of generalized achiness, all over sometimes, though no swollen joints. And we can go on from there. Other parts of the ROS could involve references to the cardiovascular system, or the genitourinary tract, or psychiatric symptoms. It can really be very extensive. The point is to inquire about any problem and see what turns up, even if the patient didn't bring it up on his own.

So, what have we got here? A previously healthy man has had a prolonged fever—two months—plus coughing and mouth sores, GI problems, rashes, fatigue, weight loss, achiness. Really, it seems like just about everything is going wrong with our patient. How do we even start to make a broad differential diagnosis to help focus the rest of the evaluation? Often, it's best to keep things simple at first. His chief complaint was fever, and that's a good place to start.

Almost all fevers are caused by one of four broad categories of illness: infection, cancer, autoimmune disease, and miscellaneous. Of these, infections are by far the most common, especially for relatively brief fevers. But the longer a fever persists, the less likely it's going to be an infection, or at least not a straightforward infection. The kinds of infections that cause prolonged fevers are unusual ones—not ordinary pneumonia or strep throat, but things like tuberculosis or fungal infections; or abscesses; or smoldering, low-grade infection in bone tissue. Almost any infection, even ordinary ones, can also cause unexpected prolonged fevers in people with a compromised or malfunctioning immune system. Cancer can also be a cause of prolonged fevers, including cancers of the blood, for example, leukemia, or cancers of solid organs, like the kidney. Also, cancers can themselves lead to immune problems, so patients can have an underlying cancer that predisposes to infection.

A third category of fevers includes autoimmune diseases, like lupus or rheumatoid arthritis. Then, in the miscellaneous category go things like drug reactions—yes, actually, antibiotics, for instance, can cause a so-called drug fever, plus hyperthyroidism, and some genetic recurrent fevers. And sometimes, even prolonged fevers can occur without any identifiable cause.

Now we're ready to move on to the physical exam. Remember, we're going to keep our eyes and ears open, and we're going to be looking for clues that can lead us towards or away from our main categories of prolonged fever: infections, cancer, or autoimmune diseases. We're also going to pay close attention to the lungs, GI, and skin exams, since our patient has symptoms in those areas.

Our patient is a thin young Caucasian man. His cheeks are sunken. His temperature is 99.8°F, pulse 98, respirations 36. In his mouth there are thick, patchy white plaques inside his cheeks and on his gums. He has some swollen lymph nodes in his neck. He looks like he is having some trouble breathing; you can see his ribs individually poking out with each inspiration, and the notch above his sternum pulls in with each breath. We call these findings retractions, and they're a sign that he's needing to use a lot of extra muscle force to move air in and out of his lungs. His lungs themselves sound crackly and wet, almost like you're listening to a bowl of Rice Crispies cereal with milk. The medical term for that sound is crackles, or sometimes it's called rales. That means there is fluid in the lungs. The remainder of the exam was normal.

Those findings on the physical exam. what do they mean? The white material in his mouth is thrush, an overgrowth of a yeast called Candida. Thrush is commonly seen in newborns and young babies, but really should not occur in healthy young men. The appearance of thrush here suggests that something has gone wrong with his immune system. He also has some swollen lymph nodes, which are most commonly seen during infections, but could occur from cancer.

The crackly sound in his chest, that's fluid bubbling around with each breath. Crackles can be caused by heart disease, because a poorly functioning heart allows blood to sort of pool behind it. It pushes out into lung tissue. But in this case, there's not much other evidence of heart disease. We're much more suspicious of infection in the lungs creating pus. That's the fluid that's bubbling.

Our patient, is quite ill. He's had fevers for two months; he has what sounds like pneumonia; and that thrush is a hint that his immune system is not working. We'll go ahead and see what some initial labs and tests show. One of the most common blood tests done is a CBC, or Complete Blood Count. This used to be done by a person looking through a microscope, counting up the kinds of cells seen. Now, a CBC is done electronically. A CBC counts the quantities of the three basic types of blood cells: the red cells, that carry oxygen; the white cells, that fight disease; and the platelets, those help blood clot. In addition, a CBC usually includes a differential; we usually just call that a diff, which breaks down the white cells into subtypes.

Our patient's CBC with diff shows that all three cell lines are low. He's anemic, with low red cells, plus he has low white count, and low platelets as well. The diff shows a striking lack of a certain kind of white cell called a lymphocyte. That typically accounts for maybe a plus or minus 50 percent of the total white cell; our patient has zero. Maybe that's related to what we're suspecting is some kind of immune disorder here, leading to infections that our patient is not shaking off.

We've also ordered a chest X-ray. This is a very common test, and one that's used in a variety of circumstances, both as a screening test and as a confirmatory test. It's essentially a photograph of the chest, but one taken using X-rays rather than visible light. X-rays can pass through body tissues, but they're blocked by denser things. When X-ray film is exposed to X-ray radiation, it turns dark. So, whiter areas are where the X-rays were blocked, and there are varying shades of grey where there has been a partial block, or scattering, of the X-rays. In the human body, air blocks X-rays least, so healthy lung tissue looks dark. Bones block X-rays well, so they look the most bright, or white, on a film. Fluid-filled things are kind of grayish, or in between. Modern X-rays are usually taken digitally, so these white-grey-dark distinctions can be shown in different ways, but most doctors prefer to look at X-rays with the traditional colors, as if we're really reading films.

When a chest X-ray is done, we can assess several things: the health of the bones in the chest, the condition of the lung fields, and the size and shape of the shadow made by the heart. Ordinary X-rays don't show anything in three dimensions and can't show a whole lot of detail when one structure is located right on top of another, but nonetheless, this remains one of the most useful, quick, and easy tests that can be done in the emergency department or in the office. Our patient's chest X-ray confirmed the physical exam. We see fluffy, white areas superimposed across both lung fields, where instead of air, there is excess fluid. That fluid blocks some of the X-rays, so you get areas that look more white than air ought to look. There is some kind of widespread problem in the lungs here. The heart and the bones, by the way, those were normal.

Now, traditionally, in the hospital, when grand rounds are presented, it's a real, recent patient case. For this course, we're usually using composite cases to help protect patient confidentiality. However, today's case is a true patient. This is the first case report of this specific illness, to which I've added just a few details. This case was originally published in the June 5, 1981 edition of the CDC's *Morbidity and Mortality Weekly Report*. I also left out a few other details, which are the last few clues. Let me give them to you now. This 1981 report included five men, all were previously healthy, and all became very ill with similar presentations. All of these men were homosexual, and all lived in Los Angeles, California.

After this report, hundreds of other cases were reported in California and New York. Many were in homosexual men, which continues to comprise the highest risk group for this illness in the United States, though worldwide, heterosexual transmission has become more likely. Other initial reported cases occurred in people with hemophilia, who were regularly treated with pooled human blood products, and in IV drug users. Later, more cases appeared in women and men who were not part of those initial high-risk groups.

Let me tell you the rest of this young man's story. He was found to have pneumonia, caused by a very unusual fungus called Pneumocystis jirovecii— At the time, it had been called *Pneumocystis carinii*—which was only seen in severely immunocompromised people. He also had an ongoing infection with a virus called CMV, which usually causes only mild symptoms, though it was making our patient very ill. Despite aggressive treatment, our patient died two months after presentation, and his autopsy showed ongoing infections and no evidence of cancer to explain his immune compromise.

This was the first case of the modern epidemic of AIDS, or Acquired Immune Deficiency Syndrome, caused by what was later found to be HIV, the human immunodeficiency virus. What we know now is tremendously more than what we knew in 1981. We know far more about the virus, and we've also learned far more about the immune system and how it functions in health and in disease. Perhaps that's the bit of a silver lining on this horrible disease—it led to an explosion of research into immune functioning and disorders, and made new classes of medications to help not only those with HIV, but many other conditions as well.

What we now know is that HIV itself is a virus; it's roughly spherical, and about 60 times smaller than the human red blood cell. That's actually rather large for a virus. It's one of a kind of viruses called retroviruses that have their own unique enzymes and proteins that can literally insert their own genetic material into that of the infected host cells. Viruses are, in a way, not really living organisms. They don't have any way to extract energy from their environment, and they can't reproduce on their own. What they do is infect the cells of living organisms and use their own genetic instructions to take over the cell's machinery, sort of like a new boss moving into a factory and telling the workers what to do.

If you're infected by a common cold virus, for instance, the viral instructions that take control of the cells lining your nose tell those cells to make lots of extra mucus and to use their own cellular energy and metabolism to make more virus particles that can be spread around. HIV is even more clever than that, taking this idea of controlling a cell one step further. As a so-called retrovirus, HIV contains a special enzyme called reverse transcriptase that turns the virus RNA into DNA that is directly inserted into the DNA of the host cell. It's not just a boss shows up and takes over, giving instructions; it's a boss that literally takes over the host DNA and makes the host's old boss give instructions from HIV.

Wait. It gets worse. HIV preferentially infects our own immune cells—the cells that are supposed to be fighting off infections. The host's own immune-fighting apparatus, instead of defending the body against HIV, is tricked into damaging our own cells and making more HIV to infect more cells.

Now, HIV doesn't necessarily make the host immediately ill. It can replicate and spread in a relatively small number of cells, leaving plenty of normal immune cells to do their job. It can take years for people with HIV infection to develop signs of serious illness. The diagnosis of AIDS is made when a person with HIV infection has clinical manifestations of disease, either caused by the virus itself or by an opportunistic infection. Without treatment, about 50 percent of people infected with HIV will develop AIDS within 10 years, although a small number of people seem to remain healthy indefinitely. In addition to destroying the host immune system, HIV infects cells in the brain, causing, eventually, a form of dementia, and sometimes cells in the gut and other tissues.

Without a functioning immune system, serious illness can occur from out-of-control, ordinary infections, for example, the thrush our patient example presented with. A fairly ordinary, innocuous infection can be much harder to clear or can have severe or prolonged symptoms. There are also less ordinary infections, sometimes called opportunistic infections. These are caused by organisms that couldn't cause any problems for a healthy individual at all. One of the typical illnesses at presentation of AIDS is the lung infection seen in our patient, Pneumocystis. This only occurs in people with depressed immune systems. Though we can still use antibiotics, antivirals, antiparasitic drugs, and antifungals to some benefit in AIDS patients, none of these drugs works as well as they would in a person with a normal immune system. Keep that lesson in mind, that drugs help our immune system fight infections; they don't knock out infections very well on their own.

There is another important role for immunity: to protect us from cancer. We're going to talk about cancer more in a later case, but just a brief preview. Cancer cells are, in fact, different from normal, healthy body cells. They often have different proteins on the cell surface, or have other molecular features that distinguish them from our own cells. Because of that, our immune systems can at least sometimes tell cancer cells from normal cells and attack them.

They're akin to a foreign invader, like a bacteria or virus that's not supposed to be there, a cancer cell is also an enemy that can be attacked. People with AIDS, like people with other severe immune deficiencies, have a dramatically increased risk of many different kinds of cancers, and their cancers can grow and spread much more quickly than expected. Many of the cancers more commonly seen in AIDS patients are themselves triggered by a viral infections, illustrating the overlap between infection, immunity, and cancer-related diseases.

There are several different ways that HIV infections can present. There is an acute phase, occurring two to four weeks after initial infection. The symptoms here are usually fever, aches, sore throat, swollen lymph nodes, sometimes a rash, or some GI symptoms. Those symptoms are not very specific, and many of these acute infections are not diagnosed as HIV. One common misdiagnosis, at this point, is infectious mononucleosis. Many people have no symptoms at all during this earliest phase. In retrospect, we're not sure when our patient had contracted the HIV, or when he had, perhaps, had symptoms like these in his acute phase. He may never have noticed this, or his symptoms could have been so mild that they weren't remembered.

After the acute phase, there's a prolonged period of latency, where the virus slowly spreads without symptoms. Depending on the viral load, that is, how many virus particles there are in the blood, a person at this stage can be more or less contagious. In some cases, very high viral loads and infectivity can be associated with minimal, if any, symptoms, at least for a while. During this stage, patients can be found by routine screening of sexually active adults or others with risk factors. If symptoms are present, they might include chronic enlarged lymph nodes, fever, fatigue, weight loss, diarrhea, or cough, and all of these can come and go and may not overlap at the same time, which may make the diagnosis easy to overlook. Catching people early, here in the latent stage, before obvious symptoms of AIDS develop, leads to a better long term prognosis.

Full-blown AIDS, which usually occurs within 10 years of exposure, includes more severe symptoms, including fevers with soaking night sweats, cough and shortness of breath, chronic diarrhea, plaques in the mouth, rashes, distorted vision, and persistent fatigue. Which symptoms predominate depends on which opportunistic infections are present. Those initial five case reports, including our patient, were all in this phase of full-blown AIDS, though that hadn't been known at the time.

The most commonly used test for HIV is a blood test for antibodies to the virus, which usually becomes positive 3 to 12 weeks after infection during seroconversion. Seroconversion is when the serologic tests—the serum tests for antibodies—become positive. This delay in positivity means that someone with acute HIV, a new infection with symptoms, may still have a negative HIV test. In cases of suspected acute HIV, before seroconversion, a test for HIV genetic material in the blood using the PCR technique can show infection. This same test, sometimes called a viral load, can also be used to see how heavily the blood is infected, and thus how contagious a person might be.

Another test commonly used in the evaluation and follow up of an HIV patient is a CD4 count, a count of the T helper lymphocytes that are destroyed by HIV infection. A normal CD4 count is around 800 or 1200. In advanced HIV and AIDS, this trends into the 100s, or eventually down to zero.

The most effective treatment of HIV starts early. We have medicines that can prevent even the initial transmission of HIV; this can be used during the birth of a baby to an HIV positive mom, or after an inadvertent needle stick blood exposure for a health care worker, or, perhaps, after an unsafe sexual encounter. When an HIV infection is diagnosed, we have about thirty different anti-HIV medicines to stop the spread of the virus. These are used in a variety of combinations to make them more effective, and also to prevent the virus from developing resistance. Current HIV medications need to be taken every day for the rest of the patient's life.

We also have a number of medications to prevent and treat the opportunistic infections that cause a lot of the suffering in HIV patients. Again, these need to be taken long term. Medication regimens for AIDS and HIV patients can be complex and very expensive, and may lead to significant side effects. It's also crucial to help people with HIV infections maintain good overall health and nutrition, and to take steps to prevent transmission to other people.

I want to step back for a moment to review a brief timeline of the story of HIV and AIDS to illustrate the remarkable progress we've made in a very short time. HIV, or a virus that later became HIV, probably first made its way into humans in the early 1900s, spreading from an infection in primates in central Africa. The first known case of HIV-related illness was in a person who died in the Congo in 1959. In about 1968, HIV probably first arrived in The United States. In 1975, the first reports of a "wasting illness," with symptoms that were likely related to HIV infection were occurring in Africa.

In May of 1981, a journalist for a local gay-oriented newspaper wrote about a strange pneumonia striking men in New York. The next month, the CDC for the first time formally reported a cluster of cases, including our patient case presented today. By the end of 1981, 121 people had died of this in the United States. By 1983, the virus was isolated, though it didn't acquire the name HIV until 1986. By then, antibody screening was routinely being used to prevent transmission by donated blood, though that was too late to save life of Ryan White and thousands of other people who depended on blood products, especially those with hemophilia.

In 1987, the first drug to specifically treat HIV was approved. This was AZT, or zidovudine, and it's still used widely today. In 1989 there were an estimated 100,000 cases of AIDS in the United States, including many babies and children who contracted the infection during birth. By 1992, AIDS had become the number one killer of men in the United States from age 25 to 44, and two years later, it became the number one killer of women of that age. Remember, this is only about 10 years after the first cases were reported. Drugs could, by then, prevent the transmission of HIV from mother to baby, and soon a drug regimen was developed for prophylaxis after exposures. New drugs and new drug strategies became widely available for prevention and treatment. Nonetheless, by 1997 an estimated 30 million adults worldwide had become infected with HIV. Most of these people were in Africa, without access to effective treatment.

Today, in the developed world, most HIV infections can be successfully managed to maintain long-term health, especially if they're caught early. Medications, usually used in combinations, can suppress the HIV virus, and treatments are available to treat most of the opportunistic infections and other complications of HIV. Still, at this point, there is no cure, and there is no effective vaccine. In the United States, there are currently about 1.2 million people infected with HIV, and many of them don't even know it yet.

The HIV epidemic has had a huge impact on medicine. It directly pushed immunology into the front stage of science and medicine, leading to the discoveries of methods of treating opportunistic infections in not only AIDS patients, but in patients with other immune-compromising diseases, following organ transplants or treatment for cancer. This knowledge has allowed the development of an entire field of bone marrow transplantation for the treatment of many deadly diseases in children and adults. A better understanding of the science of viruses has allowed us to develop retroviral tools for gene delivery systems and promising future treatments for, perhaps, almost any genetic condition. At the same time, the surge of HIV has contributed to the return of other infectious illnesses, most notably tuberculosis. That's an old infection that shortly ago could have been considered rare, at least in the developed world. It has made a resurgence, paralleling the appearance of AIDS.

HIV has also had a significant cultural and economic impact. Whole economies, especially in Africa, have been decimated, with millions of people unable to work or care for their kids. In the United States, the AIDS epidemic has contributed to shifting attitudes about sex in our lives and popular culture. What started with a report of five cases about 30 years ago is now a major part of our medical and social landscape.

Today's case was a good opportunity to learn about some of the basic tools of medical diagnosis—the history, the physical, some of the common tests and X-rays. But, really, as a doctor, you'll see that your most important tools are your senses and your brain—listening to your patient, observing, and thinking about data you've collected. Listening: that can not only help you glean the clues you need, but can also help develop a trusting, two-way relationship with your patient.

Next up, we have a good case; it's a bit of a mystery, and it's going to test those crucial skills.

Puzzling Pain
Lecture 3

The most experienced physicians know that sometimes our initial assumptions lead us astray. Keep an open mind, keep listening, and keep an eye on the patient in front of you. It's a mistake to only look for clues that support what you think you're looking for. In fact, the clues that don't fit are often the clues that are the most useful, the ones that eventually lead you to the correct diagnosis. This lecture will teach you how important the history and physical exam can be—how looking for details is essential and how we need to make sure that we do our job thoroughly.

Abdominal Pain

- Imagine that a 36-year-old woman, Louisa, comes to our outpatient clinic with a chief complaint, in her words, of: "I'm tired of being in pain all the time." Louisa says that her main problem is abdominal pain, usually in the lower part of her belly, that sometimes gets better and worse but is essentially always there. It began four or five years ago and has gotten progressively worse.

- Because of the pain, she can no longer work. She's already seen a number of specialists, including a gastroenterologist, who diagnosed her with irritable bowel syndrome. Louisa is looking to us to review the whole picture and figure out what's going on.

- Louisa says that her pain is usually in her lower belly, below her navel. It doesn't really seem related to eating or drinking, or to any specific foods. Though she's had some occasional diarrhea, that's not usually a main problem. Her stools have never been hard, but she's been treated with a mild laxative because she has reported that passing stool is often painful. The laxative didn't help. She says that the pain doesn't seem to vary with her menstrual periods.

- She got the impression from a previous doctor that maybe the pain was all in her head, and she agrees that she feels stressed all the time. Louisa says that she did see a psychiatrist, who diagnosed her with depression. However, the medicine the psychiatrist prescribed didn't help her feel better, so she stopped seeing him.

- Louisa is a woman with chronic lower abdominal pain. Though there are many causes of these symptoms, our history, review of systems, and physical exam fit best with something wrong with the lower GI system, or perhaps a gynecological problem.

- There's also been a suggestion from a previous doctor that somehow this is all in her head. Stress and psychological factors can certainly cause significant and debilitating symptoms, including chronic pain. But she already looked for help from a psychiatrist.

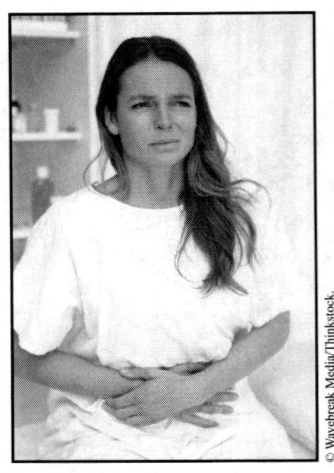

Abdominal pain is a symptom that is common to several different ailments.

- Also, there is a huge gray zone between symptoms that are physical in nature and symptoms that have a psychological basis. Belly pain will be made worse by stress, whatever the original cause of the pain might be. A classic mind-body illness that straddles this line is irritable bowel syndrome, which a previous doctor had suggested as a diagnosis for our patient.

- Our next step is to look over the laboratory information. A CBC was normal—Louisa is not anemic, meaning that she probably hasn't been losing blood from her gut. That was confirmed with a negative stool test for blood. Knowing that there is no blood in the stool goes a long way toward ruling out significant gut inflammatory disease or colon cancer.

- Louisa also had two blood tests done—an **erythrocyte sedimentation rate (ESR)**, sometimes referred to as a "sed rate," and a **C-reactive protein (CRP)**—to look for evidence of inflammation. These are very important, common tests. Both of these tests will be elevated if there is significant inflammation anywhere in the body. These tests do not tell you where the inflammation is or what's causing it.

- Louisa has had several of these done over the years of her illness, and they were always normal. Other tests done included a normal screen for celiac disease and normal urinalyses.

- Our patient has also had an ultrasound study of her abdomen and pelvis. Ultrasound uses high-frequency sound waves—too high for humans to hear—that are transmitted from a transducing probe into the body. The sound waves echo off of body tissues back to the probe. Tissues of different densities have a varying ability to reflect sound waves, so the reflected information can be processed into a visual image.

- Ultrasound is transmitted at low energies, far too low to affect tissues, and there are no known ill effects from ultrasound medical studies. There is no radiation, and typically no sedation or **IV** contrast is needed. Ultrasounds are sometimes called sonograms; an ultrasound of the heart is commonly called an echocardiogram. These terms all refer to the same imaging technology.

- Ultrasound does have some limitations. It can't peer very far into the body, so it's not as useful for deep tissues and may be difficult to use in obese patients. Ultrasound also cannot produce images through bone. Still, it's very useful for looking at the abdominal organs, including the kidneys, bladder, and liver, and it's great for gynecological assessments of the ovaries and uterus and for peeking at an unborn baby.

- Louisa's abdominal and pelvic ultrasound revealed no **pathology**. However, our patient finally disclosed that she has painful intercourse, painful passage of stool, and infertility. Those three symptoms, together, are a classic triad for a cause of chronic abdominal or pelvic pain in women: endometriosis.

Endometriosis

- Endometriosis is common. Probably about 15 percent of women have some degree of endometriosis, though the extent and severity of symptoms vary greatly. The normal endometrium is the lining of the uterus—tissue comprised of glands, blood vessels, and connective tissue that thickens and is then shed during each monthly cycle.

- In some circumstances, this endometrial tissue is found outside of the uterus—on the inside wall of the abdomen, on the ovaries, or nearby. It's unclear how this tissue gets there. It could spread during menstruation, or cells could spread though lymphatic or blood vessels. The cells of endometriosis are normal cells, just in the wrong place; this is referred to as "ectopic" tissue.

- These misplaced areas of endometrial tissue are what cause the symptoms of endometriosis. Pain is caused in part from bleeding, which may be cyclical. Recurring bleeding cycles can lead to scarring, especially because unlike bleeding in the uterus, the blood from endometriosis cannot be expelled from the body. However, the extent of endometriosis, the amount of ectopic tissue observed, doesn't always correlate with the degree of pain women experience.

- **Dyschezia**, or painful passage of stool, is a characteristic symptom of endometriosis, and it is also caused directly by the presence of endometrial tissue near the distal colon and by resulting scarring and **adhesions**. Women with endometriosis may experience painful symptoms intermittently, and they may or may not vary with their menstrual cycle.

- About 30 to 40 percent of women with endometriosis have problems with impaired fertility, perhaps also related to scarring and adhesions that alter the positioning of the ovary and fallopian tubes. However, even mild degrees of endometriosis, without significant scarring, can lead to infertility.

- The treatment of endometriosis needs to be tailored to the individual case. Medical options include the use of a variety of **hormone** strategies to reduce the development of endometrial tissue, or to stop menses altogether. There are also surgical approaches to removing or destroying the ectopic endometrial tissue through minimally invasive, **laparoscopic** procedures. While this can be effective in reducing pain and restoring fertility, the degree of success can be difficult to predict.

- Laparoscopic approaches have the advantage of a much quicker recovery, less pain, less scarring, and a reduced risk of bleeding than traditional abdominal surgery. However, they may take a little longer, and not all procedures can be done using small laparoscopic tools. The surgeon also loses the ability to feel and use his or her hands directly.

- There are also even more advanced minimally invasive techniques, using devices to robotically assist the surgeon through even smaller or fewer openings, or even by using openings through normal body orifices, such as through the wall of the esophagus.

Good Lessons
- There are some good lessons from our patient's prolonged diagnostic journey. It took several years for the correct diagnosis to be made, which is especially discouraging because there was effective therapy available. What went wrong, and what lessons should doctors and patients learn?

- Our first mistake was that there was an incomplete history. We knew that gynecological issues were a potential cause of symptoms, but we didn't ask about her sexual history. Knowing about one symptom, that intercourse had become painful, was a crucial diagnostic clue. It was overlooked perhaps in part because of embarrassment.

- Even doctors don't necessarily like to talk about these things. Still, if you're the patient, keep in mind that you need to speak up about symptoms that are bothering you. Don't wait for the doctor to ask, and don't assume that if the doctor didn't ask, he or she doesn't need to know.

- Another mistake was overlooking the necessity for a thorough and complete exam. Louisa was uncomfortable about anyone performing a rectal exam—probably because she knew it would be painful. But a gentle rectal exam could have revealed specific findings that could have helped the medical team reach the correct diagnosis sooner. A gynecological exam would have been diagnostic—but our patient had stopped seeing her gynecologist.

- Another issue was a lack of good collaboration on the part of the doctors involved. We're supposed to be a team, working together. But unfortunately, the ball got dropped, and more than once. Sometimes, the best diagnostic tool isn't a blood test or an **MRI**—it's just doctors talking to each other about the case so that everyone on the team knows what's going on.

- Another lesson is that we've all got our favorite tools and our favorite ways of looking at things. Our patient had been referred to a gastroenterologist early on, but the GI doctor was looking for GI diagnoses. In fact, the psychiatrist that the patient saw later was looking, mostly, for psychiatry diagnoses. An open mind, from all of the doctors on the team, helps avoid our putting on mental blinders that prevent us from seeing the correct diagnosis.

Important Terms

adhesion: Surfaces stuck together, typically referring to organs and tissues within the abdomen.

C-reactive protein (CRP): A blood protein that can be measured in the laboratory. An elevated CRP is an indication of inflammation.

dyschezia: Painful defecation.

hormone: A substance secreted into the blood that controls functions at a distant site—for example, insulin.

intravenous (IV): Within a vein.

laparoscopy: A surgical procedure using optical instruments inserted through the abdominal wall to view the inside.

magnetic resonance imaging (MRI): Using a strong magnetic field and radio waves to get detailed images of internal organs.

pathology: Diseased tissue, or the collective features of a disease—or the branch of medicine that studies diseased tissues.

erythrocyte sedimentation rate (often abbreviated "sed rate" or "ESR"): A blood test of inflammation.

Suggested Reading

Giudice, ed, *Endometriosis*.

Endometriosis.org, http://endometriosis.org/.

Questions to Consider

1. What kinds of medical problems, other than diseases of the stomach, cause "stomachaches"?

2. Can a doctor determine if a bellyache is caused by psychological factors? How?

Puzzling Pain
Lecture 3—Transcript

Welcome back. We have a good grand rounds case today with a common symptom and a common diagnosis, one that's probably affected some of you listening today. This particular diagnosis, though, can sometimes be tricky to make. Remember, the most experienced physicians know that sometimes our initial assumptions lead us astray. Keep an open mind, keep listening, and keep an eye on the patient in front of you. It's a mistake to only look for clues that support what you think you're looking for. In fact, the clues that don't fit are often the clues that are the most useful, the ones that eventually lead you to the correct diagnosis.

Here's what Louis Brotherson, a Scottish physician, said about today's diagnosis in 1774: "In its worst stages, this disease affects the well-being of the patient totally and adversely, her whole spirit is broken, and yet she lives in fear of still more symptoms such as further pain, the loss of consciousness and convulsions."

A 36-year-old woman, Louisa, has come to our outpatient clinic with a chief complaint, in her words, of "I'm tired of being in pain all the time." Now, traditionally, in grand rounds and formal case reports, we don't refer to patients by name; sometimes initials are used, or most commonly, we just use pronouns and awkward-sorts of sentences that avoid names altogether. But names are important, and I think, in the long run, it's better for doctors to focus on people, rather than diseases. So from here on out, in this course, I'm going to give our patients' names.

Louisa says that her main problem is pain, abdominal pain, usually in the lower part of her belly, that sometimes gets better and worse but is essentially always there. It began about four or five years ago and has gotten progressively worse. Because of the pain, she can no longer work. She's already seen a number of specialists, including a gastroenterologist who diagnosed her with irritable bowel syndrome. Louisa is looking to us, her internists, to review the whole picture and figure out what's going on.

That word, internist. What does it mean? After your graduation from four years of medical school, you can call yourself a doctor and put that MD after your name. To actually practice medicine, you need a license, which requires one year of training after you graduate; that year is called your intern year, and the people practicing during that training year are called "interns." After completing that intern year you can get a license and practice medicine, and call yourself a general practitioner, or GP, though that term is not as commonly used now, as almost all physicians choose to do further training in a residency program. Two more years of training after the intern year in a residency in general adult medicine will allow you to take the certification exam to become a board-certified doctor of internal medicine, or an internist. So an intern and an internist are two very different terms.

Back to our patient, who has been waiting patiently through that explanation to tell more about her story. Louisa says her pain is usually in her lower belly, below her navel. It doesn't really seem related to eating, or to drinking, or to any specific foods. Though she's had some occasional diarrhea, that's not usually a main problem. Her stools have never been hard, but she's been treated with a mild laxative, because she's reported that passing stool is often painful. The laxative didn't help. She says the pain doesn't seem to vary with her menstrual periods. She got the impression from a previous doctor that maybe the pain was all in her head, and she agrees that she feels stressed all the time. Louisa says she did see a psychiatrist, who diagnosed her with depression. However, the medicine the psychiatrist prescribed didn't help her feel better, so she stopped seeing him.

That's Louisa's story, in her own words. Now, let's take a mental pause to create a broad list of possible diagnoses. That'll help us know what to ask about and look for when we continue the evaluation. What we have here is a case of chronic abdominal pain. One good way to organize this would be to think about the organ systems in the abdomen, any of which could be a source of symptoms. You have the GI system itself, from the esophagus through the stomach and intestines. The respiratory system includes the lungs, which though located up in the chest can cause symptoms of belly pain. A pneumonia or infection in the lower part of the lungs can hurt in the belly. Also in the abdomen are the pancreas, spleen, liver, and gall bladder. There's also the urinary system—the kidneys and bladder—and in our female patient, the ovaries and uterus. There are bones and muscles that hold it all together, and blood vessels and nerves coursing through and around the abdomen. Any of these organs or systems can be affected by a variety of diseases, and any of them can lead to the symptom of pain.

Let's see if our review of systems turns up anything else, or, if it can help us focus a bit more on some of these organs or systems. Remember, the Review of Systems is when we have our turn to ask questions. We'll think about the organs and systems we've listed and ask further questions about each one. If the pain is from the organs of the GI system, we'd expect some other GI symptoms. Our patient reports no change in appetite, no nausea, and no vomiting; there have been no symptoms of heartburn. There's been no weight loss. She had reported some on and off diarrhea, plus painful defecation—doctors call that dyschezia. So there are some GI complaints here, though all of them are from low down in the GI tract, way at the end.

We mentioned the respiratory tract, or lungs, but our patient denies cough and denies fever. Pneumonia, or really any lung illness is unlikely in a person who has no coughing. That word—denies—for those of you who aren't yet used to medical presentations, that word might sound odd. But doctors use the word frequently, just to report what a patient says. A patient "reports" positive things, like a fever or sore throat that they have had; and a patient is said to "deny" other symptoms when they haven't occurred. Denying doesn't imply that the patient is lying or that the patient is hiding something. In a medical presentation, denies just means that the patient says that symptom has not occurred.

Pancreas, liver, and gall bladder, are there questions that can rule in or rule out those organs as a source of pain? Louisa says she's never had any jaundice. That's a yellow color, especially seen in the whites of the eyes, that can be caused by liver or gall bladder disease. Pancreas disease does cause abdominal pain, but almost always causes vomiting too, a symptom she also denies. So far, Louisa's symptoms don't fit well with disease of the pancreas or the liver. Urinary problems, including kidney stones or any other blockage of urine flow, will cause pain. But her pain, she says, has never been worse with urination, and she doesn't recall ever having seen blood in her urine. We may want to check a quick urinalysis anyway, but at least from the history, urinary issues sound unlikely.

How about pelvic pain? Her pain, she says, does not really vary with menstruation. But it is down low, and we know that the so-called visceral nerves, the nerves that actually sense pain from our internal organs, are wired to our brain in a way that doesn't make their sensations very specific. In other words, a person might feel pain from the abdomen, but the actual site of tissue disease could be somewhere else. That's in contrast to the nerves that detect pain, say, in our skin. If you feel a skin pain very specifically on your hand, chances are that there is something going on right there. But nerves from the inside of the gut don't make a pain sensation exactly over the organ sending the signals. Appendicitis pain, for instance, begins right over the belly button, even though the appendix lives in the lower, right part of the belly. Anyway, let's keep this in mind: though she senses pain low in her belly, it might be so-called referred pain, originating somewhere else.

Let's go back to our Review of Systems. Could this pain be from muscles or bones in the abdomen? When asked, Louisa denies any history of trauma and denies vigorous exercise or activities that might cause injury. Also, she says that the pain never varies with the way she moves and is never particularly worse when she presses on the bones or muscles in her belly. This really isn't sounding like a muscle or bone problem.

One of the most difficult kinds of pain to track down, and to treat, can be when pain arises from the nerves themselves. We rely on nerves to transmit information to or from the brain, but what happens when there is damage to a nerve, say from being pinched between two vertebrae in the spine, or from an infection, like shingles? The pain can feel like it's from out in a limb, or in the belly, when in fact the pathology, the disease, is somewhere else entirely. Nerve-generated pain is severe and is often described as burning or sharp and unremitting, but really, it can feel like almost anything. Sometimes nerve issues can include tingling or weakness, which Louisa denies.

That's a good review of systems to cover the systems we had suspected could have been the cause of abdominal pain. Let me give you a little teaser, though, there was one question that we could have asked that we've left out;

it's actually a question that's often overlooked. It would have been a great clue, too. We'll get back to it later.

After the ROS, traditionally comes our detailed, background history, including family history, social questions, etc. Briefly, for today, the family history doesn't offer much; there is no history of gut problems from either of her parents' side, and she has no siblings. Our patient is married and has no children. Before she became ill, Louisa had worked as a librarian. It's time to move on to the physical exam. Louisa is a Hispanic woman, who appears to be comfortable and well. Her vital signs are normal. HEENT, that is, head eyes, ears, nose, and throat, reveals nothing abnormal. Her chest is clear, and cardiac exam is normal. When gently palpated, she seems to have diffuse discomfort of her abdomen starting below her belly button, or maybe she's just apprehensive about that part of the exam. There are no masses that can be felt, and palpating externally over her bladder and ovaries doesn't elicit any complaints. A gynecologic exam was deferred. Our patient was very uneasy about a rectal examination, so none was performed. No rashes or other lesions are seen on the skin, and movement of her legs or contraction of her abdominal muscles doesn't elicit pain.

Before we move on to labs and imaging, let's briefly review what we know. Louisa is a woman with chronic lower abdominal pain. Though there are many causes of these symptoms, our history, review of systems, and physical exam fit best with something wrong with the lower GI system, or perhaps a gynecologic problem. There's also been a suggestion from a previous doctor that somehow this is all in her head. Stress and psychological factors can certainly cause significant and debilitating symptoms, including chronic pain. But keep in mind that she already looked for help from a psychiatrist. Also, there is a huge grey zone between symptoms that are physical in nature and symptoms that have a psychological basis. Belly pain will be made worse by stress, whatever the original cause of the pain might be. A classic, mind-body illness that straddles this line is irritable bowel syndrome, which a previous doctor had suggested as a diagnosis for our patient.

It's very important, though, that we not put all of our diagnostic eggs in one basket, at least, not yet. We don't yet have all of the information we need. Even if the diagnosis is looking likely to be largely psychological, it's our job to confirm that by continuing to follow up other leads to rule out other issues that need to be treated differently.

Our next step is to look over the laboratory information. Louisa has actually had quite a few lab tests already, and she thought ahead and she brought those records with her. That's a very good idea for any patient to remember. If you've seen other doctors for the same problem, bring the notes and tests and results of any x-rays or other studies with you to your new doctor. That may mean you have to ask, ahead of time, for copies of these records, but it will save everyone a lot of time and money, and can help keep the diagnostic ball rolling. A CBC, or complete blood count, was normal. Louisa is not anemic, meaning she probably hasn't been losing blood in her gut. That was confirmed with a negative stool test for blood. Knowing that there is no blood in the stool goes a long way towards ruling out significant gut inflammatory disease or colon cancer.

Louisa has also had two blood tests done to look for evidence of inflammation. These are very important, common tests, so it's worth stepping back to learn more about them. These two tests are an ESR, sometimes called a sed rate, and a CRP. Both of these tests will be elevated if there is significant inflammation anywhere in the body. That includes a significant infection, now, not a common cold or sore throat, but an abscess or pneumonia or something like that, or they'll be elevated from chronic inflammation from many auto-immune diseases, or inflammation that occurs during cancer. These tests do not tell you where the inflammation is or what's causing it. Many times, the tests are more useful when they're negative. In a way, a negative or normal sed rate and CRP rule out many serious illnesses, or at least illnesses characterized by inflammation. Louisa has had several of these done over the years of her illness, and they were always normal. Other tests done included a normal screen for celiac disease, and normal urinalyses.

Louisa has also had an ultrasound study of her abdomen and pelvis. Ultrasound uses high frequency sound waves—too high for humans to hear—that are transmitted from a transducing probe into the body. The sound waves echo off of body tissues back to the probe. Tissues of different densities have a varying ability to reflect sound waves, so the reflected information can be processed into a visual image. Ultrasound is transmitted at low energies, far too low to affect tissues, so there are no known ill effects from ultrasound medical studies. There is no ionizing radiation, and typically no sedation or IV contrast is needed. Ultrasounds are sometimes called sonograms. Also, an ultrasound of the heart is commonly called an echocardiogram, or just an echo. These terms all refer to the same imaging technology.

Ultrasound does have some limitations. It can't peer very far into the body, so it's not as useful for deep tissues and may be difficult to use in obese patients. Ultrasound also cannot produce images through bone. Still, it's very useful for looking at the abdominal organs, including the kidneys, the bladder, and the liver, and it's great for gynecologic assessments of the ovaries and uterus, and for peeking at an unborn baby. Louisa's abdominal and pelvic ultrasound revealed no pathology. Everything looked normal.

Is this case perhaps looking more psychological? Some of the previous clinicians thought so and encouraged psychiatric care. There was one kind of odd symptom mentioned, though, the dyschezia, or painful defecation. That's common with constipation, of course, but our patient denied that. The GI specialist diagnosed irritable bowel syndrome. Does that usually cause dyschezia? Actually, no. When asked, our patient says that the GI doc did want to perform a colonoscopy, but she refused, and she stopped going to see him after that. She was very uneasy about the rectal exam today, too.

It's never too late to ask more questions. Thinking about these other doctors involved in her care, we asked Louisa, "Have you discussed these symptoms with your gynecologist?" No, Louisa admits. She hasn't seen her gyn in several years, since her failed treatment for infertility. Even then, she recalls, gynecologic exams were very uncomfortable. And now, when asked gently about any other symptoms, she brings up one other uncomfortable thing; for the past several years, sexual intercourse has become very painful. That was the one question that could have been asked earlier, by any doctor, during the review of systems. But talking about sex can be uncomfortable for doctors and patients both, and these questions are sometimes overlooked.

The most important clues have come together. Our patient has painful intercourse and painful passage of stool, and now we learn that she's had infertility. Those three symptoms, together, are a classic triad for a cause of chronic abdominal or pelvic pain in women—endometriosis. Endometriosis is common. It probably about 15 percent of women at some degree, though the extent and severity of symptoms vary greatly. The normal endometrium is the lining of the uterus. It's tissue comprised of glands, blood vessels, and connective tissue that thickens and is then shed during every monthly cycle. In some circumstances, this endometrial tissue is found outside of the uterus on the inside wall of the abdomen, or on the ovaries, or somewhere nearby. It's unclear how this tissue gets there. It could spread during menstruation, or cells could spread though lymphatic or blood vessels. The cells of endometriosis are normal cells in the wrong place. We call that ectopic tissue.

These misplaced areas of endometrial tissue are what cause the symptoms of endometriosis. Pain is caused in part from bleeding, which may be cyclical. Recurring bleeding cycles can lead to scarring, especially because unlike bleeding in the uterus, the blood from endometriosis cannot be expelled from the body. However, the extent of endometriosis—the amount of ectopic tissue that can be observed—doesn't always correlate with the degree of pain women experience.

Dyschezia, or painful passage of stool, is a characteristic symptom of endometriosis, and it is also caused directly by the presence of endometrial tissue near the distal colon and by resulting scarring and adhesions. Women with endometriosis may experience painful symptoms intermittently, and they may or may not vary with their menstrual cycle. About 30 to 40 percent of women with endometriosis have problems with impaired fertility, perhaps also related to scarring and adhesions that alter the positioning of the ovary and fallopian tubes. However, even mild degrees of endometriosis, without scarring, can lead to infertility.

The treatment of endometriosis needs to be tailored to the individual case. Medical options include the use of a variety of hormone strategies to reduce the development of endometrial tissue or to stop menses altogether. There are also surgical approaches to removing or destroying the ectopic endometrial tissue through minimally invasive, laparoscopic procedures. While this can be effective in reducing pain and restoring fertility, the degree of success can be difficult to predict beforehand.

Laparoscopy has been a huge advance in medical technology and has dramatically changed the way many surgical procedures are done. Traditional abdominal surgery starts with a laparotomy, that's an incision that opens up the belly so surgeons can get their hands and instruments in there. The incision has to be fairly large to get adequate exposure for the surgeon to work. In contrast to this large incision required for a laparotomy, laparoscopy relies on one or more small incisions through which are inserted a camera and surgical instruments. The abdominal cavity is inflated so there is room to move around, and the surgeon watches a video feed taken by the camera in the belly. Simultaneously, small instruments inserted through small openings can be used to manipulate tissues. These can cut or move or suture or staple, really performing many of the same sorts of things that surgeons can do directly with their hands. Laparoscopic techniques are routinely used for abdominal surgeries, including gall bladder and appendix removal, plus many urologic and gynecologic procedures, including the surgical treatment of endometriosis.

Laparoscopic approaches have the advantage of a much quicker recovery; there's less pain; there's less scarring; and there's a reduced risk of bleeding. However, they may take a little bit longer and not all procedures can be done using small laparoscopic tools. The surgeon also loses the ability to feel and use his or her hands directly. There are also even more advanced, minimally invasive techniques using devices to robotically assist the surgeon through even smaller or fewer openings, or even by using openings through normal body orifices like through the wall of the esophagus.

Louisa decided to pursue more aggressive surgical therapy, in part, because she had been suffering for a long time, and she was eager to get relief. A laparoscopic procedure was successful in verifying her diagnosis by direct visualization of the ectopic endometrial tissue through a scope, followed by removal of most of the tissue and scars. Unfortunately, though surgical therapy was effective in reducing pain, Louisa and her husband had to continue to pursue additional treatments to assist fertility.

There are some good lessons here from our patient's prolonged diagnostic journey. It took several years for the correct diagnosis to be made, which is especially discouraging, because there was effective therapy available. What went wrong, and what lessons should doctors and patients learn? Our first mistake was that there was an incomplete history. We knew that gynecologic issues were a potential cause of symptoms, but we didn't ask about her sexual history. Knowing about one symptom, that intercourse had become painful, was a crucial diagnostic clue. It was overlooked, perhaps in part, because of embarrassment. Even doctors don't necessarily like to talk about these things. Still, if you're the patient, keep in mind that you need to speak up about symptoms that are bothering you. Don't wait for the doctor to ask, and don't assume that if the doctor didn't ask, he doesn't need to know.

Another mistake, overlooking the necessity for a thorough and complete exam. Louisa was uncomfortable about anyone performing a rectal exam, probably because she knew it would be painful. But a gentle rectal exam could have revealed specific findings that could have helped the medical team reach the diagnosis sooner.

A gynecologic exam would have been diagnostic, but our patient had stopped seeing her gynecologist, either because of discomfort with the exam, or maybe because she was discouraged by the lack of progress in treating her infertility. Some internists may not be comfortable doing a complete gynecologic exam, and that's fine, but someone should have asked if that part of the exam had been done, and if the doctor didn't feel that he or she had the right skills to do that part of the exam, he should have asked for help by referring her back to the gyn.

That brings us to another issue, a lack of good collaboration on the part of the doctors involved. We're supposed to be a team, working together. But unfortunately, the ball got dropped, and more than once. The gynecologist knew there was infertility, but that wasn't known to us until late in the game; we also didn't know that she hadn't had a good gyn exam in several years. Our patient stopped seeing GI because she didn't want a colonoscopy. That's, of course, a decision that she has a right to make, but if we knew that earlier, it could have been helpful. Sometimes, the best diagnostic tool isn't a blood test, or an MRI, or anything fancy or expensive; it's just collaboration, doctors talking to each other about the case, so everyone on the team knows what's going on.

As a patient, you can encourage that kind of collaboration. Bringing medical records and tests with you to every visit. Make sure every doctor you see knows about every other doctor you see, and that they all send each other their visit notes, so they have each other's thoughts and plans. Although it's not practical for every doctor to call each other for every case, when a diagnosis is unclear, or when things aren't going smoothly, ask your doctors to get on the phone. You'd be surprised how often a quick phone call solves problems. The telephone is a crucial and underused diagnostic instrument.

All right, one more quick lesson, there's an old saying, if all you have is a hammer, every problem looks like a nail. What this means is that we all have our favorite tools and our favorite ways of looking at things. Our patient had been referred to a gastroenterologist early on, which I think was a very reasonable step. But the GI doc was looking for GI diagnoses. And, in fact, the psychiatrist that the patient saw later was looking, mostly, for psychiatry diagnoses. That's OK, that's their job. But patients do not come with a label on their forehead that tells you what kind of specialist they ought to see. An open mind, from all of the doctors on the team, helps avoid our putting on mental blinders that prevent us from seeing the correct diagnosis.

Let's go back to our case; let's tie up some loose ends about a few alternate diagnoses that seemed plausible. There was a thought that our patient's pain could be based on psychological factors, and I think that wasn't an unreasonable possibility. Real discomfort and real pain can be caused, in whole or part, by stress and life issues, and the way that our minds respond to the challenges in our lives. People with chronic, unexplained pain should look into therapy and stress reduction to improve the quality of their lives. However, it's a mistake to hand off care of a patient with chronic pain to a mental health practitioner. Our patient's medical evaluation should not have stopped once she was referred to psychiatry. We can, and we should, offer help for the psychological impact of stressful symptoms, even while continuing our medical evaluation and treatment. In other words, it's not one or the other—psychology or physical problems. Most patients, actually, have both.

That's illustrated well by another diagnosis that was considered—irritable bowel syndrome. This is a common condition, leading to symptoms of abdominal pain, bloating, and diarrhea, or constipation symptoms. People with irritable bowel syndrome have no abnormal tests and no abnormal ultrasounds or biopsies. But their pain is quite real. What irritable bowel seems to be is an increased sensitivity to the normal sensations of the gut. Symptoms are worse with stress but don't occur only with stress. The treatment of irritable bowel syndrome primarily is focused on addressing lifestyle issues—improving the diet, working on stress reduction, and relaxation techniques, and, to a lesser degree, using medications to reduce the symptoms. Irritable bowel syndrome is a good example of an illness that kind of straddles psychology and what I suppose we should call traditional, organ-based medicine.

Today's case showed how important the history and physical exam can be, how looking for details is essential, and how we need to make sure that we do our job thoroughly. We're going to see that theme again and again. In our next case, we'll once again see that the right question at the right time can lead to the clue that cracks the case.

Just Look at Me

Lecture 4

Traditional medical education starts in the classroom. At many medical schools, the first two years are devoted to lessons in anatomy, biochemistry, physiology, etc.—to create a foundation of understanding of how the body works at times of health and what happens during times of disease. But even from the beginning of medical school, individual case histories are crucial and powerful teaching tools. For all of us in medicine, there is always more to learn. And we learn best from our own patients.

Red Rash

- Jayden, a 10-year-old boy, is brought to the emergency department with a chief complaint of "Just look at me." The remainder of the HPI was taken both from the child and his parents and older sibling, all of whom have accompanied him to the visit.

- Jayden had been in excellent health until five days ago, when he started to complain of feeling hot and tired. That night, he developed a cough and runny nose, and a fever began of 102 degrees Fahrenheit. The next day, his family noticed his eyes had turned red. His eyes have stayed red, and he has continued to run fevers from 102 to 104 degrees. Last night, his ears started to look red. Today, red spots have spread to his entire body. He says that the rash doesn't really itch or bother him.

- Additional history and review of systems don't reveal much. From his physical exam, we learn that his respiratory rate and heart rate are both elevated, and his blood pressure is normal. Overall, Jayden doesn't look well.

- There are two concerning things on his exam that we had better deal with quickly. Even before we focus on the diagnosis, we need to take some initial steps to address problems that may become life threatening if we don't act quickly.

- The first issue is his respiratory status. He's breathing quickly, at 40 breaths per minute, and fast breathing could mean that his lungs are not working as well as they should. He also has an overall kind of glassy-eyed, half-slumped appearance, which could be caused by a lack of oxygen delivery to his brain.

- We quickly use a device called a **pulse oximeter** to check the oxygen saturation in his blood. It is indeed low, at 90 percent. Before doing anything else, we should give him some extra oxygen by a special mask, and as we move along, we need to keep an eye on his respiratory status. Over the next few minutes, his pulse oximeter measurement improves.

- The second issue is that his heart rate is fast, and his mouth is dry. When asked, he doesn't remember the last time he urinated. Again, overall, he looks kind of glassy and wan and not terribly interactive. These findings suggest significant dehydration or even impending **shock**—which is when poor tissue perfusion starts to cause damage to vital organs.

- While we're asking more questions and working toward a diagnosis, we're not going to delay treatment for the dehydration. We quickly get him a small cup of juice for him to sip and refill it every few minutes to encourage him to continue drinking.

- Also, we'll ask our staff to start to make arrangements to transport our patient to the hospital. We don't know the diagnosis yet, but it seems like this child is going to need hospital care.

- There are many illnesses characterized by rash and fever. In this case, there is a rash and fever plus some additional hints. Our patient has pink eyes, fever, a cough, and what sounds like pneumonia with an abnormal chest exam. He also looks significantly ill. Put that together, and one rash-plus-fever illness seems very likely: measles.

Measles

- Because measles seems to be a likely diagnosis, we're going to immediately take some steps to control the infection. We'll make a list of anyone who had been in the waiting room with the patient and all staff that interacted directly with this family. Measles is very, very contagious—perhaps the most contagious illness known to mankind.

- When moving the patient back though the office to the ambulance, we'll have him and his family wear masks; they may have measles, too. We'll also immediately contact the health department so they can investigate the home and community for other potential exposures, beginning when the child became contagious, four days prior to the appearance of rash. Highly contagious and dangerous illnesses like measles are a public health call to arms.

- Jayden was transported from the clinic to the ICU of the local children's hospital, and placed in a negative-pressure isolation room to prevent air from his room from flowing back into the hospital. Strict isolation precautions were followed, and his family members were monitored for illness.

- In addition to measles, our patient was also suspected of having pneumonia. Jayden had a high fever and severe cough, and he also had an abnormal crackly sound in his lungs and was breathing quickly, with a low oxygen saturation. Pneumonia was confirmed by a chest X-ray.

- Measles, the virus itself, can invade lung tissue and cause pneumonia. Once there is fluid from measles infection in the lungs, frequently a **secondary** infection caused by **bacteria** can set in. This is sometimes called a **superinfection**—when one invader takes advantage of a first viral or bacterial infection, causing a second infection on top of the first. Although we have no medicine to fight the measles pneumonia directly, intravenous antibiotics were begun to treat the bacterial superinfection.

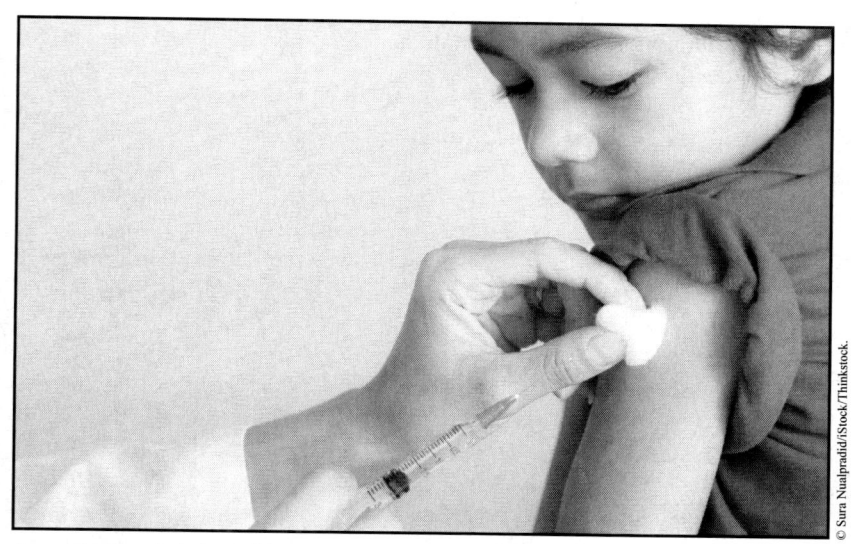

A vaccination is injected into a person to protect him or her from a specific disease.

- A confirmatory blood test for measles, called serology—which refers to blood tests on the liquid part of blood—was performed, which confirmed that Jayden did indeed have measles. Even though he was never vaccinated, our patient had high titers of anti-measles antibodies, confirming that this was a measles infection.

- There is no specific therapy for measles—nothing to kill the virus or make the infection itself milder or shorter. What we can do is provide fluids to support good blood circulation and extra oxygen, or ventilatory support, for the 1 in 20 measles patients who develop pneumonia as a complication. We also gave antibiotics, which can help if the secondary pneumonia is caused by bacteria.

- Another complication of measles is brain inflammation, called **encephalitis**. This can lead to **seizures** or permanent brain damage and occurs in about 1 in 1,000 measles patients. A much rarer complication is an untreatable, long-term degenerative brain disorder called SSPE that can start 10 years or more after natural infection. Encephalitis and SSPE are more common in the youngest patients.

- In the developed world, with access to supportive care, the mortality rate from measles is about 1 or 2 out of 1,000 people. In the third world, the mortality is up to 1 in 4. Measles, though entirely preventable with vaccines, continues to kill about 160,000 children, worldwide, each year—which is down from 2.6 million deaths per year prior to the wide availability of vaccines in the 1980s. That's good, but we still have a way to go.

- Measles is a serious illness, but it is one that can almost always be prevented by a vaccine that is very safe. Unfortunately, the rate of measles is increasing dramatically in Europe and the United States. The single factor that has led to a resurgence of measles is falling vaccination rates, driven by an entirely unfounded fear of vaccines.

Triage
- How did we know, up front, that our patient was very sick? This step is called triage—assigning a degree of severity to an ill or wounded patient so that the care team knows who needs attention fast. It's a crucial skill for all health-care workers to develop.

- Reviewing the **vital signs** is essential. This includes the heart rate, respiratory rate, and blood pressure. For all of these, numbers that are either too high or too low mean trouble, and the further from normal they are, the bigger the trouble you can expect.

- In children, the normal ranges of vital signs depend on the age of the patient. Babies normally have faster heart rates than children, who have faster heart rates than adults. Also, vital signs can be affected by factors like anxiety or pain.

- The patient's temperature is considered the fourth vital sign, and fever will also drive up both heart rates and respiratory rates.

- The pulse oximeter reading is sometimes considered the "fifth" vital sign. These devices are inexpensive and found in almost all offices and hospitals and provide a quick way to check on oxygenation.

- Children can have significant problems with respiration and oxygen delivery even with a normal pulse oximeter reading, so that reading has to be interpreted in the context of the overall picture.

- Even more important than these numbers in triage is the overall appearance or gestalt of the patient. A child who is interactive, smiling, talking, and playing is in good shape. A child who is listless, hard to wake, or just kind of "out of it" is the kind of child a pediatrician worries about the most.

Important Terms

bacteria: A unicellular microorganism lacking a nucleus.

encephalitis: Inflammation of the brain, most typically caused by infection.

pulse oximeter (often abbreviated "pulse ox" or "POX"): A device that measures the pulse and oxygen saturation in blood.

secondary: A symptom or problem caused by some other medical problem. For example, a secondary headache may be caused by a sinus infection, concussion, or brain tumor.

seizure: A sudden disruption in the normal electrical activity of the brain, accompanied by altered consciousness, movements, or other neurologic manifestations.

shock: A life-threatening state of insufficient blood flow to multiple organs.

superinfection: An infection that occurs on top of a first infection.

vital signs: Collectively, clinical measurements of pulse rate, blood pressure, respiratory rate, and temperature.

Suggested Reading

De Kruif, *Microbe Hunters*.

Offit, *Deadly Choices*.

Centers for Disease Control (CDC), http://www.cdc.gov/measles/pubs-mmwr.html.

Questions to Consider

1. What kinds of illnesses are especially prevalent in travelers, or those born overseas?

2. How can you tell if a child is very sick—so sick that he or she ought to be in the hospital?

Just Look at Me
Lecture 4—Transcript

Traditional medical education starts in the classroom. At many medical schools, the first two years are devoted to lessons in anatomy, biochemistry, physiology, and pathology. Those subjects create a foundation of understanding of how the body works at times of health and what happens during times of disease. But even from the beginning of medical school, individual case histories are crucial and powerful teaching tools. Young medical students, and even very experienced practicing physicians, don't yet know everything that can be learned about the science of health. For all of us in medicine, there is always more to learn, and we learn best from our own patients. No matter how experienced and well-read you might be, every patient is a new learning opportunity.

As we go through the cases in this course, I want you to keep three learning goals in mind. First, you'll be learning specific medical information, what symptoms mean, and how we evaluate them. Along the way, you'll learn about many specific health problems as illustrations. Second, you're going to see how doctors think, how we approach problems, and how we come up with solutions. The third goal, and perhaps the most important, is to turn that knowledge around, back to yourself. After all, we all have our own health problems and all end up on the other side of the stethoscope as patients. What's the best way to work with doctors to help improve our own health? In other words, this course will teach you how to be a better patient.

Today's case is an ancient illness. Accurate descriptions of plagues of this condition appear in histories thousands of years old, at times causing catastrophes. In 1529, this illness killed two thirds of the inhabitants of Cuba. In 1951, a single case of this illness appeared in Greenland, and over the following months, of the 4,262 inhabitants of Greenland, only five did not become seriously ill with this disease. Our patient today is patterned very closely after a real case, from the United States, from 2010. Jayden, a 10-year-old boy, is brought to the emergency department with a chief complaint of, "Just look at me."

Now, I've told you, that chief complaint is to be reported, whenever possible, in the patient's own words. In pediatrics, we do sometimes get some pretty off-the-wall chief complaints, and sometimes they're about Disney princesses or new sneakers, and have nothing whatsoever to do with the actual medical concern. Still, sometimes even a cryptic chief complaint like today's—"Just look at me"—may actually contain a little nugget of wisdom.

The remainder of the history of present illness was taken both from the child and his parents and older sibling, all of whom have accompanied him to the visit. The room was a little cramped. Jayden had been in excellent health until about five days ago, when he started to complain of feeling hot and tired. That night, he developed a cough and runny nose, and a fever began at 102 degrees. The next day, his family noticed his eyes had turned red, so they called their family physician, and he called in prescription antibiotic eye drops. Jayden's eyes have stayed red, and he has continued to run fevers from 102 to 104 degrees. Last night, before bed, his ears started to look red. He woke in the middle of the night because of coughing, and at that time, red splotches were seen on the back of his neck. Today, the red spots have spread to his entire body. He says the rash doesn't really itch or bother him. But still, that was his chief complaint—"Just look at me," referring to his rash.

As we've been doing traditionally, we'll step back briefly after the HPI to sketch out a mental list of possible diagnoses. It's an important step; it will help us think about the things to look for in our additional history questions and physical exam, keeping our minds open to multiple diagnostic possibilities. The main problems, here are fever and rash. We also have red eyes, cough, and some runny nose.

Now, fever we've talked about before in a previous case; it's usually caused by either infection, autoimmune or inflammatory diseases, or perhaps cancer. In children, especially when the fever hasn't gone on very long, almost all fevers are related to infection, so that's where we're going to focus our investigation. The cough, the runny nose, those go with infection, too. The next step in narrowing down the kinds of infection to suspect will have to do with exactly what kind of rash we're dealing with, so we'll tackle that a little later after we've examined the rash during the physical exam.

Before the physical, some additional history and a review of systems. Jayden had been in good health previously. His family travels a lot because of dad's job, and Jayden and his brother attend a non-traditional school involving a lot of internet-based classes. There is no suggestive family history, and they don't recall being around anyone else who had been particularly ill. Our patient has had no sore throat, no vomiting, no diarrhea, and the only medicine he has been taking is ibuprofen to help reduce the fever. He has an allergy to the antibiotic amoxicillin, which mom recalls caused a rash similar to this one several years ago when prescribed for an ear infection. But he's had no antibiotics of any kind recently.

On to the physical exam. Jayden is an African American young man, sitting in mom's lap. Vital signs include a temperature of 103° F, pulse 140, respirations 40 per minute, and blood pressure 98/78. Normal vital signs may be different for children than for adults. For a 10 year old, these numbers mean his respiratory rate and heart rate are both elevated, and his blood pressure is normal. Overall, Jayden doesn't look well. He's kind of half slumped in mom's lap, and his eyes look glassy and red. A test of blood perfusion, called a capillary refill, is delayed by two seconds—that's a quick test that's especially used in pediatrics, when we quickly squeeze the color out of a finger or toe and see how long it takes for the color to return. A normal cap refill is instantaneous. His refill is slow, which could mean that his blood perfusion is poor. That's often a sign of dehydration. Jayden's mouth is dry. The lung exam reveals crackly, noisy sounds in the lower lung fields. His heart exam is normal, though his heart rate is fast. The belly exam is normal too. He does have a widespread rash, and we'll describe that further in just a few minutes.

First, though, there are two concerning things on his exam that we had better deal with quickly. Even before we focus on the diagnosis, we need to take some initial steps to address problems that may become life-threatening if we don't act quickly. Number one is Jayden's respiratory status' he's breathing quickly, at 40 breaths a minute, and fast breathing could mean that his lungs are not working as well as they should. He also has kind of an overall glassy-eyed, half-slumped appearance, which could be caused by a lack of oxygen delivery to his brain. We quickly check a measurement with a device called a pulse-oximeter, to check the oxygen saturation in his blood. It is low, at 90 percent. Before doing anything else, we should give him some extra oxygen by a special mask; as we move along we need to keep an eye on his respiratory status. Over the next few minutes, his pulse-ox measurement improves.

Number two, his heart rate is fast, and his capillary refill is slow; along with that, his mouth is dry. When asked, he doesn't remember the last time he urinated. Again, overall, he looks kind of glassy and wan and not terribly interactive. These findings suggest significant dehydration or even impending shock; that's when poor tissue perfusion starts to cause damage to vital organs. So while we're asking more questions and working towards our diagnosis, we're not going to delay treatment for the dehydration. We quickly get him a small cup of juice for him to sip, and refill it every few minutes to encourage him to continue drinking. Also, we'll ask our staff to start to make arrangements to transport our patient to the hospital. We don't know the diagnosis yet, but I think this child is going to need hospital-level care. By the way, the elevated heart rate and respiratory rate could also be caused by his fever, so later on, when the fever is reduced, we'll want to reassess his breathing and pulse.

We're addressing his oxygen needs, and we've taken steps to correct dehydration, and we're continuing to monitor Jayden's status and vital signs. Now, let's look closer at this rash of his. It's flat, it's pink-red areas, in some areas the individual spots are so close together that they become one soft of large red area; we call that a confluent rash. The doctor word for a flat rash, the kind you can see but not feel, is macular. Other kinds of rashes are raised up off of the skin, or papular. There are a lot of words that can be used to describe rashes, but what's more important is to recognize the patterns of rashes that suggest certain diagnoses. The more you see, the more you know, and the more likely you'll recognize what you're seeing. Remember the chief complaint, "Just look at me." Our patient was right; with this and many other rash illnesses, the diagnosis can be found by looking at the patient.

There are many illnesses characterized by rash and fever, far too many to go through individually. For illustration, let me mention a few prototypical examples. Could our patient have chicken pox, for example? No, that rash looks very different. It's raised and includes many spots that have a small bubble, kind of visible inside the spot. That bubble becomes a little blister and later ruptures and crusts. And unlike this patient's rash, chicken pox itches, a lot. Even from the brief description, this isn't chicken pox.

Scarlet fever is another classic fever-plus-rash illness. This is usually caused by the same bacteria that causes strep throat and is usually accompanied by a sore throat, which our patient doesn't have. Also, the classic rash of scarlet fever is sandpapery, with tiny fine bumps that are accentuated under the waistband of clothing and other pressure areas. This isn't scarlet fever. Hives are a very common rash, especially in childhood, and are often triggered by infections that can also include fever. Also called urticaria, hives are large, raised, pink-to-red, warm areas that itch like crazy. This isn't hives.

A very serious and worrisome rash of childhood is called petechiae. These are small dots of red to purple blood trapped under the skin from broken blood vessels. A good test to distinguish petechiae is to press over the rash with a glass tumbler. Most rashes will fade when pressed—this is called blanching—and the rash will return after the skin is relaxed. However, petechiae, and large areas of confluent petechiae called purpura, will not blanch. Petechiae and purpura can sometimes be caused by minor viral infections but can also be caused by very serious infections, including meningitis and blood poisoning. It can also occur with leukemia and other blood disorders. So, a non-blanching, purplish or red rash needs urgent evaluation. Our patient's rash blanches easily, so it's not petechiae.

Lyme disease can also cause a rash and fever. The rash is very characteristic. It begins as a small bump at the site of a tick bite, and then it gradually expands into one large, red area or a large, red sort of bulls-eye shape. Sometimes, there is more than one red area. Accompanying this rash with Lyme disease can be fevers, aches, and chills. Our patient's rash really didn't look like this and spread much too quickly to be Lyme disease. There are several viral infections that cause a flat, pink, blanching rash. Just to mention a few: fifth disease causes a rash on the cheeks and upper arms but doesn't really cause fever or other signs of significant illness. Roseola is a flat, pink rash that occurs in young babies after a fever. Rashes can occur with many other infections, including mononucleosis, influenza, hand-foot-mouth disease; there are dozens of other possibilities.

Now, not every fever plus rash is caused by infections. For instance, Kawasaki disease is an inflammatory disorder of blood vessels—a vasculitis—that is fairly common in pediatrics. It causes prolonged high fevers and irritability, along with several other symptoms, not all of which have to be present, things like rashes, red eyes, swollen hands and feet, cracked or swollen lips, and enlarged lymph nodes. Our patient did have red eyes, remember. But Kawasaki is not common after age five. Still, it's a possibility to keep in mind.

In this case, we have the rash and fever plus some additional hints. Our patient has pink eyes, fever, a cough, and what sounds like pneumonia with an abnormal chest exam. He also looks significantly ill. Put that together, and one rash-plus-fever illness seems very likely—measles. We had a few other clues, too. The family was said to travel a lot, and it turns out that they had just been in France. Western Europe has seen a tremendous surge of measles cases in the last several years, including 16,000 cases in France in 2012. This has led the World Health Organization to issue travel advisories to ensure adequate vaccination of travelers to Europe. It also turns out that neither our patient nor his brother was ever vaccinated against measles, because, if you remember, his family didn't have them enrolled in traditional schools. They didn't think it was needed.

Since measles seems to be a likely diagnosis, we're going to immediately take some infection control steps. Remember that cramped exam room I mentioned? Maybe that wasn't a good idea. We'll make a list of anyone who had been in the waiting room with the patient and all staff that interacted directly with this family. Measles is very, very contagious, perhaps the most contagious illness known to mankind. Infectious droplets can linger floating in the air of an exam room for hours. When moving the patient back though the office to the ambulance, we'll have him and his family wear masks, For all we know, they may have measles too. We'll make sure that any of his potential contacts in our office have been fully vaccinated.

If he came into contact with babies too young to be vaccinated, protection can be offered with shots of immune globulin. We'll make sure that the ambulance crew and receiving hospital know that we're dealing with a very infectious illness so everyone can take precautions. We'll also immediately contact the health department so they can investigate the home and the community for other potential exposures, beginning when the child became contagious, which was four days before the appearance of rash. Highly contagious and dangerous illnesses like measles are a public health call to arms.

Jayden was transported from the clinic to the ICU of the local children's hospital and placed in a negative-pressure isolation room to prevent air from his room from flowing back into the hospital. Strict isolation precautions were followed, and his family members were monitored for illness. Though his parents remained well, his unvaccinated brother developed measles ten days later.

In addition to measles, our patient was also suspected of having pneumonia. Jayden had a high fever and severe cough and also had that abnormal crackly sound in his lungs and was breathing quickly with a low oxygen saturation. Pneumonia was confirmed on a chest X-ray. Measles, the virus itself, can itself invade lung tissue and cause pneumonia. Once there's fluid from measles infection in the lungs, frequently, a secondary infection caused by bacteria can set in. This is sometimes called a superinfection, when one invader takes advantage of a first viral or bacterial infection, causing a second infection on top of the first. Though we have no medicine to fight the measles pneumonia directly, intravenous antibiotics were begun to treat the bacterial superinfection.

Jayden patient required continued supplemental oxygen, IV fluids, nutritional support, and IV antibiotics. He stayed in the hospital for eight days. He went home in good condition, with instructions to get caught up on all of his vaccines as soon as possible. An aggressive public health effort identified 110 people, all potential contacts of Jayden, his brother, or secondary measles cases. All of them needed additional doses of vaccine or immunuglobulin and monitoring. Six other people developed measles from contact with Jayden, two of whom required hospitalization. The estimated total cost of this measles outbreak to the local health department was $300,000, not including any of the direct medical bills; that's just the cost of the investigation and treatment of contacts.

A confirmatory blood test for measles, called serology, was performed, which confirmed that he did, indeed, have measles. Serology refers to blood tests on the liquid part of blood. If you put a tube of blood in a centrifuge and spin it, you'll get a clot of heavier blood cells in the bottom, and a clear-to-yellowish fluid on top; that's called the serum. In the serum are immunoglobulins; those are also called antibodies. These are large protein molecules that help the immune system recognize and attack invading viruses and microorganisms.

We can test for specific kinds of antibodies, in this case, antibodies against the measles virus. Sure enough, even though he was never vaccinated, our patient had high titers of anti-measles antibodies. That confirms that this was a measles infection.

There is no specific therapy for measles, nothing to kill the virus or make the infection itself milder or shorter. What we can do is provide fluids to support good blood circulation and extra oxygen or ventilatory support for the 1 in 20 measles patients who develop pneumonia as a complication. We also gave antibiotics, which can help if the secondary pneumonia is caused by bacteria. Another complication of measles is brain inflammation, called encephalitis. This can lead to seizures or permanent brain damage and occurs in about 1 in 1,000 measles patients. A much rarer complication is an untreatable, long-term degenerative brain disorder called SSPE that can start 10 years or more after natural infection. Encephalitis and SSPE are more common in the youngest patients.

In the developed world, with access to supportive care, the mortality rate from measles is about one or two out of 1,000 people. But in the third world, the mortality is up to one in four. Measles, though entirely preventable with vaccines, continues to kill about 160,000 children worldwide each year. Now, that's down from 2.6 million deaths per year prior to the wide availability of the vaccine in the 1980s. That's good, but we still have a way to go.

When we started this case, Jayden was quite sick, and we had to kind of rush through some of the initial steps to get him stabilized and safe. Let's circle back to review what happened in more detail. How did we know, up front, that our patient was very sick? This step is called triage—assigning a degree of severity to an ill or wounded patient, so the care team knows who needs attention fast. It's a crucial skill for all health care workers to develop. What do we look for?

Reviewing the vital signs is essential. This includes the heart rate, respiratory rate, and blood pressure. For all of these, numbers that are either too high or too low mean trouble, and the further from normal they are, the bigger the trouble you can expect. In children, the normal ranges of vital signs depend on the age of the patient. Babies normally have faster heart rates than children, who have faster heart rates than adults. Also, vital signs can be affected by factors like anxiety or pain. The patient's temperature is considered the fourth vital sign, and fever will also drive up both heart rates and respiratory rates.

There is also a number we mentioned earlier that's sometimes called the fifth vital sign—the pulse oximeter reading. These devices are inexpensive and found in almost all offices and hospitals; they provide a quick way to check on oxygenation. However, children can have significant problems with respiration and oxygen delivery even with a normal pulse-ox, so that reading has to be interpreted in the context of the overall picture.

Even more important than these numbers in triage is the overall appearance, or gestalt, of the patient. A child who's interactive, who's smiling and talking and playing, that's a child in good shape. A child who's listless or hard to wake or just kind of out of it, that's the kind of child a pediatrician worries about the most.

In our measles patient, there were several overlapping reasons why he was so ill. One was his pneumonia, which prevented his lungs from efficiently oxygenating the blood. But he was also dehydrated, which decreased the amount of blood available for delivery to tissues. Think of it this way; if the circulatory system is like a bunch of trains running along tracks delivering fuel, he both had less fuel on each train—that's a lack of oxygen—and also fewer trains themselves. The treatment of severe dehydration requires intravenous fluids, but mild-to-moderate dehydration can often be treated with oral liquids, at least in a child like our patient who is conscious enough to drink and who isn't vomiting.

Jayden also had a high fever, 103 degrees. Now, fevers, themselves, are not harmful. They do not cause brain or tissue damage. Years ago, before the availability of vaccines to prevent serious infections, high fevers would often herald a serious infection, like meningitis or a blood stream infection, and those infections could cause serious harm, including brain damage. But now, among vaccinated children with good access to health care, fevers are very rarely caused by serious or harmful infections. Nonetheless, though fevers themselves are harmless, they do create problems. First, fevers make a patient feel really bad. People with fevers are achy and they're miserable.

They won't want to drink, which may contribute to dehydration. Also, fevers make people breathe more quickly, which increases the loss of water in the breath. Warm skin also loses more water to evaporation. So, fever contributes to dehydration in many ways, decreasing the ability of the circulatory system to deliver nutrients and oxygen to the tissues. Poor oxygenation, poor circulation, fever, dehydration, these are all interconnected problems that if untreated could lead to more complications and serious consequences.

There was another symptom our patient Jayden had; it was mentioned briefly, but then we focused on more immediate concerns. He had red eyes, one cause of what's commonly called pink eye, or conjunctivitis. In fact, before our patient came in so ill, the family had called the doctor to get a prescription for this. Ordinary pink eye is an infection of the eye, usually bacterial, that causes a pink eye with a lot of goo and crust. It's quite common, and although it's contagious, it's not particularly serious.

I don't disagree with a doctor calling in eye drops for suspected pink eye over the phone, but, in this case, even over the phone, it was clear that something else was going on. When the family called, the patient already had a substantial fever and a cough. These are not symptoms of ordinary pink eye. And his eyes, though pink, never had the expected gooey discharge that we see with ordinary pink eye. So, over the phone, someone could have been suspicious that there was more to the story, especially if someone had noticed that this child had not been vaccinated against measles. Parents, understandably, they like to avoid a doctor visit by occasionally calling ahead. It's the physician's responsibility, even over the phone, to ask the right questions so nothing important is missed.

Measles is a serious illness and one that can almost always be prevented by a vaccine that is very safe. So why are rates of measles increasing dramatically in Europe and the United States? The single factor that's led to a resurgence of measles is falling vaccination rates, driven by an entirely unfounded fear of vaccines. Sometimes rumors just come out of nowhere, but in this case, the distrust of measles vaccination stems from a single source, a publication in 1998 in a prestigious British medical journal, The Lancet. The lead author, Dr. Andrew Wakefield, claimed to have found evidence of MMR vaccine genetic material in the gut tissue of a handful of children with autism. In press conferences afterwards, he directly linked MMR vaccines to the development to autism, and a firestorm of concern erupted. Since then, no independent researcher has been able to replicate Dr. Wakefield's findings, and studies of millions of children have not found any evidence of an MMR-autism link. It's been revealed that Wakefield's study itself was fraudulent, and it's been retracted by the co-authors and by The Lancet. Still, the damage was done.

We're now seeing the effects of that distrust in falling vaccine rates. Measles, which was essentially eradicated from the United States in the 1980's, is back. Most cases have been linked to unvaccinated travelers, who, like our patient, bring back cases from overseas communities where measles has become common. Because measles is so contagious, secondary cases then occur among their contacts when they return home. Though measles vaccine is very effective, like any other medical intervention it's not 100 percent. Some vaccinated individuals do remain unprotected. Also, some babies are too young to be vaccinated, and some children and adults have immune deficiencies or other health problems that prevent vaccination. These individuals, babies and those with immune problems, are the most likely to have complications from measles. So it's especially important, to protect the most vulnerable among us, for everyone to get vaccinated. That protects us, our children, and our communities.

Measles commonly presents with fever, red-appearing eyes, a rash, and a cough. It is a diagnosis that many practicing physicians have never seen, but one that we had better become familiar with. The anti-vaccine movement has led to falling rates of the immunizations and a resurgence of measles, and other vaccine-preventable illnesses, too, like pertussis and mumps. We must stay vigilant to recognize potential cases of measles early on, and also to continue to encourage routine vaccinations by providing good, honest information about both the risks and benefits of immunizations and the risks of not vaccinating.

Next up, we have a very common symptom and a quote from Lewis Carroll. See you then.

Headaches in Wonderland
Lecture 5

Migraines can be a very odd disorder. Although most patients' main migraine symptom is headaches, some migraine types cause unexpected neurological or other symptoms—sometimes without any headache at all. Sometimes patients' cases are messy and complicated, and sometimes the best strategies for prevention and therapy aren't clear. The case that you will learn about in this lecture is a satisfying one. It has a clear diagnosis and a good, effective plan for prevention and treatment.

Sinus Headaches

- Gordon, a patient in the emergency department, comes in with the chief complaint of "I've got another one of these sinus headaches." The patient is a 42-year-old male, who is actually well known in the emergency department. He says that he gets sinus headaches all the time. This one began earlier in the day, with a severe headache starting kind of over his right eye, though it has now spread to both sides of his forehead. He says that when he gets these, he almost can't think straight, and his nose gets all stuffed up.

- Gordon has had six emergency department visits in the last four months. Every time, he complains about headaches and ends up getting IV fluids and pain medicines. He stays a few hours, feels better, and leaves.

- The classification of headaches starts with one question: Is this a primary or a secondary headache? Primary headaches are ones that occur without any other abnormality or specific pathology. These include migraine, tension, and cluster headaches. Although these kinds of headaches can be very painful and disruptive to life and work, they're sometimes thought of as "benign" headaches because they don't get worse and worse, and no one dies because of them.

- In contrast, secondary headaches are headaches caused by something else—something else that can be directly identified and treated. These include headaches from a brain tumor, an intracranial bleed, an abscessed tooth, meningitis, or—as our patient suspects—a sinus infection. Sudden or severe high blood pressure can also cause headaches.

- The secondary headache category also includes headaches that accompany many viral or bacterial infections, such as influenza or strep throat, or headaches caused by trauma. They can also be caused by **metabolic** disturbances, including low oxygenation or low blood sugar or from substance abuse or withdrawal.

- We are going to need more history and a physical exam. Headaches are almost always diagnosable based only on the history, with a physical exam to confirm suspicions. This is not a high-tech diagnosis. It involves going through some crucial questions with the patient to get an in-depth history.

- The most crucial headache question is as follows: Is this your first headache or your worst headache? That's very important—things like an intracranial bleed will cause a severe, worst-in-your-life headache, and that's a huge red flag for immediate action.

- More questions include the following: What happens when the headache starts? What symptoms develop with the headache? With migraines, there is often an aura—a visual or auditory phenomenon, such as flashing lights, that precedes the headache.

- Does the pain spread around? What does the pain feel like? Do you have any other medical problems? Are you stuffy all the time or just with the headaches? Is there anything that makes the headache get worse or better? Are you taking any medicines? What happens when you get a headache?

- After the questions have been answered, it's time for the physical exam. Gordon's vital signs are entirely normal, including a normal blood pressure. His neck is not stiff. A head, eyes, ears, nose, throat (**HEENT**) exam reveals cloggy, nasal-sounding speech. There is no nasal discharge and no post-nasal drip. His eye exam is normal, including normal pupils and normal pupil constriction to light. Neurologically, everything is normal.

- The recurrent, nonprogressive nature of his symptoms and the lack of any abnormal findings on the physical exam weighs against almost all causes of serious secondary headaches.

- There are just a few other red flags to review—a few more indications that a patient is at higher risk for a serious, treatable cause of headache that we don't want to miss, including the following.
    o A progressive nature—headaches that are getting worse and worse.

    o A "worst headache ever" (sometimes also called a "thunderclap headache").

    o Headaches accompanied by signs of infection, such as fever or stiff neck.

    o Headaches that change with posture or with coughing, straining, or sneezing.

    o Headaches accompanied by an abnormal physical examination.

    o Headaches in people with ongoing medical problems, such as cancer or HIV.

    o New headaches in people over 50 years old.

- Every item on this list relies only on the history and physical examination. We don't need any CT or MRI scans, or blood tests, for the vast majority of headaches that bring patients to the emergency department or to doctors' offices. There is no role for advanced imaging or other tests, as long as there are none of these red flags in the history and physical examination.

- In Gordon's case, there are no red flags, so this is very likely to be one of the primary headaches. There really are only a small handful of common primary headache types; these are almost always migraine, tension, or cluster headaches.

- Tension headaches are common. They can last from 30 minutes to 7 days and have a pressing or tightening quality; they're not throbbing. The pain is bilateral—which means that it occurs on both sides of the head—and of mild to moderate intensity. They're not aggravated by activity and lack **nausea** and vomiting. Typically, they're not made worse with lights or loud sounds. Our patient isn't having tension headaches.

- Cluster headaches are less common, but they're really quite characteristic. The pain is brief—from 15 minutes to 3 hours, without treatment. They begin and stay unilateral and are accompanied by one-sided facial symptoms on the same side as the pain: a red or watery eye, congestion or watery nose, one-sided sweating, or one-sided pupil or eyelid changes. The thing to keep in mind about cluster headaches is how these symptoms are so striking and unilateral and that the headaches are really quite brief. Our patient isn't having cluster headaches.

Migraines

- The most common primary headache disorder is migraine. These headaches last 4 to 72 hours and are unilateral (or at least begin unilaterally). The pain is of moderate to severe intensity and has a pulsating or throbbing quality. They get worse with activity, such as walking around or working.

- Migraines will always be accompanied by either nausea or vomiting or a combination of photophobia and phonophobia—which means that the headache gets worse with light and sound.

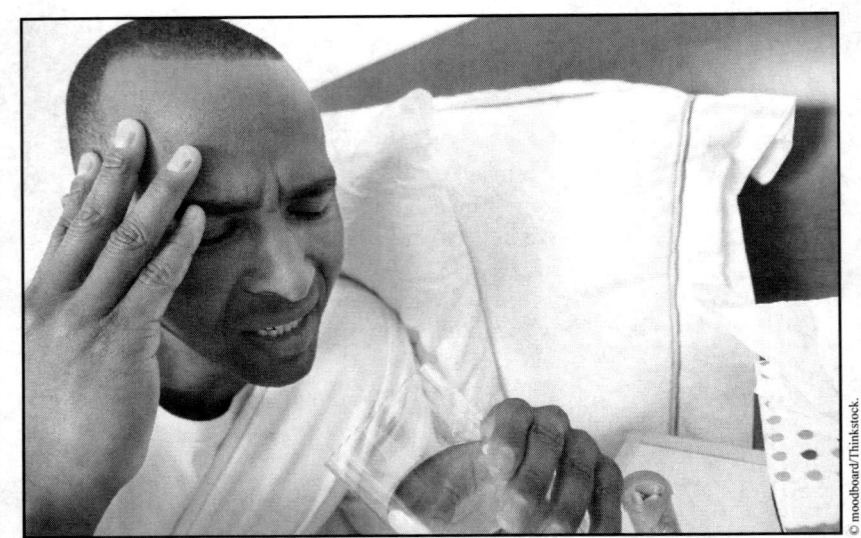

Migraines are severe headaches that occur again and again for a person.

- Though not part of the definition of migraines, they characteristically improve after sleep. Gordon mentioned sleeping off his headaches. We've ruled out secondary headaches with our history and physical, and his headache pattern fits perfectly into the definition of migraine. That's our diagnosis.

- Often, migraines are accompanied by changes in what's called the autonomic nervous system, the part of our nervous system that's automatic—the things we don't have to think about. It includes the nerves that make us sweat and the nerves that constrict blood vessels and make the skin look pale.

- Some migraine sufferers become pale and sweaty, and many feel nausea or abdominal pain from these autonomic nerve changes. Autonomic nerves also innervate the lining of the nose and can cause nasal congestion or stuffiness from increased tissue swelling—explaining why our patient thought he was having sinus headaches.

- Some, but not all, migraines are accompanied by an aura. These are reversible neurological signs or symptoms that occur before the headache, or sometimes just as the headache is beginning. Common auras include changes in vision, such as sparkling lights or a colored haze. They can also include auditory hallucinations, or weakness, or a vague feeling of dread.

Treating Migraines
- Dealing with migraines should always start with prevention. Many (though not all) migraines have specific triggers. These can include lack of sleep, hunger, dehydration, stress or illness, or sometimes bright lights or reading while in a car.

- People who have migraines should track their episodes and see if some of these common triggers seem to be part of the problem. Not all migraine sufferers have all of these triggers, but many have at least some, and some of these can be avoided through lifestyle modification, stress reduction, yoga, getting a good night's sleep, and other nonmedical steps. It's also very important for people with migraines to avoid falling into the trap of medication overuse and to modulate their caffeine intake.

- Beyond these preventive lifestyle strategies, migraine sufferers need an action plan to start as soon as possible when a migraine begins. For people who do have a warning aura, the migraine action plan needs to start as soon as the aura begins—which may be well before the actual headache. A migraine caught early is much more likely to be stoppable.

- A migraine action plan should include both medical and nonmedical steps. Usually, the patient will benefit from getting to a dark, quiet environment quickly. Sometimes a small snack, including some sugar, will help, perhaps even including some soda or coffee with caffeine. Although habitual caffeine use can lead to migraines, when taken at the start of a migraine, caffeine can help reduce its severity.

- Medicines can help, especially if taken at the start. These can include over-the-counter pain relievers like ibuprofen or acetaminophen. There are also very effective prescription migraine-stopping medicines. The best of these are in a family called the triptans. They all work similarly to block the brain receptor that is central to migraine development.

- All migraine sufferers who don't get full relief from over-the-counter products should have one of these triptans available for immediate use when a migraine begins. They come as pills and nasal sprays and in auto-injector devices that are especially useful for the many migraine patients who have vomiting with their headaches. Triptans, though very effective, can trigger rebound headaches if used too frequently.

- If, despite trigger avoidance and a good action plan, migraines are still occurring frequently, we ought to consider starting a daily migraine prevention strategy. This can involve adding a daily medication that can act as a migraine preventer. There are several of these available, though some can have side effects.

- There are also some more natural and potentially safer approaches to daily migraine prevention, including daily vitamin B_2 or magnesium supplements. Some studies have shown these to be quite effective in preventing migraines.

Important Terms

HEENT: "Head, ears, eyes, nose, and throat"—referring to these areas of the physical examination.

metabolic: Related to chemical processes that sustain life.

nausea: A feeling of queasiness, or that one is about to vomit.

Suggested Reading

Buchholz, *Heal Your Headache*.

Questions to Consider

1. What are the red flags that mean a headache is caused by a serious illness that needs treatment right away?

2. How are sinus headaches different from other headaches?

Headaches in Wonderland
Lecture 5—Transcript

Doctors are interested in people, not just what makes them sick, but also what makes them tick. In that way, they're a lot like writers, and sometimes doctors can learn some interesting things from novels and stories. We'll be doing that more than once in this course. Here's an example you might recognize: "It was much pleasanter at home," thought poor Alice, "when one wasn't always growing larger and smaller, and being ordered about by mice and rabbits. I almost wish I hadn't gone down the rabbit-hole…" That's a quote from Lewis Carroll's Alice in Wonderland, a fantastic tale published in 1865. Alice goes down the rabbit-hole for adventures with all sorts of creatures. People have speculated about how Carroll could have thought of this idea of shifting perspectives. Does Alice get small, or does the world around her get large? Or is it just her imagination, or maybe something else that makes the world seem to change size? We'll get back to that later.

First, we're in the emergency department tonight, and we have a patient who's just about fed up. Gordon's chief complaint is, "I've got another one of these sinus headaches." The patient is a 42-year-old male, who's actually well known in the emergency department. Even before we went in to see him, one of the nurses came by to give us a heads up—"That guy is always in here. He just wants drugs." Well, maybe so. Maybe not. Let's see what the story is.

Gordon, at first, he doesn't seem very happy to talk to us. The lights have been turned off in the small exam room, and he's lying there with a sheet pulled up over his head. He complains that it's the same thing, again and again, and we ought to just read his file. "It's all in there," he says. But ED docs, we're not really big on reading. We prefer to hear the story ourselves, from the beginning. We take a seat and let Gordon talk.

He says, again, it's a sinus headache, he knows what it is, he gets them all the time. This one began earlier in the day, with a severe headache starting kind of over his right eye, though it's now spread to both sides of his forehead. He says, when he gets these he almost can't think straight, and his nose gets all stuffed up. Gordon says, "I knew even this morning that I was going to get one of these. I just knew it." Then, our patient refuses to speak to us anymore. He ducks back under his covers and says it hurts to talk and tells us to leave and bring back his medicine. We decide it's time to step outside.

The nurse brings by a stack of paper from his last few ED trips; this is an old hospital, and the records aren't computerized. Sure enough, he's had six emergency department visits here in the last four months. Every time he complains about headaches and ends up getting IV fluids and pain medicines. Then he stays a few hours in the ED, feels better, and leaves. You note that he's been told to follow up at various times with his own physician, and with an ENT specialist to look into sinus disease, and with a neurologist. It's unclear whether he's followed up with anyone. By the way, real emergency physicians don't call it the ER. It's the ED. In other words, it's not a room, it's a department.

OK, let's step back and think about headaches. The classification of headaches starts with one question: Is this a primary headache, or a secondary headache? Primary headaches are ones that occur without any other abnormality or specific pathology. These include migraine, tension, and cluster headaches. Though these kinds of headaches can be very painful and disruptive to life and work, they're sometimes thought of as benign headaches, because they don't get worse and worse, and no one dies because of them.

In contrast, secondary headaches are headaches caused by something else, something else that can be directly identified and treated. These include headaches from a brain tumor, or an intracranial bleed, an abscessed tooth, meningitis, or, as our patient suspects, a sinus infection. Sudden or severe high blood pressure can also cause headaches, though the majority of people with high BP actually have no symptoms at all.

The secondary headache category also includes headaches that accompany many viral or bacterial infections, like influenza, or strep throat, or headaches caused by trauma. They can also be caused by metabolic disturbances, including low oxygenation, for example from altitude sickness, or low blood sugar, or from substance abuse or withdrawal. That's just a partial list to get started. The list of secondary headaches is really very, very broad.

Then we have one other idea. The nurse has suggested that our patient is really here because he's seeking drugs. Now, that is a possibility. We are going to need more history here, and a physical exam. It's time to head back into the exam room. In the meantime, we've ordered a dose of pain medicine, a mild narcotic. We say to our patient, "I know this has been rough for you. I see you've been here a lot for these headaches. I need to ask you some questions to see if we can get to the bottom of this, to help you feel better today but also to try to keep you from needing to come back to the emergency department so much." Gordon peeks out from under his covers. He gradually sits up and answers our questions.

Now, headaches are almost always diagnosable based only on the history, with a physical exam to confirm suspicions. This is not a high-tech diagnosis. We're going to go through some crucial questions one by one to illustrate how an in-depth history works. Our most crucial headache question: Is this your first headache, or your worst headache? That's very important; things like an intracranial bleed will cause a severe, worst-ever-in-your-whole-life headache, and that's a huge red flag for immediate action.

In this case, no, it's not the worst or the first. Gordon says this feels like every other sinus headache he's ever had. He says he's had these for the last 10 years, and he knows what they feel like. Every one of his headaches, he says, feels about the same. OK, more questions. What happens when the headache starts? What symptoms develop along with the headaches? With migraines, there is often an aura, a visual or auditory phenomenon, flashing lights or something like that, that precedes the headache. Gordon says, no, that never happens. His headache start with, well, just a headache. When the headache gets severe, he says, he gets a very stuffy nose and a stuffed up feeling in his sinuses above his right eye.

Does the pain spread around? Yes, Gordon says it's now "all over my head." But it always starts over the right eye. What does the pain feel like? It's a throbbing sort of pain, Gordon says. You ask, are you stuffy all the time, or just with the headaches? He says, no, just with the headaches. And he adds, he's seen an allergist and an ENT, and they didn't do him any good.

Is there anything that makes the headache get worse, or get better? Gordon says that they usually get better if he just lies down quietly. If he tries to work, they get worse. He says it's not the position of his body; the headaches do not get particularly worse when he stands up. It's more that any kind of work or activity, that's what makes it worse. He also denies that the headache is worse when he coughs, or sneezes, or strains to lift something.

Are you taking any medicines? No, he says. He was prescribed allergy medicine, and it didn't help. He just takes ibuprofen when it gets really bad, and then, if it's not getting better, he comes to the hospital. How many times, you ask, have you taken ibuprofen? He says he's taking it a lot lately, at least once a day for the past two weeks. Gordon denies any other medicines or street drugs. He says he hates coffee and doesn't drink tea or caffeinated sodas. He works from home as a customer service rep fielding incoming support calls.

So, we ask, what happens when you get a headache? He says most of the time he takes ibuprofen and goes to sleep, and usually, when he wakes up, he feels better and then can get back to work. Only sometimes, he says, he can't sleep, and it gets worse and worse, so he comes to the emergency department. The ED staff was leery, thinking he was a "drug seeker." Does this sound like a drug seeker? Gordon did, indeed, follow-up with an allergist and ENT. And he says, most of the time, he treats his own headaches at home and doesn't come in. You look at the ED records again. Usually, he's discharged home without any prescriptions at all. He's not asking for medicine. He's asking for relief. Ask yourself, as health care providers, have we done a good job for our patient so far?

It's time for the physical exam. Our patient is sitting up now. He looks reasonably comfortable. The vital signs are entirely normal, including normal blood pressure. His neck is not stiff. HEENT exam reveals cloggy, nasal-sounding speech. There is no nasal discharge and no post-nasal drip. His eye exam is normal, including normal pupils and normal pupil constriction to light. With an opthalmoscope, we can see all the way to the back of the eye, and we confirm that there is no increased pressure in the cranium pushing the nerves at the back of the eye forward.

We move on with the exam. Chest, lungs, heart, belly, they're all normal. In a headache evaluation, the neurologic exam is very important, especially to look for asymmetries in strength or reflexes, or anything else abnormal that could hint at a physical problem with the brain or with the spinal cord.

We make Gordon count backwards by threes as a way to test his cognition, and we make him walk on a straight line to check his balance. We check his strength by having him hold his arms out for 20 seconds. Everything here, neurologically, is normal.

Fortunately, our patient, Gordon, seems to be feeling better overall, so we step back outside to decide what to do next. Let's come back to the first decision point in the headache evaluation. Is this a primary headache, or a headache secondary to something else? We already have a lot to reassure us. We know this isn't a tumor; anything growing in the brain would cause progressive, worsening symptoms. He's had these headaches for years, and they're stable. It is not a tumor. It's also not an intracranial bleed, because it's not a worst- or first-ever headache. He doesn't have a fever or a stiff neck, so meningitis is out. Really, the recurrent, non-progressive nature of his symptoms and the lack of any abnormal findings on the physical exam weighs against any kind of serious, secondary headaches.

There are just a few other red flags to review, a few more indications that a patient is at higher risk for a serious, treatable cause of headache that we don't want to miss. We already have the information, but let's go through the most important hints again. Headaches that change with posture or with things like straining or coughing may be related to either too much or too little pressure in the cranium. This could be caused by tumors or other conditions that interfere with the normal flow of the fluid around the brain. Our patient doesn't have a history of this kind of headache.

Any patient with other health conditions, like cancer or HIV, may need additional evaluation for headaches, because they're at risk for a variety of intracranial complications, both from these diseases and also from medicines used to treat these diseases. Also, the age of the patient is important. Most primary headaches begin in the teen years, through perhaps the 30s or 40s. It is unlikely for someone in their 50s, say, to first develop migraines or any other primary headache. Our patient is 42, and he's had headaches for 10 years, so that's reassuring. But if this were new headaches in someone over 50, even with an otherwise normal history and physical, we might want to be a little more cautious of our diagnosis.

So, to summarize, our red flags for potentially dangerous or secondary headaches are, number one, progressive-nature headaches that are getting worse and worse; number two, a worst headache ever—sometimes these are also called thunderclap headaches; number three, headaches accompanied by signs of infection, like a fever or a stiff neck; number four, headaches that change with posture or with coughing, straining, or sneezing; number five, headaches accompanied by an abnormal physical examination, especially something abnormal on the neurologic exam; number six would be headaches in people with ongoing medical problems, like cancer or HIV, and probably, number seven, new headaches in people over 50 years old.

That list will reliably distinguish the primary headaches, that is, the main, common, ordinary headaches, from headaches caused by medical problems that may need urgent intervention. Let's think about that list; every single item there relies only on the history and physical examination. Do we need any CT or MRI scans, or blood tests, for the vast majority of headaches that bring patients to the ED or to doctors' offices? No, no we don't. There is no role for advanced imaging or other tests, as long as there are none of these red flags on a good, thorough, careful history and physical examination. Now, even though imaging is not necessary or recommended, it is often done, perhaps with a goal of reassuring the patient, or perhaps as a form of defensive medicine to prevent lawsuits. Or maybe, it's because doctors think patients expect some kind of scan.

Whatever the reason, advanced imaging is frequently performed during a headache evaluation, even if there are no red flags that make positive findings likely. In that case, imaging with CT or MRI is much more likely to find something incidental, or completely meaningless, than it is to find something that doctors need to know about. One more subtle point, distinguishing a primary from secondary headache depends on a thorough, relaxed, complete history and physical exam. That takes time and patience. Rushed doctors are unlikely to do a thorough job, which means that rushed doctors end up ordering more tests and scans to confirm what's going on.

OK, our patient Gordon needs no tests, no scans. We have all of the information we need to make a definite diagnosis now. We have no red flags at all, so this is very likely to be one of the primary headaches. There really are only a small handful of common, primary headache types; these are almost always migraine, tension, or cluster-type headaches. Let's go through them and see if the history and physical fit into one of those diagnoses.

Tension headaches are common. They can last from 30 minutes to a week or so and have a pressing or tightening sort of quality; they're not throbbing. The pain is bilateral—that means on both sides of the head—and of mild to moderate intensity. They're not aggravated by activity, and lack nausea and vomiting. Typically, they're not made worse with lights or loud sounds. Our patient, Gordon, has a unilateral, a one-sided headache, or at least, it begins unilateral, with an intense, throbbing sort of pain. This is not a tension headache.

Cluster headaches are less common, but they're really quite characteristic. The pain is brief, from 15 minutes to about three hours. They begin and stay unilateral and are accompanied by one-sided facial symptoms on the same side as the pain, perhaps a red or watery eye, congestion or watery nose, one-sided sweating, or one-sided pupil or eyelid changes. The thing to keep in mind about cluster headaches is how these symptoms are so striking and always unilateral, and that the headaches are really quite brief. Our patient isn't having cluster headaches.

There's another headache type that may be contributing here, and it has to do with medicines. Many medicines can themselves cause headaches. If you read those product inserts, the ones with the teeny, tiny mouse type, you'll see that headaches are among the most common side effects of many medications. But there are also some medications that when overused can trigger what are called rebound headaches. This, ironically, includes all of the over-the-counter and prescription medicines used to treat headaches in the first place! That's right, ibuprofen and acetaminophen as well, if used regularly, will lead to rebound headaches as they wear off. Often, headache sufferers find themselves taking their medicines for several days in a row, continuously, because the headaches keep coming back. That perpetuates the cycle. Headache treatment medicines should not be used more than a few days in a row, and not more than three days a week, to avoid these rebound headaches. Gordon says lately he had been using ibuprofen frequently, and that may have started to contribute to at least some of his headaches.

Caffeine is also a common headache contributor, especially in people who are used to consuming coffee and other caffeine sources every single day. A day, then, without the caffeine that you're used to may well become a day with headaches. The withdrawal of habitual caffeine, that's the common headache trigger.

Back to our primary headaches, the most common primary headache disorder is migraine. These headaches last 4 to 72 hours and are unilateral, or at least, begin unilaterally. The pain is of moderate to severe intensity, and has a pulsating or throbbing quality. They get worse with activity, like walking around or working. Migraines will always be accompanied by either nausea or vomiting, or a combination of what's called phonophobia and photophobia. That means that the headache gets worse with light and sound. Our patient, Gordon, didn't use those words, phonophobia and photophobia, but he did hide under the covers with the lights out.

Though not part of the definition of migraine, characteristically, they improve after sleep. Remember, Gordon mentioned sleeping off these headaches, too. So, all of this fits. We've ruled out secondary headaches with our history and physical, and Gordon's headache pattern fits perfectly into the definition of migraine. That is our diagnosis.

Often, migraines are accompanied by changes in what's called the autonomic nervous system. This is the part of our nervous system that's automatic, the things we don't have to think about. It includes the nerves that make us sweat, and the nerves that constrict blood vessels and make the skin look pale. Some migraine sufferers become pale and sweaty, and many feel nausea or abdominal pain from these autonomic nerve changes. Autonomic nerves also travel to the lining of the nose, and can cause nasal congestion or stuffiness from increased tissue swelling, explaining why Gordon thought he was having sinus headaches.

Think about this case. Gordon is stuffy in the ED and says he always gets stuffy with headaches. But doesn't that sound kind of backwards? After all, if the headaches are caused by sinus pressure, shouldn't the sinus symptoms come before the headaches? You'd also expect other symptoms of a sinus infection, like cough or persistent pus-like nasal drainage. And even the location of the pain, over his eye, that's not actually where human sinuses are located. We have sinuses in the lower, middle forehead, and right behind our eyes, and right under our cheeks, but not really above our eyes.

Gordon is not having sinus headaches. The appearance of congestion with the migraine had fooled him and his doctors into thinking that the sinuses were the cause of the headaches. In fact, most people who are having what's been diagnosed as sinus headaches are having migraines. A few other diagnostic pearls, headaches related to sinus infection often feel worse when bending forward or lying down, and are often accompanied by a decreased ability to smell or to taste. Gordon reported none of these findings.

OK, back to migraines. Some, but not all, migraines are accompanied by an aura. These are reversible neurological signs or symptoms that occur before the headache, or sometimes, just as the headache is beginning. Common auras include changes in vision, such as sparkling lights or a colored haze. They can also include auditory hallucinations, or weakness, or a vague feeling of dread. I suspect our patient did have an aura; he mentioned that he could tell when a headache was going to occur, even before it started. Maybe that was one of these vague aura sensations that are difficult to describe, but Gordon certainly knew when he had that feeling and what it meant. Gordon said, way at first, that he knew in advance before a headache was going to strike.

About those visual changes, a unique phenomenon that can occur with migraine is a visual hallucination where things look much bigger or smaller than they really are. Some people experience this as if they, themselves, have dramatically shrunk in size, and that everything around them has grown very large. Remember that quote from Alice in Wonderland. It's thought that Lewis Carroll himself suffered from migraines that included this kind of hallucination; this is based on some suggestive drawings he made and records of him seeing what was then called an oculist, or eye doctor. Perhaps Alice's Adventures in Wonderland were inspired by the author's migraine headaches. We'll never know for sure, but we've adopted a special name of these special visual hallucinations that make things look smaller, or larger, or closer, or farther than they really are. These are called Alice-in-Wonderland Syndrome.

Back to Gordon. We have a firm diagnosis now, and we're ready to talk treatment. Dealing with migraines should always start with prevention. Many, though not all, migraines have specific triggers. These can include lack of sleep, or hunger, or dehydration, sometimes stress, or illness, or bright lights, perhaps reading while in the car. There's actually overlap between migraines and car sickness, especially in children. Many children who have car sickness go on to become adults who have classic migraines.

People who have migraines should track their episodes to see if some of these common triggers seem to be part of the problem. Not all migraine sufferers have all of these triggers, but many have at least some, and some triggers can be avoided though lifestyle modification, stress reduction, yoga, getting a good night's sleep, and other simple, non-medical steps. It's also very important for people with migraines to avoid falling into the trap of medication overuse, and to control their caffeine intake.

Beyond these preventive lifestyle strategies, migraine sufferers need an action plan to start as soon as possible when a migraine begins. For people who do have a warning aura, the migraine action plan needs to start as soon as the aura begins, which may be well before the actual headache. That's good! A migraine caught early is much more likely to be stoppable. A migraine action plan should include both medical and non-medical steps. Usually the patient will benefit from getting to a dark, quiet environment quickly. Sometimes, a small snack, including some sugar, will help, perhaps even including some soda or coffee with caffeine. That's right, though habitual caffeine use can lead to migraines, caffeine itself, when taken at the start of a migraine, can help reduce its severity.

Medicines can help, especially if taken right at the start of the headache. These can include over-the-counter pain relievers, like ibuprofen or acetaminophen. There are also very effective prescription migraine-stopping medicines. The best of these are in a family called the triptans. They all work similarly to block a brain receptor that's central to migraine development.

All migraine sufferers who don't get full relief from over-the-counter products should have one of these triptans available for immediate use when a migraine begins. They come as pills, nasal sprays, and an auto-injector devices that is especially useful for the many migraine patients who have vomiting with their headaches. Note, these triptans, though very effective, they can themselves trigger rebound headaches when used too frequently.

If despite trigger avoidance and a good action plan migraines are still occurring frequently, we ought to consider starting a daily migraine prevention strategy. This can involve adding a daily medication or sometimes a dietary supplement that can act as a migraine preventer. There are several of these available, though some have some side effects.

And now that we have a definite diagnosis, our patient was very happy to learn that there are things he can do to prevent these headaches and to more effectively treat them while staying at home. With a more regular sleep schedule and increased exercise, Gordon was able to reduce his life stress, preventing some of the migraines. We also prescribed effective medicine to stop migraines at home and asked Gordon to follow up with his primary care doctor to explore whether a daily prevention medicine or supplement would be a good idea. Over the following six months, he did not return to the emergency department for care.

Migraines can be a very odd sort disorder. Though most patients' main migraine symptom is headaches, some migraine types cause unexpected neurologic or other symptoms, sometimes without any headache at all. Just a few examples, migraines can cause episodes of intense confusion, or a stroke-like paralysis of half of the body, or sometimes intense, repetitive vomiting with or without abdominal pain, or, perhaps episodes of blindness, dizziness, vertigo, or trouble walking. Some of these migraine symptoms run in families. What distinguishes all of them is that the symptoms are sudden and brief and follow a similar pattern every time, and that in between episodes all symptoms resolve.

That was a good, satisfying case. We have a clear diagnosis, and we have a good, effective plan for prevention and treatment. Sometimes, though, cases are a little bit more messy and complicated. And sometimes the best strategies for prevention and therapy aren't so clear. See you next time.

The Tennis Player
Lecture 6

Cancer is a common disease—one that we've learned a tremendous amount about in the last few decades. It is a complex illness that can present in many ways, and we still have a lot to learn about prevention, screening, and treatment. In this lecture, you will learn about a case that illustrates the shortcomings of our knowledge. But even when a patient's story turns bleak, there's always something a physician can do to help the patient, even if the disease cannot be stopped.

Non-Acute Pain

- Julie, a 52-year-old woman, comes to our general medicine outpatient clinic with a chief complaint of "I can't play tennis anymore." Julie says that she used to be a very active athlete, but about 10 years ago, she started having mostly right-sided hip and knee pains. She was diagnosed with osteoarthritis.

- She tried medical therapy with painkillers, injections, and steroids, but these were not very effective. Julie really wanted to get back to her active lifestyle, so she had right-hip replacement surgery eight years ago.

- She was able to return to active sports but continued to have some pain, now more on her left side, kind of in the front of her hip, or sometimes more in her left thigh. She complains now that this left-sided pain has gotten much worse, and she thinks she needs a referral back to orthopedics for left-hip replacement surgery.

- **Arthritis** would be on the top of our list of possible diagnoses. Arthritis of a joint means that there is more than just pain, but also evidence of inflammation with redness, warmth, stiffness, or changes on an X-ray. In adults, the most common cause of arthritis is chronic overuse (osteoarthritis) or infection in the joint or by autoimmune conditions like rheumatoid arthritis or lupus.

- We may also be dealing with a fracture—probably not a sudden, acute fracture, but perhaps a stress fracture, which is bone damage that develops more gradually, from overuse. There are other orthopedic and mechanical conditions that can cause hip pain, including bursitis and tendonitis. These, as well as muscle and tendon strains, are also caused by overuse. Our patient's active lifestyle has put her at risk for all kinds of injuries.

- In addition to orthopedic and joint conditions, gynecological problems, such as endometriosis, can cause pain in the front of the pelvis, near the hip joint. Also, anything that presses or pinches a nerve that goes toward the hip can cause pain to be sensed in the hip area. Hip or bone pain can also be caused by cancer, including primary cancers of bone or bone marrow, or the spread of cancers from other sites.

- A physical exam reveals a bit of a fast heart rate, along with a firm mass, about the size of an almond, under her left armpit. It's under the skin and freely moveable and feels like an enlarged lymph node.

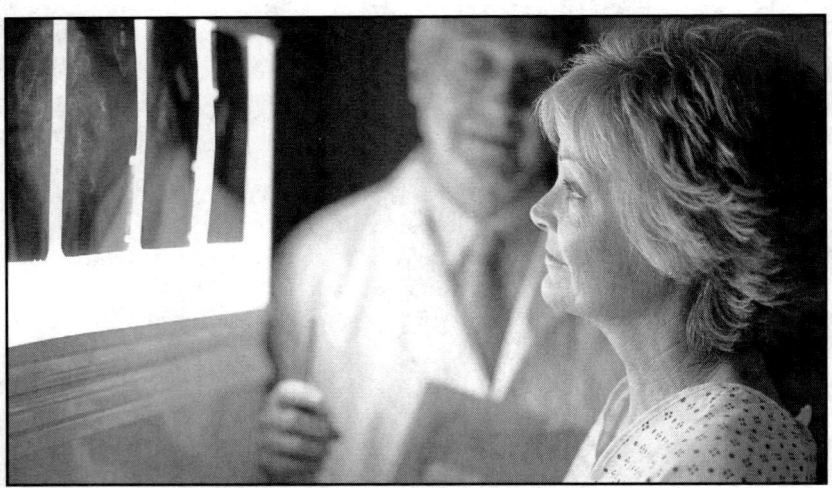

It is very difficult for a doctor to tell a patient that he or she has cancer, but there are treatments that might help, and science is advancing every day.

- Our first, simplest test is a set of X-rays. There's an area of bone at the top of the femur, near the hip joint, that looks kind of irregular and splotchy. It's not a simple fracture; this is an area of abnormal bone—maybe a cyst of some kind, chronic bone infection, or some kind of cancer. It is not arthritis.

- The CBC shows anemia, with a decreased amount of red blood cells. In general, this can be caused by either blood loss or by decreased production of red cells. The remainder of the cell lines, the platelets and white cells, are normal. The labs also reveal an increased sed rate, meaning that some kind of inflammation is going on, somewhere.

- A great diagnostic tool—and sometimes underappreciated—is collaboration between doctors. Our patient, it turns out, has never had a mammogram. An oncologist does one the next day, revealing a suspicious breast mass on the left.

- After consultation between Julie, the primary care doctor, oncologist, and surgical teams, the decision is made to proceed immediately with an open biopsy of the breast mass. Although a needle biopsy could have been done first, doing a less-invasive test before surgery, Julie felt that whatever was going on, she wanted to know for sure—and as soon as possible.

- Tissue during surgery is examined by the pathologist, who confirmed seeing the abnormal cells of breast cancer. The surgical procedure is extended to remove the chains of nearby lymph node, several of which also turn out to be positive for containing cancer cells.

Cancer
- Our final diagnosis is breast cancer with **metastatic** spread to the local lymph nodes and bone, both near the hip and other sites. Sharing news like this isn't a one-time event; it isn't one big talk at which all questions are answered. Discussions like this should always end with plans for the next discussion and open-ended time for families and doctors to share how they feel.

- Cancer, at its core, is a genetic disease—that is, it's a disease that affects the genetic material of the cells. Every cell is governed by the instructions carried on its chromosomes, the genes that encode the proteins that control every function of every cell. Cancer cells are cells that have lost the ability to control their own growth and differentiation, and they grow and spread far beyond the tissues that they ought to call home.

- There are two kinds of genetic changes that can lead to cancer. First, there are germ line mutations, which are genes that are present way back in the embryo, passed on from mother or father, and are present in every cell in the body. These mutations are hereditary, meaning that you're born with them. Hereditary mutations account for about 10 percent of all cancers.

- The second kind of genetic change occurs only in a single cell—a mutation or mistake that's created when the cellular genetic material is copied to make new cells. Sometimes this happens just randomly, but for many kinds of cancers, we know what things cause at least some or most of these cellular changes.

- Radiation, including solar radiation, can disrupt or damage DNA, as can environmental toxins or smoking. Certain infections can also directly cause certain cancers, or chronic infections can lead to chronic cell damage that can eventually lead to cancer.

- Although there are both somatic and germ line kinds of mutations, many cancers are related to not one genetic change, but several overlapping conditions. Although cancer is always genetic, it usually arises from a combination of contributions from multiple genes, sometimes (but not always) including hereditary genes carried in families.

- One very common risk factor for almost all cancers is age. The longer our cells have been alive, the more years they've had to sustain the damaging hits on their genetic material that lead to cancer. Almost all cancers increase in frequency with age, and in fact, it may be true that if we live long enough, eventually we will all get some kind of cancer.

- Cancer isn't one disease. Any tissue can develop cancer, and often, there are potentially multiple types of cancer even in one kind of body tissue, all of which have different health consequences and treatments. But whatever the initial cause and whatever the kind of cancer, what all cancers have in common is that the genetic mechanism that should have controlled the growth and spread of the cell fails, and the cell keeps dividing and growing and spreading.

- The signs and symptoms of cancer can be almost anything. They depend on where the cancer is, how fast it's growing, and whether it's pushing on blood vessels, nerves, or other crucial tissues. Some cancers themselves release chemicals into the blood that cause symptoms in any part of the body. Cancers can also cause symptoms if they spread or metastasize to other areas.

- There are sometimes constitutional symptoms of cancer. There may be prolonged and difficult-to-explain fever, weight loss, or marked fatigue. These symptoms may occur because of the metabolic demands of the growing cancer tissue or in part because of the body's immune system trying to attack and fight off the cancer. However, breast cancer often occurs with none of these constitutional symptoms.

- Immunity, or a lack of immunity, is an important part of cancer biology. Our immune systems are there to fight off foreign invaders, and we think of invaders as infections like bacteria or viruses that barge into our bodies from outside. But cancer cells are also, in a sense, foreign invaders—invaders from the inside.

- Our immune systems have developed to be very good at sniffing out and destroying these cancer cells. People with immune deficiencies, or altered immune systems for other reasons, are at higher risk for developing many kinds of cancer.

Treating Cancer
- Surgery is the primary, main therapy for breast cancer, and surgery alone can be curative when breast cancer is caught early. After surgery, many women with early cancer pursue what's called adjunctive therapy, which refers to things done in addition to the primary therapy—surgery—to increase the chance of cure or long-term survival.

- Although theoretically an early cancer shouldn't have spread to outside tissue, we can't know if a few cancer cells have snuck out—and even a few cells, or one cell, can continue to grow and allow cancer to spread. Adjunctive therapy for breast cancer includes mainly chemotherapy, hormonal therapy, and radiation.

- Chemotherapy refers to drugs given to kill cancer cells or halt their spread. It's most effective on rapidly dividing cells, and different kinds of breast cancer may be more or less sensitive to chemo. The chemotherapy drugs are often more effective when used in combinations. Although side effects may be very difficult, we have gotten better at managing many of them.

- Many, but not all, breast cancer cells have receptors for female hormones. If they do, medications to block hormones can prevent cancers from spreading.

- Radiation therapy can also be used to destroy rapidly dividing cancer cells, though there are side effects and dose limitations. These adjunctive therapies can be used to increase the chance of long-term survival or as palliative therapy to extend life and provide comfort, even in patients who cannot be cured.

Important Terms

arthritis: Joint inflammation, typically manifested by stiffness and pain accompanied by swelling.

metastatic: Cancer appearing at a site distant to the original cancer, caused by migrating and then proliferating cells.

Suggested Reading

Link, *The Breast Cancer Survival Manual*.

Mukherjee, *The Emperor of All Maladies*.

Weinberg, *The Biology of Cancer*.

American Cancer Society, http://www.cancer.org/.

Questions to Consider

1. What is the best way for doctors to communicate bad news to patients?

2. How do you know if a screening test is a good idea?

The Tennis Player
Lecture 6—Transcript

We have a puzzler today, a scary case. This is a common disease, and one that we've learned a tremendous amount about in the last few decades. On the one hand, this is a disease that can kill a healthy 36 year old woman in just a few months; while in a 90 year old, it may not need to be treated at all.

Julie, a 52-year old woman, comes to our general medicine outpatient clinic with a chief complaint of "I can't play tennis any more." Julie says she used to be a very active athlete. She was on the first women's lacrosse team at her college, and this was many years ago when there wasn't nearly as much women's athletics for students. She was also a competitive swimmer, and almost made the Olympic team. She has continued to play softball and tennis and works as a teacher and coach for several girls' teams at a high school.

However, about 10 years ago, Julie started having mostly right-sided hip and knee pain. She was diagnosed with osteoarthritis. She tried medical therapy with painkillers, injections, and steroids, but these weren't very effective. Julie really wanted to get back to her active lifestyle, so she had right hip replacement surgery eight years ago. She was able to return to active sports but continued to have some pain, now more on her left side, kind of in the front of her hip, or sometimes more in her left thigh. She complains now that this left sided pain has gotten much worse, and she thinks she needs a referral back to orthopedics for left hip replacement surgery.

It's time to create a brief differential diagnosis. We have a case of gradually increasing, non-acute hip pain in an active woman with a history of arthritis. Seems pretty straightforward, but let's not fall into that trap of assuming we already know what's going on. Arthritis would of course be top of the list. The word comes from the Greek; arthro- meaning joint, and -itis, meaning inflammation. That suffix, itis, it comes up a lot in medicine. Appendicitis is inflammation of the appendix, gastritis is inflammation of the stomach. Arthritis of a joint means that there is more than just pain, but also evidence of inflammation with redness, warmth, stiffness, or perhaps changes on an X-ray. In adults, the most common cause of arthritis is chronic overuse, sometimes that's called osteoarthritis. That becomes much more common with age, and is more common in athletes. Arthritis can also be caused by infection in the joint or by autoimmune conditions, like rheumatoid arthritis or by lupus. By the way, another term, arthralgia, that's the medical term for joint pain without evidence of inflammation.

We might also be dealing with a fracture here, probably not a sudden, acute fracture, since the symptoms have evolved gradually, but perhaps what's called a stress fracture. This is bone damage that develops more gradually from overuse. Stress fractures, they're more common in athletes, and especially common in people at risk for decreased bone mineral density. They also often appear at the beginning of a training season, or when an athlete changes to a new sport or a new workout routine.

There are other orthopedic and mechanical conditions that can cause hip pain. These include bursitis, that's inflammation of the little fluid-filled sac that there to protect muscles and tendons; or tendonitis, or inflammation of the thick bands of tissue that connect the muscle to the bone. These, as well as muscle and tendon strains, they're usually caused by overuse, so we're seeing here that our patient's active lifestyle has put her at risk for all kinds of injuries.

One other orthopedic sort of problem that can cause hip pain is avascular necrosis, caused by decreased blood flow to the bone or joint. This happens most commonly at the hip, and one of the causes is prolonged oral steroid therapy. Now, Julie was treated with an oral steroid, prednisone, for several months for her arthritis years ago. That's probably too long ago to have caused avascular necrosis now, but it's worth keeping in mind.

OK, let's start thinking kind of outside of the box a little. We have a good list of orthopedic and joint conditions, but hip pain doesn't have to be related to the actual bones or the joint. Gynecologic problems, like endometriosis, can cause pain in the front of the pelvis, near the hip joint. Also, anything that presses or pinches a nerve that goes towards the hip can cause pain to be sensed in the hip area, even if that pinch is up higher on the nerve. So, for example, a slipped disc pressing on a nerve root in the spine can cause hip pain down low. Pressure on a nerve as it passes through the pelvis is called sciatica, and that can cause hip, or thigh, or sometimes knee pain. You can also have pain in the hip area from a hernia, where abdominal contents poke out of a weak area of the lining of the abdomen. Hip or bone pain can also be caused by tumors, including benign cysts or tumors of bone, or cancer of the bone or the bone marrow, or the spread of cancer from other places. Infections of bone, called osteomyelitis, those can also cause pain that can begin suddenly or gradually, depending on the kind of infection.

Now, let's get some more history and a physical exam. The pain, Julie says, it gets worse as the day goes on and is especially bad on active days. That actually doesn't really fit with most causes of arthritis. Really, arthritis causes stiffness and pain that is worse first thing in the morning, upon waking up. Arthritis may also get worse again later in the day with activity. Julie denies any fever or swelling or redness over any joint, which kind of weighs against this being some kind of infection. She denies having had any easy fatigue, weight loss, fevers, or night sweats. That's reassuring and points us away from many more serious illnesses, like leukemia or lupus.

Julie says her pain is at times dull or at times sharp. It's usually in the front of her left hip and doesn't shoot up or down or reach towards her spine. We would have called pain that moves or shoots down a radiating pain, and that can be a sign of nerve compression. Nerve-based pain is often burning in quality, and it often is accompanied by changes in sensation or strength that Julie isn't complaining about. So, there's no radiation, there's no burning, there's no changes in strength or sensation. This really isn't sounding like pain from a pinched nerve in her pelvis or in her back.

Since some gynecologic conditions were on our differential, we ask about a gyn history. Julie is now postmenopausal and had a long history of irregular or infrequent periods. This could have been related to her lean physique and her active lifestyle. There is a so-called female athlete triad that includes menstrual disturbances, disordered eating habits, and bone mineral loss. Often, athletic women have all or part of that triad, and in this case, it could have put her at risk for stress fractures from poor mineral density. Julie denies having had pelvic pain, or painful periods, or any sexual health concerns.

We've learned what we're going to learn from the history, so it's time for the physical exam. Vital signs include a heart rate of 86, respirations 16,

Blood pressure 106/78, and temperature 98.9. What do you think of those? They look pretty normal, and if you look up the normal ranges for a woman of Julie's age, they are normal. But, she's an athlete, and has been for years. I'd sort of expect a lower resting heart rate than 86. Of course, she is in pain, that might explain a bit of that relatively fast heart rate right now.

More exam, HEENT, that stands for head, eyes, ears, nose, and throat; that exam is normal, her lungs are clear, her heart exam is normal too. We find a firm mass, about the size of an almond, under her left armpit. It's under the skin, and it's freely moveable, and it feels like an enlarged lymph node. Her belly exam is normal, and nothing unusual is found on Julie's skin; gyn and breast exams are normal as well. Her hip joints seem to have a normal, full range of motion, though we find some pain when rotating her left hip outwards.

Before we go forward, let's just briefly think back to our differential. Are we convinced that Julie has ordinary osteoarthritis? I don't know about that. She's at risk for stress fractures, and the timing of her pain isn't exactly what's expected from arthritis. Plus, we have a little bit of a high heart rate, and this single lymph node in her armpit or axillary area. I think our orthopedic colleagues would appreciate our digging a little more before sending her onwards to their clinic.

Our first, simplest test is a set of X-rays. Though her pain is on the left, we'll get films of her entire pelvis, both hip joints, and both femurs. Being able to compare the right and left sides can be helpful in finding subtle sorts of things. We can easily see the titanium hardware from her right hip replacement surgery; that looks fine. But on there on the left there's an area of bone at the top of the femur, near the hip joint, that looks kind of irregular and splotchy. It's not a fracture; the bone isn't just broken. This is an area of abnormal bone, maybe a cyst of some kind, or chronic bone infection, or some kind of cancer. It is not arthritis.

Let's get some blood work. The CBC shows anemia, with a decreased amount of red blood cells. In general, this could be caused by either blood loss or by decreased production of red cells. The remainder of the cell lines, the platelets and white cells, are normal. The labs also reveal an increased sed rate, meaning some kind of inflammation is going on, somewhere.

OK, we now know that there's abnormal bone at approximately the site of Julie's pain. It's unlikely to be a benign or simple cyst of the bone, because we've got that increased sed rate and anemia to explain. There was also that small lymph node on Julie's exam. Always keep your eye on those funny, unexpected findings. They're often good clues.

A great diagnostic tool, sometimes underappreciated, is collaboration between doctors. Since we happen to work in a multispecialty outpatient clinic with its own radiology department, let's walk down the hall. let's see what our radiologist says about those films. Sure enough, she says that what she's seeing isn't normal bone. It looks like maybe a chronic bone infection or maybe primary bone cancer, or metastatic cancer spreading from somewhere else.

Our next step is to call our orthopedic surgery colleague. He agrees that something's fishy on that X-ray and says he'd be happy to jump in and biopsy it. But maybe, he says, we ought to speak with the oncologist first. So another phone call. The oncologist shares the team's concern and points out that though primary bone cancer is possible, that lymph node might mean there is something brewing in the chest area. Our patient, it turns out, Julie has never had a mammogram. So one is done the next day, revealing a suspicious breast mass on the left.

Now, Julie herself has been told the results of the blood tests, the X-ray, and now the mammogram, and we need to make sure that we're taking the time to explain to her what's going on, to give her a chance to ask questions, and to make sure that she's involved in the medical decision process.

After consultation between Julie, the primary care doc, the oncologist, and the surgeon, the decision is made to proceed immediately with an open biopsy of the breast mass. Although a needle biopsy could have been done, Julie felt that whatever was going on, she wanted to know for sure, and she wanted to know as soon as possible. Tissue during surgery is examined by the pathologist, who confirmed seeing the abnormal cells of breast cancer.

The surgical procedure is then extended to remove the chains of nearby lymph nodes, several of which also turn out to contain cancer cells.

Next, a bone scan is performed. This is a study that involves the administration of an IV chemical that bind especially to sites of active bone turnover. The chemical is also radiolabeled, meaning it releases a tiny amount of a radiation tracer that can be picked up by a scintillation camera. The bone scan shows increased uptake of tracer at the site of abnormal bone from the X-ray near the hip joint, but also along several sites in the spine and on the skull.

Our final diagnosis is breast cancer with metastatic spread to the local lymph nodes and bone, both near the hip and other sites. Julie was told the news, at first briefly in recovery after her surgery, but then again at a longer sit-down discussion with the oncologist who could best explain the prognosis and options for the next steps in evaluation and care. Exactly how to do this depends on the situation and depends on the patient. In Julie's case, she wanted to hear all of the news as soon as possible, though in other cases, it may have been better to wait a day or two so arrangements could be made for family to attend that meeting or to give the patient a few days to clear her head after anesthesia.

And doctors also know this; sharing news like this isn't a one-time event. It isn't one big talk at which all questions are answered. There's never enough time to answer all questions, and sometimes people just can't absorb all of the information the first time. Discussions like this should always end with plans for the next discussion, and plans for what issues will be discussed, as well as open-ended time for families and doctors to share how they feel.

We have some big decisions to make now about further evaluation and treatment. But before we get back to Julie's case, let's back up to talk about cancer and breast cancer screening. Cancer, at its core, is a genetic disease. That is, it's a disease that affects the genetic material of the cells. Every cell is governed by the instructions carried on its chromosomes—the genes that encode the proteins that control every function of every cell. Cancer cells are cells that have, in a sense, gone bad. They've lost the ability to control their own growth and differentiation and grow and spread far beyond the tissues that they ought to call home. They've gone bad because of changes in their genes.

There are two kinds of genetic changes that can lead to cancer. First, there are so-called germline mutations. Now, these are genes that are present way back in the embryo, passed on from mom and dad, and they're present in every cell in the body. These mutations are hereditary; you're born with them, and hereditary mutations account for about 10 percent of all cancers.

The second kind of genetic change occurs only in one cell, only in a single cell; It's a mutation or mistake that's created when the cellular genetic material is copied to make new cells. Sometimes this happens just randomly; it's bad luck. But for many kinds of cancers, we know what things cause at least some or most of those cellular changes. Radiation, including the solar radiation from the Sun, can disrupt or damage DNA, as can environmental toxins or smoking. Some infections can also directly cause certain cancers, like cervical cancer, which is caused by infection with the human papilloma virus, or in another example, chronic infections like certain kinds of hepatitis lead to chronic cell damage that can eventually lead to cancer. One more example, chronic severe reflux into the top of the esophagus can eventually damage the cells there, leading to esophageal cancer.

It gets even more complicated. Though there are both somatic and germline kinds of mutations, many cancers are related to not one genetic change, but several overlapping conditions. For instance, someone may have a genetic predisposition in their cells that leads to a decreased ability to repair the damage from sunshine. So, in that person, relatively modest sun exposure can lead to cancer. Cancer usually arises from a combination of contributions from multiple genes, sometimes, but not always, including hereditary genes that are carried in families.

One very common risk factor for almost all cancers is simply age. The longer our cells have been alive, the more years they've had to sustain damaging hits on their genetic material that lead to cancer. Almost all cancers increase in frequency with age, and in fact, it's probably true that if we lived long enough, eventually all of us will all get some kind of cancer.

Cancer, of course, it isn't one disease. Any tissue can develop cancer, and often there are potentially multiple types of cancer, even in one kind of body tissue, all of which have different health consequences and different treatments. But whatever the initial cause and whatever the kind of cancer, what all cancers have in common is that the genetic mechanism that should have controlled the growth and spread of those cells, that mechanism fails, and the cell keeps dividing and growing and spreading. So how does cancer make a patient sick?

The signs and the symptoms of cancer can be almost anything. They depend on where the cancer is, how fast it's growing, and whether it's pushing on blood vessels, or nerves, or other crucial tissues. It may also depend on whether the cancel is blocking the flow of bile, for instance, or expanding in the bone marrow and pushing on bone, which can cause pain. A cancer pressing on the brain could cause headaches, or weakness, or seizures. Some cancers themselves release chemicals into the blood that cause symptoms in any part of the body, like flushing or diarrhea. Cancers can also cause symptoms if they spread or metastasize to other areas.

There are sometimes constitutional symptoms of cancer. These may be prolonged and difficult to explain, including fever, or weight loss, or marked fatigue. These symptoms may occur because of the metabolic demands of the growing cancer tissue, or in part because of the body's immune system is trying to attack and fight off the cancer. However, breast cancer often occurs with none of these constitutional symptoms.

Let's focus back in now on Julie's breast cancer. Is there anything she could have done to prevent it? Many of the risk factors for breast cancer are what we call unmodifiable, that is, there's nothing Julie or anyone else could have done. Gender, of course is a big risk factor. Breast cancer is 100 times more common in women than in men. Age, as we mentioned—the risk of breast cancer continues to increase with every decade of life, though in general, the most aggressive, the most deadly breast cancers occur in younger women.

Breast cancer presenting in elderly women may grow very slowly, and may not need aggressive therapy. There are also genetic risk factors, including several known familial germline mutations that, if present, may cause a cancer risk as high as 80 percent. Women who come from families with a striking history of either breast cancers in young women, multiple cases of ovarian cancers, or men who have breast cancer, those women should be screened for these sorts of mutations.

What about lifestyle factors, and other ways to help prevent breast cancer? Actually, having children seems to be a little protective, but taking birth control pills may increase the risk. Those aren't huge influences. Prolonged use of combined hormone-replacement therapy, common in the 1980s and 1990s, also contributed to increased breast cancer risk. Alcohol use is clearly a risk factor for breast as well as other cancers, as is obesity and a lack of physical activity. Smoking, including passive tobacco exposure, may also increase breast cancer risk, at least in some genetically susceptible individuals.

What about screening? Early detection of life-threatening illnesses, like cancer, is a cornerstone of public health, because cancer detected early, prior to spread, is much more treatable than advanced cancer. Screening to detect early breast cancer is especially important for women with genetic or other risk factors. There are several ways to screen for early breast cancer. The first is regular self-exam, checking for lumps, or masses, or changes in the skin or anything else new that could be an early warning sign. Now, no study has actually found that regular breast self-exams prevent death from breast cancer, but it's cheap, and it's safe, and it's generally recommended, as are breast exams from doctors or nurses at regular health visits.

But the most effective screening method is the use of mammograms. Mammography is a breast X-ray looking for changes in the tissue density that can occur with early cancers. They can detect breast cancer early, and they do save lives. But there is controversy over when they ought to be done. Breast cancer in younger women is rare, but it can be more aggressive, so mammography in younger women may be more likely to show false results from denser tissue, leading to more unnecessary repeat tests and biopsies. The consensus now is for screening mammography to be done every one or two years, starting at age 40 to 50. Women at higher risk ought to be screened more often, and starting younger. As women live into their 80's or 90's, the question of whether to continue mammography should be individualized according to risk and overall patient health and expected lifespan.

I want to use this example of mammography to illustrate one potentially under-recognized facet of cancer screening, and actually, of the entire assumption that it's always a good idea to do screening tests. We assume that is always a good idea to catch every breast cancer as early as possible, but is that really true? A 2012 study looked at the rates of cancer detection and late-stage breast cancer before and after the era of mass mammography screening. The number of very early breast cancers detected doubled once women began routine mammos. That is good. But the rate of late-stage breast cancer presentations, those didn't drop nearly as much, They fell only by about 8 percent. So, if every early breast cancer was going to go on to become an advanced breast cancer, then this doubling of early pick ups should have led to a similar drop, by half, in advanced cases. When the numbers are analyzed and adjusted for other known variables, it looks like about 30 percent of breast cancers, when picked up by mammography and treated early, would never have gone on to become serious, invasive illness. Many of those would never have caused any symptoms at all and would have gone away on their own.

So that's a limitation of early screening, We can't assume early pick ups always prevent late, serious illness. Though we've learned more about the genetic makeup of cancers and are better able to predict their behavior, we still don't really know which early cancers are most likely to spread. Add to that the other big down side to screening—false positives that lead to further expensive tests and a lot of worry.

Julie didn't have any family history of cancer; she was active, she didn't smoke, and actually, her history of infrequent periods would have predicted a lower risk of breast cancer. Because of that, Julie decided not to pursue routine mammography, and in retrospect, this did not turn out to have been such a good idea. Sometimes we just don't have a perfect answer.

Over the few meetings, the oncologist and surgeon discussed treatment options with Julie. Surgery is the primary, main therapy for breast cancer, and surgery alone can be curative when breast cancer is caught early. In

Julie's case, surgery was pursued to remove the bulk of the tumor, the main part, even though there was already spread to other sites. For Julie, we know surgery will not be curative, but it can help extend her life by decreasing the further spread of cancer.

After surgery, many women with early cancer pursue what's called adjunctive therapy. This refers to things done in addition to the primary therapy, that was the surgery, to increase the chance of cure or long-term survival. Though theoretically, an early cancer shouldn't have spread to outside tissues, we can't know if a few cancer cells may have snuck out; and even a few cells, or even one cell, can continue to grow and allow cancer to spread. Adjunctive therapy for breast cancer includes mainly chemotherapy, hormonal therapy, and radiation.

Chemotherapy refers to drugs given to kill cancer cells or halt their spread. It's most effective on rapidly dividing cells, and different kinds of breast cancer may be more or less sensitive to chemo. The chemotherapy drugs are often more effective when used in combinations. Though side effects may be very difficult, we have gotten better at managing many of them. Many, but not all, breast cancer cells have receptors for female hormones. If they do, medications to block hormones can prevent cancers from spreading.

Radiation therapy can also be used to destroy rapidly dividing cancer cells, though there are side effects and dose limitations. These adjunctive therapies can be used to increase the chance of long-term survival, or as palliative therapy to extend life and provide comfort, even in patients who cannot be cured.

Julie, who was an active, healthy person, she chose very aggressive therapy. A modified radical mastectomy was performed, immediately followed by chemo; radiation therapy was directed at her chest at the areas of metastases. She then had breast reconstruction surgery. For 14 months, apart from feeling ill for several days after each cycle of chemo, Julie felt well and was able to play some tennis and golf. However, she then developed sudden seizures, lethargy, and neurologic problems, and was found to have metastatic disease in her brain. Following the wishes she had discussed with her family and oncology, as well as radiation and her surgical teams, chemo was discontinued and radiation treatment for her brain disease was planned. However, before that treatment was begun, Julie became comatose, and further support was only given with fluids and pain medication. Julie died two days later.

William Osler, who is in many ways the father of what we think of as modern medicine, he said, "The good physician treats the disease; the great physician treats the patient who has the disease." Cancer is a complex illness that can present in many ways, and we still have a lot to learn about prevention, screening, and treatment. Julie's story is humbling, and it's a little scary. But even when things turn bleak, there's always something a physician can do to help the patient, to help with comfort, and to help ease a patient's journey, even when we cannot stop her disease.

Sudden Collapse
Lecture 7

The person in front of you collapses to the floor. You have no time for a chief complaint or history. There is a woman lying on the floor in front of you, and she looks to be about 50 years old. She is pale, and she's taking what are called **agonal** respirations: just the barest gasps that occur when a person is near death. Within moments, even these respiratory efforts stop. What do you do?

Layman/Bystander CPR
- Depending on your expertise, it may be appropriate to take different steps, but the following are basic lifesaving steps that anyone can do. The first few minutes are critical.

- Most importantly, it is much, much better to do something than to do nothing while you try to remember what you're supposed to do. You don't need to be perfect and 100 percent follow the guidelines and the exact methods of CPR, but you'd better act fast.

- When you come across someone who appears to be dead, follow these steps.
    1. Make sure the person isn't just sleeping or lying still. Give him or her a shake. Yell, "Are you okay?" In our example, this person just collapsed in front of our eyes. You can probably skip step 1.

    2. Yell for help. Call out, "Someone call 911." If there are people nearby, point to one person specifically and tell him or her to make that call.

    3. If you're in a public place, such as a mall or sporting event, and someone is around to help you, tell someone to go get you an automated external defibrillator (**AED**). Many places—including gyms, department stores, schools, and churches—

now have these devices available. If one of these is available, using one as quickly as possible is the single best way to improve survival.

4. While waiting for someone to call 911 and get the AED, start rescue CPR. Roll the person onto his or her back. Start pushing right in the middle of the chest, hard and fast. Use two hands, one on top of the other, and after every push, relax so that the chest can bounce back up. You shouldn't stay leaned into the chest—it's down, up, down, up. A good rhythm is the beat from the song "Stayin' Alive" by the Bee Gees (think "push, push, push, push, stayin' alive, stayin' alive").

5. Keep going, pushing hard and fast, until either trained emergency rescue personnel show up or someone runs over with the AED.

6. If you have an AED, follow the instructions on the device. Studies have shown that even school-aged children can use these correctly. There will be a cartoon on the front showing the steps and a big "ON" button—pushing that is the first step. After that, the machine will have voice prompts to tell you exactly what to do. You will put a big sticky pad on the front of the chest; then, make sure no one is touching the victim. The computerized device will monitor what the heart is doing, and if appropriate, the device will tell you to push the "shock" button to deliver a jolt of electricity to start the heart beating again. An AED is a smart and safe device—it will not suggest

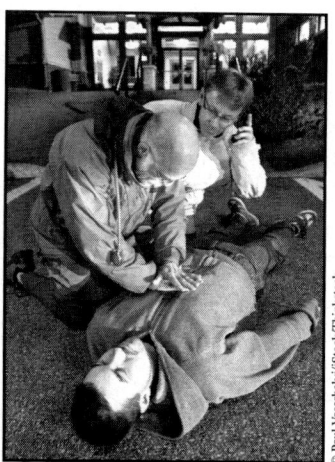

If you notice that someone collapses near you, you might need to perform CPR in order to save his or her life.

117

giving a shock to a normally beating heart, and in fact, the "shock" button won't do anything if you push it unless it's safe to give a shock to the victim. After the shock, the machine will analyze the heart rhythm again and continue to tell you what to do.

- If at any time during the rescue process the victim starts to respond—that is, starts to move or takes breaths—stop what you're doing, roll the patient to lie on his or her side, and wait for rescue personnel.

- The newest guidelines for bystander CPR have de-emphasized some of the traditional parts of CPR that had been taught. Rescuers are no longer encouraged to even check for an open airway and breathing; that used to be the first step, but that's been dropped, because it turns out that the faster you start pumping by pressing on the chest, the better chance the victim has. Don't check pulses; don't mess with the airway. Don't even bother with mouth-to-mouth resuscitation or rescue breaths. Just jump in, push hard, and push fast—while calling for help and for someone to get you an AED.

- There are some situations where other approaches to CPR are needed. First, you have to be safe yourself to do CPR. If a victim is in a busy street or is drowning, it may not be safe for you to approach. Do not endanger yourself to do CPR.

- Also, children and babies need a different kind of CPR. For young people, it's unlikely that a cardiac problem has caused their collapse; much more likely, it's something like choking or a problem with breathing. For children, you should open the airway and give rescue breaths before pressing on the chest.

- For any choking victim, adult or child, remove any visible blockage from the airway before proceeding with CPR—but even if you can't inflate the lungs, continue those chest compressions.

- Some people might hesitate to help a stranger who has a sudden collapse because they might worry about malpractice lawsuits that might occur if resuscitation is unsuccessful. Every U.S. state and many countries have so-called Good Samaritan laws that protect people from lawsuits if they stop to help someone who appears to be in mortal danger.

Heart Attacks

- Almost all causes of sudden collapse are from the heart, from some condition that suddenly stops the heart from beating. The most common cause of this is what is colloquially called a heart attack, or myocardial infarction (MI). This is when a lack of blood flow to the heart muscle itself causes the death of heart muscle cells. It's often accompanied by a sudden change in the heart rhythm, a so-called **arrhythmia**. Instead of the heart beating in an organized way that effectively pumps blood, it just kind of quivers.

- No blood flow to the brain means that the body will collapse and die quickly. Sudden arrhythmias can also occur because of other conditions, including genetic predispositions to sudden death that can run in families.

- Historically, heart attacks have been thought of as a disease of a certain kind of person: usually, a successful, driven, type A kind of man. However, heart attacks are in fact the leading cause of death among women.

- Although our ability to deal with and treat a heart attack has become increasingly effective, we're still seeing an increasing impact of heart disease. This is mostly because it is so difficult to effectively modify well-known risk factors for atherosclerotic heart disease.

- The heart is, essentially, a muscle—a not-too-large muscle, but one that has to contract and relax and contract and relax, continuously, without a rest. Like any other muscle or living tissue, the heart needs oxygen, carried by blood though the coronary arteries that course along the surface of the heart. If these coronary arteries get blocked, there won't be enough blood flow or oxygen, and parts of the heart muscle itself will be damaged or killed.

- The most common reason for blockage of flow though the coronary arteries is atherosclerosis: the buildup of plaques along the walls of the coronary blood vessels. A similar process can occur in blood vessels leading to the brain, causing stroke, or to other blood vessels affecting other organs. Therefore, the risk factors for stroke and heart attack overlap in many ways.

- It's commonly thought that atherosclerotic plaques are made of fatty deposits, but that is an oversimplification. Although fats, or lipids, do contribute to these plaques, there are also inflammatory cells, scarring, and clotting cells and proteins that contribute to the plaques.

- These so-called atheromas start to develop in the teens and twenties and slowly proliferate. Longstanding, stable blockages can lead to the natural development of collateral vessels—new vessels that can bypass the blockage to deliver blood. Atherosclerotic plaques can lead to symptoms in several different ways.

Prevention and Screening

- The prevention of heart attacks is really the prevention of the development of atherosclerotic plaques. There is a tremendous amount of research, looking at multiple overlapping and additive risk factors. The most important ones are as follows.
    1. A healthy lipid profile. We don't just look at the total cholesterol; the specifics are important. But the bottom line is that a healthy diet, healthy weight, and an active lifestyle lead to more healthful blood lipids and decrease cardiovascular risk. Even with great lifestyle habits, some people will still have unfavorable lipids because of genetic predispositions. For these patients and for patients who are unable to sustain healthy life habits, medications may help reduce lipid risks.

2. Healthy blood pressure. Increased blood pressure contributes to the development of plaques and also forces the heart muscle to work harder and need more oxygen. A healthy blood pressure depends on both lifestyle and genetic factors.

3. Healthy weight. Excessive fat tissue contributes to inflammation and atherosclerosis, and risk factors for obesity overlap with those for unhealthy lipids and increased blood pressure.

4. Preventing and treating diabetes. Primarily, this is a matter of healthy eating and healthy weight—but there is a big contribution of genetics as well. It is not fair to assume that all of these risks are only because of lifestyle choices.

5. Avoiding smoking, which dramatically increases the risk of heart attacks, especially when combined with other risk factors.

- To help identify problems early, it is important to screen for heart disease risk in healthy people. Current recommendations stress low-tech screenings that are safe and effective. These include measuring blood pressure at least every two years, measuring blood lipids every five years, following body weight, and screening for elevated blood glucose (a manifestation of diabetes) starting at age 45. Regular counseling regarding smoking cessation and maintaining healthy diet and exercise habits is also recommended.

- There are also some higher-tech tests that may be helpful for people at higher risk for cardiovascular disease. A stress test forces the heart to work harder—while running on a treadmill, a continuous **EKG** reading looks for early signs of insufficient oxygen to the heart muscle, called ischemia.

- A newer test is a cardiac **CT scan** to measure calcium deposits around the heart (calcium being one constituent of atherosclerotic plaques). These are sometimes advertized heavily to the general public, and it's unclear exactly who should get these tests or how to interpret the results. They're not recommended for routine use.

Important Terms

AED: Automated external defibrillator.

agonal: Occurring just before death.

arrhythmia: An irregularity in the heart rhythm. Although this term is used commonly, a more exact term that is preferred is "dysrhythmia."

computed tomography scan (CT scan): A study that uses a series of X-rays to construct two-dimensional images of internal structures.

EKG: Electrocardiogram—sometimes abbreviated ECG.

Suggested Reading

Mayo Clinic, *Mayo Clinic Healthy Heart for Life*.

American Heart Association, http://www.heart.org.

Questions to Consider

1. What is the first thing to do if someone next to you collapses on the floor?

2. What are the best ways to prevent heart disease—and why is there so much heart disease in the United States?

Sudden Collapse
Lecture 7—Transcript

During this course, we've had our patient encounters in the Emergency Department, in a doctor's office, and in the hospital. We've been busy. Today is a day off to do some shopping, and so far it's been a relaxing day. You're in line, and you're ready to check out at Target. The person in front of you collapses to the floor. We've got no time for a chief complaint or history. There's a woman lying on the floor in front of you. She looks to be about 50 something. She is pale, and she's taking what are called agonal respirations, just the barest gasps that occur when a person is near death. Within moments, even these respiratory efforts stop. What do you do?

Because we have a mix of people here at grand rounds with varying degrees of medical experience, I'm going to proceed with the best instructions for what's called layman bystander CPR. Depending on your expertise, it may be appropriate to take different steps, but there are certain basic lifesaving steps that anyone can do. These first few minutes are critical. Most importantly, it is much, much better to do something than to stand there and do nothing while you try to remember what you're supposed to do. We don't need perfect, we don't need to 100 percent follow the guidelines and the exact methods of CPR, but we'd better act fast.

When you come across someone who appears to be dead, this is what to do. First, make sure the person isn't just sleeping or lying still. Give them a shake. Yell, "Are you OK?" Now, in our example, this person just collapsed in front of our eyes. You can probably skip this step. Then, yell for help. Call out, "call 911." If there are people nearby, point to one of them specifically and tell them to make that call. If you're in a public place, like a mall or a sporting event, and someone is around to help you, tell someone to go get you an "AED." Many places now have these devices available—gyms, department stores, schools, churches, many places. If one of these is available, using one as quickly as possible is the single best way to improve survival.

While waiting for someone to get that AED, start rescue CPR. Roll the person onto their back. Start pushing right in the middle of the chest, hard and fast. These are called chest compressions. Use two hands, one on top of the other, and after every push, relax so the chest can bounce back up. You shouldn't stay leaned into the chest—it's down, up, down, up. A good rhythm is the beat from the song "Stayin' Alive" by the Bee Gees: push, push, push, push, stayin' alive, stayin' alive. Then keep going, pushing hard and fast until either trained emergency rescue personnel show up, or someone runs over with the AED. If you're getting tired, and you will, try to swap out doing those chest compressions with another bystander.

If you have an AED, use it as soon as you can. Follow the instructions on the device. Studies have shown that even school-aged children can use these correctly. There will be a cartoon on the front showing the steps, and a big "ON" button, Pushing that is the first step. After that, the machine will have voice prompts to tell you exactly what to do. You will put a big sticky pad on the front of the chest, then make sure no one is touching the victim.

The computerized device will monitor what the heart is doing, and if appropriate, the device will tell you to push the "shock" button to deliver a jolt of electricity to start the heart beating again. An AED is a smart and safe device; it will not suggest giving a shock to a normally beating heart, and in fact, the "shock" button won't do anything if you push it unless it's safe to give a shock to the victim. After the shock, the machine will analyze the heart rhythm again and continue to tell you what to do. If at any time during the rescue process the victim starts to respond, that is, she starts to move or takes breaths,, stop what you're doing, roll the patient to lie on her side, and wait for rescue personnel.

There are a few finer points about CPR to review, and for completeness, we'll get back to those by the end of this lecture. For now, we'd better continue to focus on this stranger, who has now become our patient. It was a crowded day at Target, and people quickly went to get help. You had started pushing on the middle of her chest, up and down fast, and within a minute, someone came running up with a bright green box, an AED. You immediately push the ON button. You rip through the buttons of her shirt, and apply the AED pad—that's just a big sticker with wires that connect it to the AED.

You apply the pad right over the middle of her chest, plug the cord from the pad into the AED. The device lights up, and you hear a loud electronic voice: ANALYZING ... STAND BACK. DO NOT TOUCH THE VICTIM. SHOCK RECOMMENDED. You yell out, "STAND CLEAR" and push the big red SHOCK button. The victim jerks as current surges across the pad. There's a moment of silence. Then the victim curls up her arms up towards her chest. That's when the ambulance pulls up, and the EMTs rush in to take over. She's moving now, kind of writhing and gasping, and the EMTs put an oxygen mask on her face, some monitors on her chest, and rush her away.

So, what happened? We didn't really get much of a history or physical, so our differential diagnosis at this point is brief. Almost all causes of sudden collapse are from the heart, from some condition that suddenly stops the heart from beating. The most common cause of this is what's colloquially called a heart attack, or myocardial infarction; it's abbreviated MI. This is when a lack of blood flow to the heart muscle itself causes the death of heart muscle cells. It's often accompanied by a sudden change in the heart rhythm, a so-called arrhythmia. Instead of the heart beating in an organized way that effectively pumps blood, it just kind of quivers. No blood flow to the brain means that the body will collapse and die quickly. Sudden arrhythmias can also occur because of other conditions, including genetic predispositions to sudden death that can run in families.

Now, in this case we're not really the patient's doctor; care will be taken over by the ED, by the emergency department physician. Still, we're curious about the case, and a quick phone call gets us an informal update. We later learn that our patient had a second cardiac arrest; that is, another episode when her heart stopped beating effectively, requiring another shock in the ED. Blood tests and an EKG revealed that she had likely had an MI, and she was quickly whisked off to the cath lab. A study confirmed blockage of two of her coronary arteries, which were successfully reopened with a balloon procedure. She'll probably spend a few more days in the hospital and is expected to make a full recovery from her myocardial infarction.

Historically, heart attacks have been thought of as a disease of a certain kind of person: a man, usually, a successful, driven, type A kind of man. However, heart attacks are, in fact, the leading cause of death among women; 1 in 30 women will die of breast cancer; 1 in three will die of heart disease, most commonly, the kind of coronary artery disease that leads to heart attacks, though our ability to deal with and treat a heart attack has become increasingly effective. Our patient actually died and was resuscitated twice. We're still seeing an increasing impact of heart disease. This is mostly because it is so difficult to effectively modify well-known risk factors for atherosclerotic heart disease.

The heart is, essentially, a muscle—a not-too-large muscle, really, but one that has to contract and relax and contract and relax, continuously, without a rest, ever. In an average human lifespan, the heart will beat over two billion times. Like any other muscle or living tissue, the heart itself needs oxygen, carried by blood though the coronary arteries that course along the surface of the heart with small vessels penetrating perpendicularly, into the meat of the heart muscle itself. If these coronary arteries get blocked, there won't be enough blood flow, there won't be enough oxygen, and parts of the heart muscle itself will be damaged or killed.

The most common reason for blockage of flow though the coronary arteries is atherosclerosis, the buildup of plaques along the walls of the coronary blood vessels. A similar process can occur in blood vessels leading to the brain, causing stroke, or to other blood vessels affecting other organs. So the risk factors for stroke and heart attack overlap in many ways.

It's commonly thought that atherosclerotic plaques are made of fatty deposits, but that is an oversimplification. Though fats, which we usually call lipids, do contribute to these plaques, there are also inflammatory cells, scarring, and clotting cells and proteins that contribute to the plaques. In any case, we know that these so-called atheromas start to develop in the teens and twenties and slowly proliferate. Longstanding, stable blockages can lead to the natural development of collateral vessels, new vessels that can bypass the blockage to deliver blood.

Atherosclerotic plaques can lead to symptoms in several different ways. They can rupture, releasing inflammatory chemicals that quickly create a big clot, completely occluding flow; that would typically lead to a big, sudden heart attack. Or small bits of them can break off, flowing downstream to potentially cause a sudden blockage in a smaller vessel. Or, they can just slowly limit blood flow to adjacent heart muscle. In that case, symptoms could be milder and could come and go, especially becoming symptomatic during times of increased heart work—during exercise or stress.

Angina pectoris is the name for these reversible episodes of chest pain. They're not mini heart attacks—there's no cellular death. But rather, they can be thought of as warning signs of a possible big heart attack later. The character and kind of pain and other symptoms experienced by people with angina is similar to the pain of a heart attack, but it is temporary and usually less severe.

So, the prevention of heart attacks is really the prevention of the development of these atherosclerotic plaques. There is a tremendous amount of research here, looking at multiple overlapping and additive risk factors. There are five important ones risk factors that we stress to prevent heart disease:

First, maintain a healthy lipid profile. We don't just look at the total cholesterol. The specifics are important, but the bottom line is that a healthy diet, healthy weight, and an active lifestyle lead to more healthful blood lipids and decrease cardiovascular risk. Even with great lifestyle habits, some people will still have unfavorable lipids, that's probably because of genetic factors. For these patients and for patients who are unable to sustain healthy life habits, medications may help reduce lipid risks.

Second, keep blood pressure in a healthy range. Increased blood pressure contributes to the development of plaques, and also forces the heart muscle to work harder and need more oxygen. As with lipids and cholesterol, a healthy blood pressure depends on both lifestyle and genetic factors.

Third, keep weight healthy. Excessive fat tissue contributes to inflammation and atherosclerosis, and risk factors for obesity overlap with those for unhealthy lipids and increased blood pressure.

Number four, prevent and treat diabetes. Primarily, again, this is a matter of healthy eating, exercising, and healthy weight, but there is a big contribution of genetics as well. It is not fair to assume that all of these risks are only because of lifestyle choices.

And finally, avoid smoking, which dramatically increases the risk of heart attacks, especially when combined with other risk factors.

So, that's prevention. What about screening for heart disease risk in healthy people, to help identify problems early? Current recommendations stress low-tech screenings that are safe and effective. These include measuring blood pressure at least every two years; measuring blood lipids every five years; following body weight; and screening for elevated blood glucose, that's a manifestation of diabetes. That should be started at age 45. Regular counseling regarding smoking cessation and maintaining healthy diet and exercise habits is also recommended.

There are also some high-tech tests that may be helpful for people at high risk for cardiovascular disease. A stress test forces the heart to work harder. While running on a treadmill, a continuous EKG reading looks for early signs of insufficient oxygen to the heart muscle, called ischemia. A newer test is a cardiac CT scan to measure calcium deposits around the heart, calcium being one constituent of atherosclerotic plaques. These are sometimes advertised heavily to the general public, and it's unclear exactly who should get these tests or how to interpret the results. They're not recommended for routine use.

In our case today, our patient had a sudden collapse in front of our eyes, so there wasn't time to take a history or even talk about the symptoms. I don't think we even found out her name. But it's still important to go through the history and typical physical exam of someone having a less severe heart attack, so we know what to look for to help decide which patients are likely, or less likely, to need immediate therapy. Let's go through a second case today.

Bob, a 60 year old man, comes into our internal medicine clinic with a chief complaint of "My chest hurts." This is not an uncommon complaint—could be a heart attack, could be heartburn, could just be a pulled muscle or bruised rib. In other words, Bob could have something that will kill him in a few minutes, or he might have something completely unimportant. How can we tell the difference?

First, we'll do a quick, informal assessment just of Bob sitting there. He's an African American man, and he looks comfortable. He's not pale, he's not sweating, he's not having any difficulty breathing. In other words, he looks, and this is a good medical term, OK. If he didn't look OK, you'd probably want to jump to putting some EKG leads and oxygen on him, and maybe even calling 911. But since he's looking good, we can stay cool and work through this in our usual, organized way, starting with more history. By the way, in these grand round presentations, I'll sometimes mention a patient's ethnicity. Sometimes, a person's race can be a valuable clue; some health problems are more common among people of certain ancestry. Other times, the ethnicity really isn't relevant at all. You never know, at first, which clues are important.

OK, back to Bob, he says he gets these chest pains now and then. They're mid chest—he points right in the middle here—and feel squeezy or like pressure. To show you, he holds his hand over his chest and makes a fist. That's actually a pretty good description of the pain of angina or a heart attack. The pain sometimes comes out of nowhere, or sometimes when he walks the dog, or sometimes when he argues with people at work. It usually goes away with rest within an hour or so. That timing is important. Chest pain that lasts seconds or a few minutes is unlikely to be cardiac; neither is chest pain that lasts several hours without getting much, much worse. It's the middle-timing pain, an hour or so, that's mostly likely to be angina.

The radiation of pain and other symptoms can be good clues. Bob says that sometimes that pain will shoot to his right arm or shoulder, or is accompanied by nausea or sweatiness. This is really sounding like he's been having bouts of anginal pain. Though some people having a heart attack have never had angina previously, Bob's history is very suspicious for potentially serious heart disease.

We'll want to ask about risk factors too, including other health history, smoking, family history of heart disease. The physical exam, though, should start with a general, overall assessment. Does it look like this person is in imminent danger? A very fast or slow or irregular heart rate is very concerning during chest pain, and blood pressure and respiratory rate should be checked as well. People having heart attacks often look scared or sweaty or pale, and may have an new murmur or other irregularities on the heart exam. Bob looked well, his vital signs were normal, and the remainder of his exam was unrevealing.

Still, need to move quickly, but we ought to take a moment to make sure we've thought of a broad enough differential diagnosis for Bob's chest pain. Cardiac causes top the list, including those we've mentioned, like angina pectoris. By the way, that word, angina, is Latin for strangling or throttling, and refers specifically to a squeezing sort of pain; pectoris just means chest. Bob also could be having a full-blown MI. Other cardiac causes include pericarditis, an inflammation around the heart; or a rupture or tear of the aorta, the large vessel exiting the heart. The coronary arteries come right off the base of the aorta, so disruption of the aorta itself can block the coronaries and cause an MI.

Pulmonary embolism is caused by a big blood clot in the lungs and can cause chest pain and shortness of breath. If this is large, cardiovascular collapse or sudden death can occur. Chest pain, along with shortness of breath, can also be caused by a pneumothorax, where air is trapped outside of the lung, against the chest wall. Pneumonia can cause chest pain, particularly with cough and fever; and reflux can cause a burning pain typically in the mid-chest. Chest pain can also be caused by neuromuscular conditions, including chostochondritis, or inflammation of the edge of the breast bone. GI conditions, like ulcers or reflux, can also cause chest pain. And, finally, chest pain is a not-uncommon manifestation of anxiety or panic attacks.

Bob's workup from here will go quickly. One practical tidbit, with any patient who may be heading to the operating room, and yes, we're suspicious that Bob is having a heart attack and may need to go right into the cath lab, it's best to not allow the patient to eat or drink anything. If sedation is needed, it's safest to be done on an empty stomach. Now, if it's a big emergency and it's not safe to wait, sedation can be done right after a meal, but it's best to think ahead to minimize risk. Bob is now, as we say, NPO, nothing per oral, or, in normal-words, nothing to eat.

We get an EKG. This records the electrical activity of the heart and can show changes suggestive of either angina or an evolving myocardial infarction. It's quick and it's easy. Yes, here in our office, the EKG looks very suspicious. We make a quick call and get an ambulance over here to get him to the ED as soon as possible. There, blood tests are done to specifically look for elevations in what are called heart muscle enzymes. When heart cells die, they release specific compounds into the blood that we can test for. If those enzymes on the blood tests are up, that confirms a heart attack.

Bob, at this point, says he really doesn't even feel that bad. It's been said, by the way, that the first two symptoms of a heart attack in a man are chest pain and denial. His chest still hurts, but he says, really doc, this isn't what I thought would a heart attack. That's an important lesson. Though the chest pain of an MI can be severe, some people find that it doesn't really have to hurt so much. Be suspicious of chest pain not only when it's severe, but also in cases like Bob's, when the character is squeezey or pressury; or when it radiates to the left arm; or when there is sweating, nausea, or vomiting. The surrounding symptoms and character of the pain are more predictive of heart disease than the intensity of the pain itself.

The treatment of a heart attack is started quickly; often treatment begins before the diagnosis is actually confirmed. Basic things are done as soon as possible. Oxygen is administered—more oxygen breathed in provides more oxygen for the blood to carry, at least potentially increasing oxygen delivery to heart muscle if there isn't a 100 percent closed artery. Aspirin is typically be given to prevent further clotting, along with a medicine called nitroglycerin to widen the arteries, bringing in more blood. Medicine to treat the chest pain itself should also be given.

There are also more definitive treatments used to treat a confirmed MI. One is the administration of a thrombolytic drug. Thrombus means clot, and lytic refers to destruction, so thrombolytic drugs are our "clot busters." These work best if given quickly, before the clot gets thick and hard to break down. Also, the quicker blood flow can be restored to the heart muscle, the less heart tissue will be damaged.

Another option that's widely used is to quickly perform both a diagnostic angiogram, and then if possible, an angioplasty. These procedures are done in the cath lab, that's short for catheter, and involve using a thin tube that snakes up from the artery in the top of the leg towards the heart. Through this catheter, a small amount of dye can be injected so the inside of blood vessels can be seen under a kind of moving picture X-ray called fluoroscope. With this technique, the exact blocked area of coronary vessel can be seen, and if it's in a suitable position, a small balloon can be snaked up through the same catheter, put near the blockage, and expanded to allow blood flow. Sometimes, a small metal tube, called a stent, is left in place to hold the vessel open.

If an angiogram confirms one or more blockages, but balloon angioplasty is not possible or not successful, an open surgical procedure can be done to move blood vessels, usually from the leg, to the outside of the heart to bypass the blockages. This called a coronary artery bypass graft, sometimes it's abbreviated CABG, so it's pronounced "cabbage." Recovery from this kind of surgery takes much longer than after angioplasty. Whether by thrombolytic drugs, angioplasty, or coronary bypass surgery, restoring blood flow will only prevent further cellular damage; it will not revive dead heart tissue. Some heart repair is possible, but it takes a long time for muscle tissue to grow and adapt.

Care during and after an MI also involves monitoring for, and treating, any problem with the heart rhythm, either using medications or a pacemaker. Blood thinners are also used to prevent the spread of clots or the creation of new clots in the blocked vessel, or where angioplasty or a CABG was performed. Medications are also used to control blood pressure, pain, and anxiety. After leaving the hospital, after care includes not only medications, but also a plan for returning to or developing a reasonable exercise plan, as well as education and counseling to avoid lifestyle risk factors.

I want to go back to our first patient, the one at the department store, to expand on some of the instructions for bystander CPR. The newest guidelines have de-emphasized some of the traditional parts of CPR that had been taught. Rescuers are no longer encouraged to even check for an open airway and breathing. That used to be the first step, but that's been dropped, because it turns out that the faster you start pumping by pressing on the chest, the better chance the victim has of surviving. Don't check the pulses, don't mess with the airway, don't even bother with mouth-to-mouth resuscitation or rescue breaths. Now, jump in and push hard and fast, while calling for help and while calling for someone to get you an AED. An AED is an automatic external defibrillator. It is the single, best way to restore a normal heart rhythm, and it can be used by almost anyone. The faster the heart beat can be restored, the better the chance of life and recovery.

There are some situations where other approaches to CPR are needed. First, you have to be safe yourself to do CPR. If a victim is in a busy street or is drowning, it may not be safe for you to approach. Do not endanger yourself to do CPR. Also, children and babies need a different kind of CPR. For young people, it's unlikely that a cardiac problem has caused their collapse. Much more likely, it's something like choking or a problem with breathing. For children, you should open the airway and give rescue breaths before pressing on the chest. For any choking victim, adult or child, remove any visible blockage from the airway before proceeding with CPR, but even if you can't inflate the lungs, continue those chest compressions.

I would hope that no one would hesitate to help a stranger who has a sudden collapse, but some people might worry about malpractice lawsuits that might occur if resuscitation is unsuccessful. Every U.S. state, and many countries, have so-called good Samaritan laws that protect people from lawsuits if they stop to help someone who appears to be in mortal danger.

There's a side topic here, just to mention briefly. So far, we've mostly concentrated on heart attacks from atherosclerosis, which mostly affects older people. Much more rarely, sudden death can occur in a young, competitive athlete. Though it's possible that this was an MI, sudden cardiac death in a young person is much more likely to be related to an inherited, genetic condition that predisposes the heart to arrhythmia. Risks to look for, most importantly, are a family history of sudden death for any reason less than 40 years old. Even something like a drowning or a car accident may have, in fact, been triggered by a unrecognized cardiac event. Also, any athlete with a history of fainting or chest discomfort during exercise is at elevated risk. Individuals with personal or family risk factors should certainly have a screening EKG, and perhaps a comprehensive exam from a cardiologist, prior to competitive sports participation.

A suspected cardiac arrest should immediately trigger several events, all as soon as possible: activation of the emergency response system; CPR, starting with chest compressions; and getting an AED in place and activated as soon as possible for rapid defibrillation to restart the heart. Immediate care should be followed by transport, advanced life support, and then definitive cardiac care. Bystanders should not hesitate to jump in when help is needed. Next time, it may be your life that a stranger saves. Part of your medical school experience will be formal training in advanced cardiac life support, but I encourage everyone to take, at least, a basic CPR course.

Our next case is a younger patient, a teenager, he's surly and angry; he's not doing very well in school. Could this be just a normal teenager, or is there something else going on? We'll find out next time.

School Failure
Lecture 8

What do these three people have in common: a teenager failing school, a 40-year-old woman who has lost 10 pounds in the last few months, and a 70-year-old man who is becoming more and more forgetful? These are all presentations of depression. To a teenager, depression is presented by irritability and school failure; to an adult, perhaps disinterest in eating and taking care of herself, leading to weight loss; in an elderly person, disrupted thinking that may seem very much like forgetfulness. The good news is that depression is a treatable condition. These are not things that people just have to learn to live with.

Not Doing Well in School
- A 15-year-old patient, Trevor, is brought to our office by his father. When asked, he has no chief complaint, or at least he's not willing to say one. His father says that Trevor is failing school and is maybe falling asleep in class.

- A brief **differential diagnosis** can be broken down as follows.
    - Group 1 includes psychiatric problems, including depression or other mood disorders, plus substance abuse and attention deficit disorder. Less commonly, something like schizophrenia can begin at this age.

    - Group 2 would be what we'll call primary school problems, including bullying or social issues at school, or a learning disability.

    - In group 3 go primary medical problems, including disorders that prevent adequate quality of sleep or things like narcolepsy that cause excess drowsiness. You'd also include any primary brain disorder that could prevent learning or focusing. Hypothyroidism, among many other symptoms, can cause cognitive slowing and perhaps excessive sleepiness.

- What's especially tricky in this case is that there is a lot of overlap between the groups. For example, if for some "medical" type of reason he's having trouble focusing on his lessons, that might be leading to poor self-esteem and perhaps even bullying—which could lead to social isolation and symptoms of depression. There could be multiple, interconnected things going on for us to untangle.

- Trevor's past medical history is entirely unremarkable. The family history is positive for bipolar illness in an uncle on the father's side. The father says he himself has taken medicine for depression in the past, but he says that he "really didn't need it."

- Trevor presented several complexities. In addition to symptoms of depression, there was some evidence of a preexisting learning disorder, dyslexia; there was also the possibility that his cognitive problems could have been at least partially blamed on his history of **concussions** from playing football.

- A comprehensive psychological evaluation was performed to separate these factors. His primary diagnosis was confirmed to be major depression, with a secondary diagnosis of dyslexia.

- For the depression, Trevor was initially treated with medication alone; after some improvement, cognitive behavioral therapy was added a few months into treatment. Although he did have to repeat part of the school year, within about four months, he we doing well socially and academically.

- We do know that adolescents who experience depression have a high rate of relapse as adults, so it will be important for Trevor to continue to be monitored. There is some evidence that early recognition and aggressive therapy of adolescent depression may lessen the chance of adult relapse—or at least make recurrences milder.

- An important lesson to remember is that children are not little adults, and health issues in children and teenagers present differently from health conditions in adults. Depression in young people may have as major symptoms school problems and irritability instead of the sadness and hopelessness seen in adults.

- Another key lesson is that a variety of things can cause children to do poorly in school. These can include medical problems (such as a sleep disorder), school issues, or psychiatric conditions.

- Psychiatric conditions, such as depression, can present with a variety of vegetative, mood, and physical symptoms. In other words, psychiatric diagnoses should always be on the list of the differential diagnoses of any physical problem, and our differential diagnoses of psychiatric complaints should always include medical diagnoses, too. The boundaries are often fuzzy and sometimes misleading.

Major Depression
- It's important to make the distinction between depression—that is, the common word meaning "sadness"—and depression, the pervasive emotional disorder with specific symptoms that span far outside the realm of sadness. Of course, we all experience sadness related to life's disappointments, bereavement, and ordinary turmoil.

- When we speak of depression as a diagnosis, we're referring to something not only more intense in quality, but also broader in its effect on lives and families. Sometimes, the medical diagnosis is referred to as "major depression" to underscore this difference.

- The first primary symptom of depression is depressed mood. This can be something reported by the patient—for example, "I feel sad a lot"—or something noticed by the family. In teenagers, a depressed mood can come across as more of an irritable mood, with frequent fighting and outbursts. To qualify as major depression, the depressed mood occurs most of the day, nearly every day. Our patient was at times sad and at times quite irritable.

- The second main symptom is a lack of interest in pleasurable activities. In teenagers, this often presents as social withdrawal, dropping out of activities, or spending very little time with friends or hobbies that used to be enjoyable. One or the other, or both, of these two main symptoms of withdrawal and depressed mood are always present in major depression. Our patient had both.

- There are also a number of other symptoms, and for a formal diagnosis, at least four of these must be present to confirm the diagnosis of depression.

- So-called vegetative symptoms affect our basic life functions. There can be significant changes in appetite leading to either weight loss or weight gain. Depression can also affect sleep cycles, leading to either reduced or increased sleep. Even when there is a lot of sleep, fatigue or loss of energy is reported.

- There are also qualitative and quantitative changes in thinking patterns. Many patients with depression experience cognitive slowing, or a lack of ability to think or focus. Thoughts that do occur are often preoccupied with feelings of guilt or worthlessness that may even border on delusional—sometimes patients blame themselves for many things that are clearly not their fault. There can be pervasive hopelessness and recurrent thoughts of death, which may include thinking about suicide or planning or performing a suicidal act.

- Although the symptoms of depression in children and adults are similar in many ways, there are some significant differences. Teenagers are as likely to present with irritability, anger, or abusive language as with sadness. They more often have somatic complaints, such as bellyaches, headaches, nausea, or dizziness. In fact, chronic unexplained pain should always raise the suspicion of depression as a possible diagnosis.

- Depressed teens often complain of being bored and have low energy. They may become extremely sensitive to perceived rejection or lack of success. School absences and/or decreasing school performance are nearly universal findings in childhood depression.

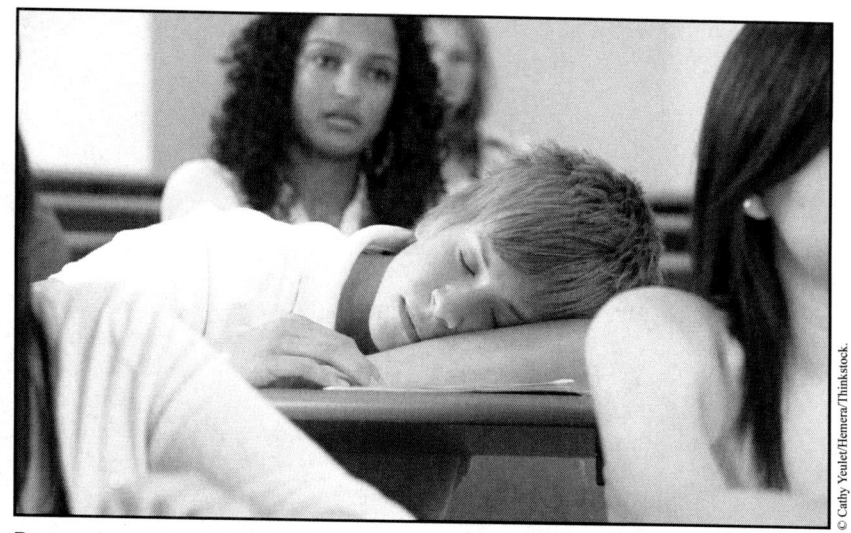

Depression manifests itself in many ways, especially for adolescents.

- Depression is a serious problem. About four to eight percent of adolescents experience a major depressive episode each year, leading to substantial problems at school and at home. Depressed teens may fail in school, lose their jobs, or turn to drugs of abuse. In addition, depression contributes to most cases of suicide, which is now the number one killer of young adults in the United States.

Risk Factors and Treatment

- There are clearly both environmental and genetic factors that contribute to the development of depression. Risk factors for children can include a history of neglect, abuse, loss of a parent (especially the same-sex parent), psychosocial deprivation, or chronic illness. However, although these factors increase the risk of depression, most children with, for example, chronic illness do not become depressed.

- In addition, whether stresses are accompanied by a supportive family may influence the possible development of depression.

- Familial or genetic factors also play a role in how resilient people can be to life's stress.

- There are several ways to treat adolescent depression. Certainly, helping to create a supportive home and school environment is essential, as is trying to gradually get the patient involved again with pleasurable activities and exercise. Sleep habits and daily routines may need to be normalized.

- Any coexisting anxiety or other mental problems, substance abuse, learning problems, or medical issues need to be evaluated and addressed, even while pursuing active therapy for depression.

- Psychotherapy can be effective, especially for mild-to-moderate depression. The most well-studied form of therapy is called cognitive behavioral therapy, which at its core is an application of the idea that our thoughts cause our feelings and behaviors.

- Although talking is of course involved, cognitive behavioral therapy isn't just talking about feelings—it's a focused approach to help patients learn to recognize their own thoughts, learn how they lead to distressing symptoms, and most importantly, how to change the way they think about things. Psychotherapy isn't as effective for more severely affected patients and may take weeks or months to help.

- The other effective therapeutic option is antidepressant medications. These aren't in any way "happy pills." They do not work quickly, but over the span of weeks, these medications can help with the mood and physical symptoms of depression.

- The most widely used group of these medications are called SSRIs. Overall, SSRIs are quite safe and well tolerated. However, some studies have showed an increase in suicidal thoughts (though not actions) in the first weeks of therapy, leading to an FDA warning on the label concerning the suicide risk. Ironically, the drop in SSRI usage caused by concerns raised by this warning has led to a net increase in teen suicide, probably because fewer teens could get effective therapy.

Important Terms

concussion: Brain trauma leading to symptoms of brain dysfunction.

differential diagnosis: A list of candidate diagnoses to explain a medical problem.

Suggested Reading

Barkley, *Taking Charge of ADHD*.

Burns, *Feeling Good*.

Solomon, *The Noonday Demon*.

WebMD, http://www.webmd.com/depression/.

Questions to Consider

1. Why do some teenagers do poorly in school?

2. How are teenagers and adults different? Why should their medical problems be evaluated differently, and how?

School Failure
Lecture 8—Transcript

What do these three people have in common: a teenager failing school; a 40-year old woman who has lost 10 pounds in the last few months; and a 70-year-old man who is becoming more and more forgetful? There's one diagnosis that can account for all of these symptoms. Here's another hint: it is the most common cause of death of young adults aged 25 to 35 in the United States.

We have a 15-year-old patient today, Trevor, he's brought into our office by his father. When asked, he has no chief complaint, or at least he's not willing to say one. "What can we do for you today?" you ask. Trevor patient looks down at his feet, and he doesn't answer. His father fills in. He says Trevor is failing school, and he and the boy's mother don't know what to do with him any more. They've taken him off the football team, and that didn't seem to matter. They've taken away all privileges, and they even offered to buy him a car for his 16th birthday if he passes all of his classes, but Trevor just doesn't seem to care.

The remainder of the history is taken almost entirely from dad. Once or twice Trevor speaks up to mutter a few words to correct something his father says. Later, we'll ask dad to step out of the room to hopefully get some more information directly from our patient. But for now, it seems we're going to have to rely on dad to tell us this story.

Trevor had been a pretty good student in the past, kind of in the mostly B range, an occasional C. Reading had always been especially difficult, but he's made his way through to 9th grade more or less on level. He attends the local public school. Over the summer, he had seemed excited about moving into high school and joining the football team, but towards the end of summer, he seemed to become more withdrawn. He made the junior varsity team and did OK academically at the start of the year, but by October he was bringing home failing grades on tests and was missing a lot of homework. Sometimes he'd do it and not bother to turn it in, and other times he just wouldn't do it. His teachers have sent comments home that he wasn't paying attention in classes and that sometimes he would fall asleep.

You ask the patient directly, "What's going on?" He looks up; he says, "eh." For those of you who are less used to teenagers, that probably means "I don't know." Dad chimes in, "He's always up in his room, I think he's sleeping all the time. Or maybe he's doing drugs." That gets a rise out of his son. Trevor actually looks up, and he says, "I am not doing drugs. You always think that." Then he looks down at his feet. Well, at least he said something, right?

OK, it's time to step back and think about what's going on. We need a brief differential diagnosis. We have a teenager who's doing poorly in school, and who is maybe falling asleep in class. I'd break the differential down this way. Group one includes psychiatric problems; here would go depression or other mood disorders, plus substance abuse and attention deficit disorder. Less commonly, something like schizophrenia can begin at this age. Group two would be what we'll call primary school problems. I'd include bullying or social issues at school here, or perhaps a learning disability. In group three go primary medical problems. Here could go disorders that prevent adequate quality of sleep, or things like narcolepsy that cause excessive drowsiness. You'd also include any primary brain disorder that could prevent learning or focusing. Hypothyroidism, among a lot of other symptoms, can cause cognitive slowing and perhaps excessive sleepiness.

What's especially tricky here in this case is that there's a lot of overlap between the groups. For instance, if for some "medical" type of reason he's having trouble focusing on his lessons, that might be leading to poor self esteem and perhaps even bullying, which could lead to social isolation and symptoms of depression. And there could be multiple, interconnected things going on here for us to untangle. So let's see what we can find out from some additional history.

Our patient had been an active football player for several years on the middle school team. He was good, and aggressive, and loved playing, and he had really been looking forward to high school-level ball. He had had a few injuries during play, including a broken wrist towards the end of last year and two concussions that kept him out of several games. Other than those injuries, he's had no significant health issues. He's taken essentially no medications, and other than regular checkups, he's barely been into the doctor's office.

Trevor has two older half brothers from his father's first marriage, who are both playing football in college. His parents are now divorced, that's his father's second divorce, though it sounds like he has a pretty good relationship with both of his parents. During the school year he lives at his father's apartment because it's closer to school.

Delving into a review of systems, Trevor denies fever or weight loss or any aches or pains of any kind. He says he's bored a lot and feels tired most of the time. Even when he wakes up, Trevor says he still feels tired. His father denies that he snores or wakes up at night, and says he thinks that his son is sleeping well. There's no history of headaches, red eyes, trembling, forgetfulness, or running away or unexplained disappearances. He rarely goes out with friends, and in fact, sees very little of his friends from middle school or the football team any more.

After all of this talking, our patient seems to be a little more engaged; he's listening to at least some of the questions, and answering some of them with one or two words. We ask dad to step outside. Let's see what the teenager has to say in private. Trevor says, "I don't know what's wrong. I just can't focus any more. Maybe I have ADD. I took a friend's Adderall, and it seemed to help." We specifically ask about substance abuse, which he denies, though he admits to taking his friend's ADD medicine, that Adderall.

A quick side comment, here, later on, we're going to talk with Trevor about that having been a bad idea. He needs to know that taking someone else's medication can be dangerous. But we'll not interrupt Trevor's story right now.

He says he sleeps OK, falls asleep fairly quickly at night, and gets up fairly easily in the morning, even though he still feels tired. He never falls asleep suddenly without warning, and has never had an episode of sleep or loss of muscle control brought on suddenly by emotions or laughter. Those last few items are symptoms of narcolepsy; that's a rare neurologic disorder that can cause excessive daytime sleepiness.

Trevor says his dad is "fine," and they get along "fine." And he denies any sort of bullying or problems with his friends at school. He says his mom is "OK." I don't know if that ranks above or below "fine," but that's the word he used. We ask, what's something you've enjoyed doing in the last few weeks, something that you like to do? And Trevor says, "eh-eh." I don't think we're going to get much more information from our interview.

Past medical history is entirely unremarkable. The family history is positive for bipolar illness in an uncle on the father's side. The father says he himself has taken medicine for depression in the past, but he says he "really didn't need it."

On to the physical exam. Trevor is a slender, young, Caucasian male, and his vital signs are normal. His affect, that's a way of saying the way he's acting, or the way he's expressing emotions, is kind of flat and uninterested. He's just kind of Blah, not really upset or worried or anxious or, really, anything. The remainder of a general medical exam is entirely normal. Specifically, his pupils are normal and normally reactive to light, and he has no trembling in his hands; those might be a few things you could look for for evidence of substance abuse. When asked to repeat digits back to you, his answers are slow and hesitant, but they are correct. We do an in-depth neurologic exam and find that his gait, strength, and coordination are all normal.

Before we come back to the differential, we'll grab a few quick lab studies. Thyroid tests are normal, a CBC is also normal, and we do chemistries; those are normal too. We do a urine drug screen that comes up positive for amphetamines; we already knew that would happen, because he admitting taking his friend's Adderall, which is an amphetamine medication. No other drugs of abuse were identified.

So now, do we have all of the information we need to make a diagnosis? I think so. Let's revisit that original grouping we presented earlier. Recall that group one was psychiatric diagnoses, group two included school-based problems. Group three, that was our primary medical disorders. Let's start with those. He says he feels fatigued or tired a lot, so we need to consider a sleep disorder that could affect the quality or quantity of sleep. Now, inadequate sleep itself is very common among adults and teens. We don't know the exact amount of sleep that is necessary, but clearly, many of us aren't getting enough, and that could adversely affect concentration at home or work. One very common cause of insufficient sleep for children and adults are those ubiquitous screens we've all become so attached to.

For most of humanity's existence, the sun provided the cue that helped us know when it was time for sleep. Though indoor gas and then electric lighting allowed the period of useful daytime to be extended, it's only very recently that we've begun staring into light sources in the evenings. All of those LCD devices—TVs, computers, smartphones, tablets—all of them are light sources, and we know that staring into them tricks our brains into thinking it's daytime. Another sleep stealer: caffeine. Its use has surged among teenagers, and that's another common contributor to poor sleep. Children and teens metabolize caffeine differently than adults, and the effects of coffee and sodas may last longer. Also, modern coffee shop coffee has far more caffeine than what many of us are used to drinking.

Another common sleep disorder is sleep apnea, sometimes called sleep disordered breathing. Loud or interrupted snoring interferes with sustained quality sleep, and children and adults can have problems with headaches, irritability, somnolence, or poor concentration. Our history, though, doesn't suggest our patient has a problem with insufficient quantity or quality of sleep or of his having a sleep disorder, like sleep apnea or narcolepsy.

Another medical problem we had mentioned earlier was thyroid disease, but the labs have shown normal thyroid function. However, our history did uncover one risk factor for another potential medical cause of cognitive problems. We know he had been an aggressive and active football player who reported that he had had two concussions. Parenthetically, I'd just say here that if a football player says he remembers two concussions, it's quite likely that he's actually had quite a few more.

Concussions are an important diagnosis to make, because we know that in the period after a concussion, the brain is vulnerable to a second injury that can be much more severe, or even catastrophic. Sudden deaths have occurred after even relatively mild tackles during the recovery phase of a first concussion. It's crucial that after a concussion, a player come off the field and not continue playing until completely free of symptoms and medically cleared.

Sometimes, there are lingering symptoms during a so-called post concussive phase that can last days or weeks or even longer. These can include cognitive slowing, difficulty with sleep, or a depressed or irritable mood. The length and intensity of this post-concussive phase does not directly correlate with the intensity of the original injury.

We're also learning more about the long-term effects of concussions, especially multiple concussions. There is a risk of permanent cognitive impairment, as well as an increased risk of depression, other mental disorders, and problems with coordination and movement. Our patient's history of concussions could be contributing to his school problems either by directly causing cognitive difficulties, or by contributing to a risk of depression.

OK, we've been going into more detail with our group three diagnoses, the ones that are essentially medical problems, like concussion or sleep disorders, that contribute to school difficulty. Let's continue working backwards numerically into group two, our "school diagnoses." This includes social and learning problems that have an adverse effect on performance. Among the most common school problems is bullying, and I can't stress enough how significant a problem that can be for our kids. Bullied children and teens do not feel safe in school. They have trouble concentrating and often develop both depressive and anxious symptoms. They may themselves lash out and end up with conduct problems, sometimes they're labeled as the bully. And they're at an increased risk of suicide, as well as substance abuse. Our patient denied bullying, but it's important to ask and pry about these issues with any child who's having a drop in school performance.

Another school issue that could be part of this picture would be a learning disability or LD. These are neurologic conditions that interfere with a student's ability to store or process information. Kids with LD have good intelligence and can perform well in some tasks, but often have one or more specific areas of weakness. For instance, dyslexia is a specific learning disability that affects language skills, including reading. LDs can be treated best if caught early, by providing additional educational support and strategies to enhance learning while working on catching up the deficient skills.

Trevor was said to have always had trouble with reading. We ought to keep in mind that that could mean Trevor has a specific learning disability that hadn't been recognized yet. This may be a part of why high school isn't going well.

On to group one, our primary psychiatric diagnoses. You're probably already getting a sense that these groupings are somewhat artificial. For instance, we know that concussion can contribute to depression; we know that learning disabilities can lead to bullying and anxiety and poor sleep; and those can themselves lead to poor concentration and memory. We've grouped our diagnoses into separate medical and psychiatric and school diagnoses to help us as doctors remember to think about those contributors. But in the real world, these problems overlap in multiple ways, and there's a huge grey zone that encompasses contributions from all of the categories into one unique patient. Categories and labels help us think, but shouldn't be straightjackets that prevent us from appreciating the complex interactions of how our minds and bodies work. Nonetheless, there are some specific psychiatric diagnoses that are important to consider, especially because an appropriate diagnosis can help lead us to effective treatment.

Attention deficit disorder, or ADD, probably affects 5 or 10 percent of teenagers. It includes one or more symptoms that include poor attention, hyperactivity, and impulsive behavior. The symptoms occur in multiple realms, not just at home and not just at school, and have been present since a child was young. ADD is a characteristic pattern of thinking and behavior that has to have been present, essentially, throughout a person's life. It is not a new condition that starts as a teen or adult. Perhaps it wasn't diagnosed earlier; that can certainly happen. But the characteristic symptoms have to have been present since childhood. Also, to qualify as ADD these symptoms have to be severe enough to affect functioning and performance.

Our patient tried one of his friend's pills for ADD, and he says it worked. But it is a myth that this means he has ADD. Anyone who takes ADD medicine will see the effects of the medication, including improved attention. Unfortunately, we know that sharing and selling of ADD medicines in high schools and college campuses is common, because young people know that the medications work. We need to do a better job ensuring that these medicines help the people who genuinely have ADD, and aren't diverted for offhand or recreational use.

Does Trevor have ADD? I don't think so. His symptoms of poor attention have really been of recent onset, and talking with him and his family, it's clear that he did not have these symptoms during his early years in school. Is our patient perhaps having problems with substance abuse, taking drugs that are interfering with his concentration in school? There are a very broad range of drugs that both teens and adults take for mood- and mind-altering purposes. This includes what were once known as street drugs, including marijuana and cocaine, plus the possibility of stolen or purchased medications, including the ADD medication that our patient admitted using. Many adults keep a number of medications in their medicine cabinets, and unfortunately, those can become a target for their own teenagers or visitors to their home.

Other substances of abuse could include alcohol, or huffing or inhaling volatile substances from plastic bags. Our patient did have a urine drug test that confirmed the presence of amphetamines, but these sorts of tests don't always turn up every possible drug of abuse. One new problem we're seeing is the increasing availability of so-called synthetic marijuanas, including chemicals that can be adapted to elude detection by drug screens. Some of these modern synthetics can be much more medically dangerous and more addictive than marijuana itself. In our history and physical, we didn't find evidence of any specific findings that suggest substance abuse, but we'll continue to keep that possibility in mind.

There is one psychiatric diagnosis that fits very well, and I think in this case accounts for a big proportion of our patient's presentation. Our top diagnosis, based on the history and physical examination, is depression. It's important to make the distinction between depression, that is, the common word meaning sadness, and Depression (with a capital D), the pervasive emotional disorder with specific symptoms that span far outside the realm of sadness. Of course, we all experience sadness related to life's disappointments, bereavement, and ordinary turmoil. When we speak of depression as a diagnosis, we're referring to something not only more intense in quality, but also more broad in its effect on lives and families. Sometimes, the medical diagnosis is referred to as major depression to underscore that difference.

The first primary symptom of depression is depressed mood. This can be something reported by the patient; they'll say, "I feel sad a lot," or something noticed by the family. In teenagers, a depressed mood can come across as more of an irritable mood, with frequent fighting and outbursts. To qualify as major depression, the depressed mood occurs most of the day, nearly every day. Our patient was at times sad, and at times very irritable.

The second main symptom of depression is a lack of interest in pleasurable activities. In teenagers, this often presents as social withdrawal, or dropping out of activities, or spending very little time with friends or hobbies that used to be enjoyable. One or the other, or both, of these two main symptoms of withdrawal and depressed mood are always present in major depression. Our patient had both.

There are also a number of other symptoms, and for a formal diagnosis, at least four of these must be present to confirm the diagnosis of depression. So-called vegetative symptoms affect our basic life functions. There can be significant changes in appetite leading to either weight loss or weight gain. Depression can also affect sleep cycles, leading to either reduced or increased sleep. Even when there is a lot of sleep, fatigue or loss of energy is often reported

There are also changes in thinking patterns. Many patients with depression experience cognitive slowing, or a lack of ability to think or to focus. Thoughts are often preoccupied with feelings of guilt or worthlessness that may even border on delusional. Sometimes patients blame themselves for many things that are clearly not their fault. There can be pervasive hopelessness and recurrent thoughts of death, which may include thinking about suicide or planning or performing a suicidal act.

Though the symptoms of depression in children and adults are similar in some ways, there are some significant differences. Teenagers are as likely to present with irritability, anger, or abusive language as with sadness. They more often have unexplained body complaints, like belly aches, headaches, nausea, or dizziness. In fact, chronic, unexplained pain should always raise the suspicion of depression as a possible diagnosis. Depressed teens often complain of being bored and have low energy. They may become extremely sensitive to perceived rejection or lack of success. School absences and decreasing school performance are nearly universal findings in childhood depression.

Depression is a serious problem. About 4 to 8 percent of adolescents experience a major depressive episode each year, leading to substantial problems at school and at home. Depressed teens may fail in school, lose their jobs, or turn to drugs of abuse. In addition, depression contributes to most cases of suicide, which is now the number one killer of young adults in the United States.

There are clearly both environmental and genetic factors that contribute to the development of depression. Risk factors for children can include a history of neglect; abuse; loss of a parent, especially the same-sex parent; psycho-social deprivation; or chronic illness. However, though these factors increase the risk of depression, most children with, say, chronic illness do not become depressed. Familial or genetic factors also play a role in how resilient people can be to life's stress.

There are several ways to treat adolescent depression. Certainly, helping to create a supportive home and school environment is essential, as is trying to gradually get the patient involved back into pleasurable activities and exercise. Sleep habits and daily routines may need to be normalized. Any co-existing anxiety or other mental problems, including substance abuse or learning problems, those need to be evaluated and addressed, even while pursuing active therapy for depression.

Psychotherapy can be effective, especially for mild-to-moderate depression. The most well-studied form of therapy is called cognitive behavioral therapy, which at its core is an application of the idea that our thoughts cause our feelings and behaviors. Though talking is, of course, involved, cognitive behavioral therapy isn't just talking about feelings, it's a focused approach to help patients learn to recognize their own thoughts, learn how they lead to distressing symptoms, and most importantly, how to change the way they think about things. Psychotherapy isn't as effective for more severely affected patients and may take weeks or months to help.

The other effective therapeutic option is antidepressant medications. These aren't at all happy pills. They don't work quickly, but over the span of weeks, these medications can help with the mood and physical symptoms of depression. The most widely used group of these medications are called the SSRIs. Overall, SSRIs are quite safe; they're well-tolerated. However, some studies have shown an increase in suicidal thoughts, though not actions, in the first weeks of therapy, leading to an FDA black box warning on the label concerning the suicide risk. Ironically, the drop in SSRI usage caused by concerns raised by this warning has led to a net increase in teen suicide, probably because fewer teens are getting effective therapy for depression.

Our patient today, Trevor, he was not a straightforward case. In addition to symptoms of depression, there was some evidence of a pre-existing learning disorder, dyslexia; and there was the possibility that his cognitive problems could have been at least partially blamed on his history of concussions. A comprehensive psychologic evaluation was performed to separate out these factors.

His primary diagnosis was confirmed to be major depression, with a secondary diagnosis of dyslexia. For the depression, Trevor was initially treated with medication alone; and after some improvement, cognitive behavioral therapy was added. Though he did have to repeat some of that school year, within about four months, he was doing well socially and academically. We do know that adolescents who experience depression have a high rate of relapse as adults, so it will be important for Trevor to continue to be monitored. There is some evidence that early recognition and aggressive therapy of adolescent depression may lessen the chance of adult relapse, or at least make recurrences milder.

Today's lessons to remember, first, children are not little adults, and health issues in children and teenagers present differently from health conditions in adults. Depression in young people may have as major symptoms school problems and irritability instead of the sadness and hopelessness seen in adults.

Remember, at the start of this lecture, I posed this puzzle: What do these three people have in common: a teenager failing school; a 40-year-old woman who has lost 10 pounds in the last few months; and a 70-year-old man who is becoming more and more forgetful? These may all be presentations of depression. To a teenager, irritability and school failure; to an adult, perhaps disinterest in eating and taking care of herself; and in an elderly person, disrupted thinking that may seem very much like forgetfulness. They are all depression, and the good news is, depression is a treatable condition. These are not things that people just have to learn to live with.

Another key lesson from today, a variety of things can cause kids to do poorly in school. These can include medical problems, like a sleep disorder: school issues; or a psychiatric problem. One last lesson, psychiatric conditions, like depression, can present with a variety of both mood and physical symptoms. In other words, psychiatric diagnoses should always be on the list of the differential diagnoses of any physical problem, and our differential diagnoses of psychiatric complaints should always include medical diagnoses, too. The boundaries are often fuzzy and sometimes misleading. We'll hear more about that next time, when what was thought to be a psychiatric diagnosis ended up being something else entirely. What was causing our next patient's peculiar dizzy spells? Wait and see.

Dizzy Attacks
Lecture 9

The last three lectures have been common diagnoses—breast cancer, heart disease, and depression. This lecture requires a little more of a mental stretch. The case in this lecture strikes about 1 in 1,000 adults per year. In a typical, busy medical practice, full-time doctors probably have about 1,500 patients they see regularly, so each year, they're likely to see a few cases of this. So it's not common, but it's not so uncommon either. The presenting symptom, dizziness, is very common.

Dizziness

- In our general medicine clinic, a 42-year-old woman named Tina says that for the last few months, she gets these "attacks" where all of a sudden she gets dizzy. She can't stand up straight, and sometimes she hears a buzzing or high-pitched sort of noise. She says that she sort of staggers around and has to eat a candy bar. Once she has some sugar, in about a half of an hour, she starts to feel better.

- These episodes are getting more intense, more frequent, and are lasting longer—now, she says, sometimes she has to eat two candy bars. Her friends have told her that she's either having **hypoglycemia** or that she's just crazy.

- Dizziness can be a challenging symptom because different people use that term to refer to different things. Dizziness can mean **vertigo**—which is a sensation of spinning, as if the environment is moving around you. True vertigo is usually caused by problems with the inner ear, where the sense organs of balance are.

- Dizziness can also refer to a lightheaded feeling, like you're going to faint. That's a completely different problem, with different physiology to think about. Dizziness in this sense is usually caused by insufficient blood flow to the brain.

- Less frequently, a feeling of dizziness can be related to feeling unsteady or off balance, caused by problems with the brain, nerves, or muscle. This can be related to a loss of either nerve input to the brain—conditions where there's a loss of sensory input, so a person can't sense, essentially, where their feet are; or a condition that affects motor function, causing weakness and unsteadiness. These are neurological problems and are most often present in elderly people.

- Finally, dizziness can be a psychological or psychophysiological effect, when a person feels kind of disconnected or disassociated with the world's sensory signals. In that case, a psychological assessment is most helpful.

- Tina clarifies by saying that the feeling she keeps having is a spinning feeling—like the room is spinning, round and round. She says she doesn't feel faint, and she's never passed out, but she is afraid she'll fall down. This is true vertigo.

- Because she also mentioned that she hears an unexplained buzzing or high-pitched sound, we can be pretty sure that this is an ear problem, specifically with the inner ear, where hearing and balance sense organs are located. That would explain the combination of vertigo and a hearing issue.

- Tina's history and physical exam support a clinical diagnosis of episodic vertigo. The main symptom of problems along the pathways of the balance system, from the balance organs through the nerves to the brain area that interprets the data, is vertigo—a sensation of movement in space when there is in fact no movement.

- The most common cause of vertigo is called benign paroxysmal positional vertigo (BPPV). It causes brief (less than one minute) episodes of vertigo triggered by a position change, such as turning over in bed or quickly looking up.

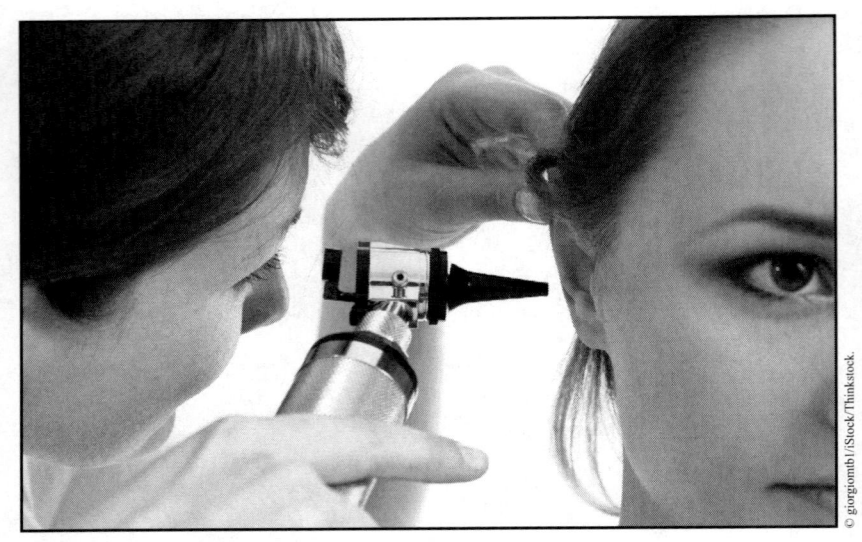

The inner ear is involved in regulating our sense of balance.

- It's caused by a problem in the balance sense organs themselves, by debris in the semicircular canals. The symptoms and **nystagmus** can be recreated in the office by moving the head in the plane of the effected canal. Tina's vertigo attacks last too long to be typical of BPPV.

- Labyrinthitis refers to inflammation in the balance and hearing organs. The vertigo can be made worse by positional changes and usually last days to weeks. Tina's symptoms have come in recurrent, isolated attacks that have come and gone repeatedly—which really doesn't fit the typical presentation of labyrinthitis.

- Another problem that can occur in the sense organs of balance is called Ménière's disease. Although we don't know exactly why it occurs, it seems to be caused by excessive endolymph fluid that interferes with the functioning of the balance organs. Ménière's patients, in addition to having periods of intense vertigo, often also suffer from hearing problems, because that same excessive endolymph affects the functioning of the cochlea.

Ménière's Disease

- For Tina, it sounds like Ménière's disease fits best because it causes attacks of vertigo that come and go, like Tina reports, and also affects hearing. Other diagnoses, such as a tumor or multiple sclerosis, seem much less likely, but after discussing these possibilities with Tina, she decides that she would like to pursue a very thorough workup.

- To definitively rule out a tumor, we need a brain scan—one that looks along the entire pathway, from the sense organs along the nerve to the brain. A CT scan is a very good study; it's relatively quick to get and can show pretty good detail, especially of bones.

- However, there are drawbacks. CT scans are basically a series of plain X-rays that are stitched together by computers to make composite images. Like other X-rays, they rely on ionizing radiation to get an image. Though the risk is small, any study involving radiation will expose the patient to some risk of damage from the radiation itself, increasing the lifetime risk of cancer.

- In contrast, an MRI scan of the brain doesn't use any ionizing radiation. It also has the advantage of imaging soft tissues like the brain with much more precision than a CT scan. MRIs are also better able to get images through the dense bones of the base of the brain, where CT scans don't penetrate as well—and, with balance problems, we need to look at the base of the brain, where the balance and sense organs are.

- The main disadvantages of MRI compared to CT are that they take much longer to do, and they are more expensive. In Tina's case, we decided to get an MRI to rule out even a small tumor, and it was normal. The MRI scan also showed that there were no brain **lesions** to suggest multiple sclerosis.

- After the MRI, we referred Tina to an **ENT** specialist, who reviewed the clinical exam and MRI and did a hearing test (which did confirm some low-frequency hearing loss). The ENT evaluation confirmed that Tina does indeed have Ménière's disease.

- The specific cause of Ménière's disease isn't completely understood. There is increased endolymph fluid, as well as differences in the glycoprotein content of the fluid; there's also evidence for alterations in the way that the fluid flows through the canals and is reabsorbed. Some studies have supported an infectious agent, genetic influences, or allergies—or a combination of these factors.

- Whatever the cause, the main symptom is episodic attacks that last for one or more hours. During attacks, there is vertigo, often accompanied by a ringing, rushing, or buzzing sort of sound (called tinnitus). There may also be a feeling of pressure or fullness in the ear.

- Accompanying these attacks is a gradual, fluctuating level of low-frequency hearing loss that can become severe and is only reversible if caught early. The pressure feeling and hearing loss usually affects only one ear, but it can affect both.

- Ménière's disease is a clinical diagnosis; there is no one specific test that confirms it. Tests are done, sometimes, to rule out other diagnoses (like the MRI Tina had). Blood tests are really of limited usefulness in the workup, though they can again rule out other problems if there are suggestive symptoms. Doing a thorough hearing evaluation is essential, and hearing will need to continue to be monitored during treatment.

- There are also high-tech tests that can support the diagnosis or monitor treatment. These include tests that directly monitor the electrical output of the organs and nerves of the inner ear when they're triggered by sounds or nearby reflex muscle contractions.

Treatment and Prognosis
- There are several treatment options for Ménière's disease, though none is really ideal. The main first therapy is dietary—restricting sodium—sometimes along with taking a diuretic to reduce body water. This simple treatment can reduce vertigo attacks but may not effectively slow hearing loss.

- Medications can be used during acute attacks to reduce the uncomfortable sensations of vertigo and nausea, but these don't reduce hearing loss, and they are also ineffective in preventing further attacks. Still, conservative management and monitoring of hearing is probably good enough therapy for many people with Ménière's disease.

- Another option for treatment is the use of steroids, which may reduce the pressure in the endolymph fluid. These can be given orally, by injection, or even by injection through the eardrum into the middle ear. There are some serious potential side effects of steroid use, especially if they're needed for a long course.

- More aggressive therapy, especially for frequent and severe vertigo attacks, can include direct injections of medicine into the middle ear. An antibiotic called gentamicin is used—not because it is an antibiotic, but because it can decrease the number of **vestibular** hair cells that are sending the incorrect balance information to the brain. Although it can effectively reduce or eliminate vertigo attacks, gentamicin can actually make the hearing loss worse, so this therapy isn't suitable for everyone.

- There are some surgical options for therapy as well. A shunt can be placed in the inner ear to drain some of the excess fluid; however, how well this works is controversial. This kind of surgery is nondestructive and can at least theoretically preserve hearing.

- Another surgical technique is to divide and destroy part of the vestibular nerve. This can achieve good control of vertigo in most patients, and usually hearing is preserved, but it is irreversible.

- The most aggressive approach of all is to remove the entire labyrinth on one side, permanently stopping symptoms of vertigo and tinnitus from one ear, but also eliminating hearing from that side. This may still be appropriate for patients with severe unilateral disease, especially if hearing is already severely affected.

- However, loss of the balance sense can affect gait in many patients, and about 30 percent of patients with unilateral disease will later develop Ménière's disease in the other ear.

- Ménière's disease is often characterized by fluctuating symptoms, with remissions and exacerbations, so it's difficult to predict the long-term prognosis. In most patients, the vertigo attacks subside within 10 to 20 years, and hearing loss remains in the moderate range.

Important Terms

ENT: A surgical specialty standing for "ear, nose, and throat"—sometimes referred to as otorhinolaryngology.

hypoglycemia: Low blood sugar concentration. Contrast with hyperglycemia (high blood sugar) or euglycemia (normal blood sugar.)

lesion: A region of an organ or tissue that has been damaged.

nystagmus: A rapid, flicking movement of the eyes.

vertigo: A spinning sensation, or feeling that one's environment is spinning around.

vestibular: Related to the sense of balance and position sense.

Suggested Reading

Kapit, *The Physiology Coloring Book.*

Meniere Man, *The Self Help Book for Meniere's Disease.*

Vestibular Disorders Association, http://vestibular.org/.

Questions to Consider

1. What organ systems, when not working properly, can cause a feeling of dizziness?

2. Are there risks to having a CT scan?

Dizzy Attacks
Lecture 9—Transcript

The last three lectures have been common diagnoses—breast cancer, heart disease, and depression. Now it's time for a little more of a mental stretch. Today's case strikes about 1 in 1,000 adults per year. In a typical, busy medical practice, full-time doctors probably have about 1,500 patients they see regularly, so each year we're likely to see one or two cases of this. So it's not common, but it's not so uncommon either. And the presenting symptom, we'll get to that, that's very common indeed.

Here's your clue: This disease may have affected many historical figures. Although we don't know for sure, Julius Caesar may have had it; he was noted in various sources to have something referred to as falling sickness. It's also suspected to have affected Martin Luther, who ascribed his symptoms to the work of the Devil, and Charles Darwin, who among other health problems had intense seasickness during his years exploring the world on the *Beagle*. More recently, Marilyn Monroe's hearing and balance problems are suspected to have been caused by this disease. So it's been around a long time.

We're in our general medicine clinic today, and our patient, Tina, is a 42-year-old woman whose chief complaint is "I'm having hypoglycemia." OK, well, that's a handy chief complaint; the medical diagnosis is right there, hypoglycemia. We can write that down on the fee ticket, there's the diagnosis, it's an early day to get to the golf course! Right? No, just kidding.

What we have here isn't uncommon, a patient who believes she already knows what the diagnosis is. And she may well be correct, and you don't want to disregard what she's saying, but at the same time, don't fall into the mental trap of starting with a false assumption. It may be that our patient was diagnosed with a specific medical condition, like hypoglycemia, by a doctor, or that she figured it out by herself, but at this point, we need more information about what's going on, and we need to keep an open mind about the diagnosis.

So let's say to Tina, "I understand you're concerned about hypoglycemia. Let's step back, though, so I understand the full picture. What symptoms are you having, what's going on that doesn't feel right?" So here's Tina's story. She says that for the last few months, she gets these attacks—that's her word—where all of a sudden she gets dizzy. She can't stand up straight, and sometimes there's a buzzy or high pitched sort of noise she hears. She says she sort of staggers around and has to eat a candy bar. Once she has some sugar, in about a half hour, she starts to feel better. These episodes are getting more intense, more frequent, and are lasting longer. Now, she says, sometimes she has to eat two candy bars. Her friends have told her that she's either having hypoglycemia, or she's just crazy. OK, time for our brief differential. Our patient has episodic symptoms, including dizziness and a funny noise that she hears. What could be going on?

Dizziness can be a challenging symptom, because different people use that term to refer to different things. Dizziness can mean vertigo; that's a sensation of spinning, as if the environment is moving around you. It's that feeling that people experience with alcohol intoxication, or after a spinning carnival ride, after the ride ends and the world seems to keep spinning around. True vertigo is usually caused by problems with the inner ear, where the sense organs of balance are.

Dizziness, though, can also refer to a lightheaded feeling, like you're going to faint. That's a completely different problem, with different physiology to think about. Dizziness meaning a faint or lightheaded kind of feeling is usually caused by insufficient blood flow to the brain. Less frequently, a feeling of dizziness can be related to feeling unsteady or off balance, caused by problems with the brain, nerves, or perhaps muscle. This might be related to a loss of nerve input to the brain—those are conditions where there's a loss of sensory input, so a person can't sense, essentially, where their feet are. Or this can be from a condition that affects motor function, causing weakness and unsteadiness. These are neurologic problems, and most often present in elderly people. Finally, dizziness can be a psychologic or psychophysiologic effect, when a person feels kind of disconnected or disassociated with the world's sensory signals. In that case, a psychological assessment can be helpful.

So, one symptom, dizziness, but four potential specialists to help. Could be an issue with the inner ear, so go to the ENT. Or a cardiologist, or a neurologist, or a psychologist. Yet here we are, in the general medical clinic. It's bad form to refer a patient to four specialists. I mean, five, really, remember, Tina came in with a chief complaint of hypoglycemia. Does she need an endocrinologist? It's our job to help narrow this down.

Back to the history. "Tina," you say, "we need your help here. What exactly do you mean by dizziness?" She says it's a spinning feeling, like getting dizzy the way kids do when they spin around a while and then stop, and it feels like the world keeps spinning. She says she doesn't feel faint, and she's never passed out, but she is afraid that she'll fall down. There's no problem with the strength in her legs; she's not weak; that's not the issue. It's just that the room feels like it's spinning around and round.

So we have true vertigo, here, this sensation that the world is spinning around her. Remember, she also mentions that she hears a buzzy or high pitched sound, an unexplained noise. So, already, after three minutes of history, we're pretty sure this is an ear problem, specifically with the inner ear, where hearing and balance sense organs are located. That would explain the combination of vertigo, the spinning sensation, as well as a hearing issue.

Let's look at some additional history and a review of systems. There's been no fever, no headaches, no nausea or vomiting, and no persistent symptoms; she gets these episodes, but in between them, she feels fine. Could this be a brain tumor? Probably not, you'd expect more persistent symptoms. An infection? Again, probably not. I mean, why would an infection cause these discrete, isolated sorts of episodes? Tina has essentially no important past medical history, no history of head trauma or concussion, no history of hearing loss or ear problems, and she takes no medicines at all.

Don't forget to ask that last question—are you taking any medicines, over-the-counter or prescription, or taking any herbal or other supplements? People often see multiple doctors, and we shouldn't assume that someone else hasn't prescribed something we don't know about. Patients should always be able to list all of the medicines they're taking, or better yet, just bring them along to every doctor's appointment.

Dizziness is a common side effect of many medications, including blood pressure medicine, anti-depressants, seizure medications, medicines to help with sleep and medicines to treat anxiety, as well as over-the-counter cold and allergy medications. Our patient says she doesn't take any of these medicines, but it's always important to ask. Tina also denied alcohol consumption or recreational drug use.

Our physical exam, Tina is a well-appearing woman with normal vital signs. Her HEENT exam is normal; there is no visible middle ear disease. By the way, when we look in the ear with an otoscope, we can easily see the external ear, the ear canal. We can also see, at the end of the ear canal, the eardrum itself—that's what separates the external ear from the middle ear cavity. Beyond the middle ear, where we can't see directly, that's where the inner ear is, and that's where hearing and balance sense takes place. Tina's cardiovascular and lung exams are normal, and a neurologic exam shows normal balance and normal gait. At the moment, she has no symptoms, and her exam is entirely normal.

Let's just say, though, for the sake of this case, that we were able to do an exam actually during an episode. Then, Tina would look fearful and unsteady, and would typically be very apprehensive about standing and walking. If we did make her walk, she might hold her feet widely apart and take small steps. One other very specific finding that's seen with vertigo, her eyes would show nystagmus, a movement where they drift in one direction, then snap back. If you want to see nystagmus, put a child in a desk chair, the kind on wheels, and spin him around a few times. Then stop the spinning, and stare at his eyes. He'll say he's dizzy, and his eyes will show nystagmus. Nystagmus isn't always present in vertigo; some patients can suppress it by staring hard at something in the distance, but it's usually there. You can also look for nystagmus through closed eyelids by watching the bulge of the eye flick back and forth, slow then fast.

So our history and physical exam support a clinical diagnosis of episodic vertigo. Now let's develop a more detailed, specific differential diagnosis. Before we do that, though, we need a brief review of the anatomy and physiology of one of our senses. This is maybe one that we don't think about much, our sense of balance.

Now, we learned in kindergarten about the five senses, but this is a sixth one. It usually operates in the background, keeping us upright and oriented in space, and we really don't even notice it much unless something goes wrong. The sense of balance relies on specific sense organs in the inner ears. There are five of these organs on each side. The utricle and saccule sense translational movement, back and forth or up and down; the semicircular canals sense rotation. There are three semicircular canals on each side, each oriented along the x, y, or z axis, so we can detect rotation around any direction.

The balance organs all operate on a similar principle. The utricle and saccule are filled with fluid, it's called endolymph, and contain a membrane that rests on little hair cells. Atop that membrane are tiny, dense stones, the otoliths. When you move or turn, these little stones lag behind, because they're denser than the surrounding endolymph. The hair cells detect the difference in motion between the otoliths and the fluid, and send signals to the brain via the vestibular nerve. The semicircular canals don't have otoliths but use similar hair cells to detect movement of the endolymph fluid.

The five balance sense organs together can detect changes in motion and rotation in any plane, basically telling you in what direction your body is moving. This information is integrated in the brain with other sensory input, including visual cues and information from your extremities about where your arms and legs are located in space. All of that information, together, is used to adjust your muscles to keep you upright and oriented.

By the way, a similar sense system, using hair cells bathed in endolymph, is how the cochlea works to detect sound vibrations. Together, the balance sense organs and cochlea are called the labyrinth, referring to the little canals and tunnels through which endolymph flows. The information from the balance organs and hearing system are all transmitted to the brain by the vestibular nerves, one on each side of the head.

We don't spend a lot of time thinking about our sense of balance, but when it goes wrong, it's very noticeable. The main symptom of problems along the pathways of the balance system, from the balance organs thru the nerves to the brain area that interprets the data, the main symptom is vertigo, a sensation of movement in space when there is, in fact, no movement. So let's get back to Tina, to develop our detailed differential diagnosis.

It can be helpful, especially when thinking about neurologic symptoms, to remember the anatomy. Tina's symptoms could be arising anywhere along the chain, from the sense organs, to the nerve that conducts the information, to the brain that interprets the nerve input. Where along that chain is the problem? Let's look at some specific diagnoses, starting with ones that affect the balance sense organs.

The most common cause of vertigo is called Benign Paroxysmal Positional Vertigo, abbreviated BPPV. It causes brief, less than one minute, episodes of vertigo triggered by a position change, like turning over in bed or quickly looking up. It's caused by a problem in the balance sense organs themselves, by debris in the semicircular canals. The symptoms and nystagmus can be recreated in the office by moving the head in the plane of the affected canal. Tina's vertigo attacks last too long to be typical of BPPV.

Another thought, labyrinthitis, referring to inflammation in the balance and hearing organs. There are many causes of this, ranging from trauma to the ear; viral infections; some bacterial infections, including infection of the middle ear, or otitis media; as well as some medications, like aspirin or ibuprofen. All of these, if they contribute to inner ear inflammation, can cause vertigo, along with other symptoms. The vertigo can be made worse by positional changes, and usually lasts days to weeks. Tina's symptoms have come in recurrent isolated attacks that have come and gone repeatedly; that really doesn't fit the typical presentation of labyrinthitis.

Another problem that can occur in the sense organs of balance is called "Meniere Disease". Though we don't know exactly why it occurs, it seems to be caused by excessive endolymph fluid that interferes with the functioning of the balance organs. Meniere's patients, in addition to having periods of intense vertigo, often also suffer from hearing problems, because that same excessive endolymph affects the functioning of the cochlea. Remember, Tina complained of a buzzy sound during her vertigo. Could something be going on with her hearing as well?

What about the nerve, the vestibular nerve, that brings information about balance from the inner ear to the brain? Vestibular neuritis refers to inflammation of this nerve, usually triggered by a viral infection. Patients with vestibular neuritis have vertigo, plus nausea and vomiting, that lasts several days to weeks. The symptoms don't come in attacks or spells, but begin all at once and then gradually fade. Since that's not really Tina's pattern of symptoms, vestibular neuritis is unlikely. Another nerve problem could be a tumor or mass pressing on the nerve, hough again, you'd expect constant symptoms or symptoms that overall are getting worse over time, rather than episodes like Tina has.

Let's move up to the brain, where balance information is decoded. A stroke could cause balance problems, though you'd expect other symptoms as well. If vertigo occurs along with any loss of function, say, trouble moving a limb, or difficulty speaking, immediate medical evaluation is warranted to quickly diagnose a potential stroke.

Older people are prone to what's caused "vascular insufficiency," where atherosclerotic disease in the blood vessels supplying the brain and inner ear lead to decreased blood flow. This can cause episodes of vertigo, usually along with nausea and vomiting. Tina, she's is too young for the typical presentation of vascular insufficiency, and her symptoms don't include nausea or vomiting.

A brain disorder that can begin at Tina's age is multiple sclerosis. Though this can cause vertigo, there are typically other symptoms and signs of neurologic dysfunction. Another brain disorder that can cause vertigo is a migraine headache. Usually, in adults, migraine-associated vertigo is accompanied by a headache and nausea. There is actually a migraine variant seen in children that causes only brief attacks of vertigo without any other symptoms. Attacks of migraine usually subside with sleep, which is not what Tina reports.

That's our differential. How do we confirm which diagnosis is correct? It does sound like Meniere's disease fits best; it causes attacks of vertigo that come and go, like Tina reports, and also affects hearing. Other diagnoses, like a tumor or multiple sclerosis, they seem much less likely, but after discussing these possibilities with Tina, she's decided that she'd like to pursue a very thorough workup to make sure we don't miss something that's unlikely, but needs to be caught early.

To definitively rule out a tumor, we need a brain scan, one that looks along the entire pathway, from the sense organs along the nerve to the brain. A CT scan is a very good study—it's relatively quick to get, and can see pretty good detail, especially of the bones. However, there are drawbacks. CT scans are basically a series of plain X-rays stitched together by a computer to make composite image. Like other X-rays, they rely on ionizing radiation to get an image. Although the risk is small, any study involving radiation will expose the patient to some risk of damage from the radiation itself, which increases the lifetime risk of cancer.

Now, I don't want patients to worry too much about this. After all, some radiation exposure occurs constantly, to all of us. Just living on the Earth exposes us to radiation from both cosmic rays and from radioactive elements in the earth's crust. One way to think about the added radiation from medical studies is to compare the amount of radiation to the background radiation we're all exposed to. For instance, a plain chest X-ray is similar to about three days of ordinary background radiation. That isn't much, and patients really shouldn't be fearful of a single chest X-ray. But CT scans are like multiple X-rays. A brain CT scan is probably similar to a few months of background radiation. An abdominal and pelvic CT is an even bigger study, comparable to about three years of background radiation.

The radiation risks from studies like CT scans are additive; the more exposures, the higher the risk. Also, risks are higher for younger patients, because they're growing and they have more years of life expectancy. Modern radiology equipment is designed to use digital signal processing to help minimize radiation exposures, in many cases using less than a tenth of the ionizing radiation that had been necessary to expose ordinary plain films. Patients and doctors should minimize radiation exposure but shouldn't be fearful of using medical studies when they're appropriate and necessary.

In contrast, an MRI scan of the brain doesn't use any ionizing radiation. It also has the advantage of imaging soft tissues, like the brain, which are more precise than a CT scan. MRIs are also better able to get images through the dense bones at the base of the brain, where CT scans don't penetrate as well, and, with balance problems, that's exactly where we need to look, at the base of the brain where the balance and sense organs are.

The main disadvantages of MRI compared to CT are that they take much longer to do, and they're more expensive. In Tina's case, we decided to get an MRI to rule out even a small tumor, and it was normal. The MRI scan also showed that there were no brain lesions to suggest multiple sclerosis. Note that depending on the story, exam, patient preferences, and clinical suspicion, an MRI is not always necessary in the workup of vertigo.

Just to mention for completeness, another kind of imaging study, an ultrasound, also doesn't use any ionizing radiation. However, the precision of ultrasound images is inferior to CT and MRI, and ultrasound cannot be used through bones like the skull. So ultrasound really wouldn't be useful at all for Tina's evaluation. We also referred Tina to an ENT specialist, who reviewed the clinical exam and MRI and also did a hearing test, which did confirm some low frequency hearing loss. The ENT evaluation confirmed that Tina does indeed have Meniere Disease.

A quick aside, a modern trend in medicine is to drop that possessive part of a disease name. Instead of calling it Meniere's Disease, we're encouraged to drop the apostrophe-s and just call it Meniere Disease. That way, we're not implying that somehow Dr. Meniere owns the disease, or even has the disease. So we sometimes say Down Syndrome, or Crohn Disease. In many cases, this just hasn't really caught on; we're just used to saying, for instance, Down's Syndrome. One disease that keeps its apostrophe is Lou Gehrig's Disease, because the baseball player Lou Gehrig had that disease.

Anyway, back to Tina and Meniere Disease. The specific cause of Meniere Disease isn't completely understood. There is increased endolymph fluid, as well as differences in the glycoprotein content of the fluid; there's also evidence for alterations in the way that the fluid flows through the canals and is re-absorbed. Some studies have supported an infectious agent, or genetic influences, or allergies, or a combination of these factors.

Whatever the cause, the main symptom is episodic attacks that last for one or more hours. During attacks, there is vertigo, often accompanied by a ringing, rushing, or a buzzing sort of sound called tinnitus. There may also be a feeling of pressure or fullness in the ear. Accompanying these attacks is a gradual, fluctuating level of low-frequency hearing loss that can become severe, and is only reversible if caught early. The pressure feeling and hearing loss usually affects only one ear, but it can affect both.

Meniere's disease is a clinical diagnosis; there is no one specific test that confirms it. Tests are done, sometimes, to rule out other diagnoses, like the MRI Tina had in this case. Blood tests are really of limited usefulness in the workup, though they can, again, rule out other problems if there are suggestive symptoms. Doing a thorough hearing evaluation is essential, and hearing will need to continue to be monitored during treatment.

There are several treatment options for Meniere Disease, though none is really ideal. The main first therapy is dietary, restricting sodium, sometimes along with taking a diuretic to reduce body water. This simple treatment can reduce vertigo attacks, but may not effectively slow hearing loss.

Medications can be used during acute attacks to reduce the uncomfortable sensations of vertigo and nausea, but again, these don't reduce hearing loss, and they are also ineffective in preventing further attacks. Still, conservative management and monitoring of hearing is probably good enough therapy for many people with Meniere Disease.

Another option for treatment is the use of steroids, which may reduce the pressure in the endolymph fluid. These can be given orally, or by injection, or even by injection through the eardrum into the middle ear. There are some serious potential side effects of steroid use, especially if they're needed for a long course.

More aggressive therapy, especially for frequent and severe vertigo attacks, can include direct injections of medicine into the middle ear. An antibiotic called gentamicin is used, not because it's an antibiotic, but because it can decrease the number of vestibular hair cells that are sending the incorrect balance information to the brain. Though it can effectively reduce or eliminate vertigo attacks, gentamicin can actually make the hearing loss worse, so this therapy isn't suitable for everyone.

There are some surgical options for therapy as well. A shunt can be placed in the inner ear to drain some of the excess fluid, though how well this works is controversial. This kind of surgery is non-destructive and can at least, theoretically, preserve hearing.

Another surgical technique is to divide and destroy part of the vestibular nerve. This can achieve good control of vertigo in most patients, and usually, hearing is preserved, but it's irreversible. The most aggressive approach of all is to remove the entire labyrinth on one side, permanently stopping symptoms of vertigo and tinnitus on that one ear, but also eliminating hearing from that side. This may still be appropriate for patients with severe unilateral disease, especially if hearing is already severely affected. However, loss of the balance sense can affect gait in many patients, and about 30 percent of patients with unilateral disease will later one develop Meniere in the other ear.

Tina has been treated conservatively with medication for acute attacks and a low-salt diet. Her hearing loss is limited to one ear, and so far, is not severe. She's also been cautioned against using medications that can worsen hearing loss, and to protect her hearing by avoiding loud noises and concerts, and keeping her headphones set low.

Meniere disease is often characterized by fluctuating symptoms with remissions and exacerbations, so it's difficult to predict the long-term prognosis. In most patients, the vertigo attacks subside within 10 to 20 years, and hearing loss remains in the moderate range.

Now, remember, Tina came in with a chief complaint of hypoglycemia. Could that have been a possible diagnosis? Hypoglycemia is something that often comes up as a patient concern, though the symptoms are often misunderstood. What is hypoglycemia, who gets it, and what symptoms does it really cause? Hypoglycemia means low blood glucose. Glucose being the main kind of sugar molecule involved in energy metabolism in people. True, measurable hypoglycemia, meaning you measure the blood glucose, and it's low, is very, very rare. Hypoglycemia is most commonly seen in people with diabetes who take too high a dose of insulin—it's the insulin administered to treat diabetes that drives down blood sugar. Other medicines can contribute to hypoglycemia, as can rare metabolic and endocrine disorders and severe malnutrition. But unless a person is taking insulin or is very ill, hypoglycemia is quite uncommon. People having symptoms of true hypoglycemia, like confusion, difficulty thinking, seizures, or coma, will not improve until glucose is administered.

Though true measurable hypoglycemia is rare, many people do seem to have mild symptoms related perhaps to shifts in blood sugar, or to a blood sugar level that though it's normal, is decreasing. Symptoms like irritability, lightheadedness, dizziness, or headache can occur, and these improve rapidly with a snack. Though blood tests in these people will not show true hypoglycemia, a good diet will improve the symptoms.

Tina's sudden, severe attacks of vertigo, along with buzzing in her ears, are not caused by any problems with blood sugar. However, problems with metabolism can contribute to other, even more significant health problems. We'll hear more about that next time.

Weight Loss
Lecture 10

In some ways, we've made great strides against diabetes. We understand far more about the physiology of both type 1 and type 2 diabetes, and we have the tools to aggressively keep blood sugars normal. We've also gotten much better at treating the complications of diabetes. However, we haven't really been able to make any strides in preventing diabetes in the first place, and the vastly increasing number of diagnoses of diabetes has dwarfed the advances to identify and treat diabetes.

A Scheduled Checkup
- In the general internal medicine clinic, a 46-year-old woman named Charlene comes in for a scheduled checkup. When asked what's on her mind, she says, "I feel fine." Charlene is either 1) perfectly healthy or 2) has something wrong with her that she hasn't noticed yet, or at least hasn't told us about yet.

- Charlene is 5 feet and 4 inches tall and weighs 180 pounds, which corresponds to a body mass index of 31, which is in the overweight or obese zone. You bring that up, in order to encourage improved diet and exercise habits. Charlene responds, "Actually, that's pretty good. I think I've lost a lot of weight this past year."

- You take a brief lifestyle history, then of diet and exercise habits, and are left with an *unexplained* 30-pound weight loss. That's a problem. Significant weight loss without effort means something is wrong.

- Moving on to labs and tests, markers of inflammation like a sed rate are normal, and the CBC is also normal. With no signs of infection, inflammation, or anemia on these simple tests, whole categories of disease have become unlikely—there's very little chance of cancer, inflammatory bowel disease, or chronic infection. A chemistry profile shows no liver disease and normal kidney function.

- But the blood glucose from the chemistry panel is high at 210. Though the range of normal glucose is wide and depends on when the last meal was eaten, blood glucose level in an adult should almost always be less than 180 and is usually less than 140. How would a high blood glucose cause weight loss? The hint will be in the urine.

- An ordinary, in-office urinalysis is done using a dipstick—a thin strip of plastic with little pads glued onto it. Each pad contains chemicals that change color when they react to different things in the urine. One pad will turn darker if there are red blood cells and another for **white blood cells**; one will change color if there are urine chemicals that are produced by bacteria, indicating a possible urine infection.

- On Charlene's urine dipstick, one pad lit up—the one for glucose. She's spilling a lot of sugar into her urine and may have been doing this all year. This can cause weight loss.

- Normally, the kidneys filter out glucose, so there is none in the urine at all. If blood sugar concentrations are high enough, as they are in Charlene, some of the sugar will spill out into the urine.

- There are no immediate symptoms of this, but in time, that lost sugar is equivalent, in a way, to being on a diet (though not a healthy one). People who spill sugar into their urine may be losing the equivalent of 400 to 500 calories each day. As dieters know, that's a big number, and unless you consistently eat extra to make that up, you will lose weight.

- With increased blood sugar and sugar in the urine, we can diagnose Charlene with diabetes, specifically diabetes mellitus.

Diabetes Mellitus

- The term "diabetes" comes from a Greek word referring to a siphon or something that passes a great deal of water. The term "mellitus" refers to the sweet taste of the urine, as if it is sweetened with honey. In 1776, the glucose concentration of the urine of diabetic patients was first measured, confirming the central role of so-called **glucosuria**—glucose in the urine—as a defining feature of diabetes.

- Understanding diabetes means understanding glucose and carbohydrate metabolism and how altered glucose metabolism causes illness. All foods contain one or more of the three so-called macronutrients—the common molecules that we eat and absorb for energy. These three macronutrients are carbohydrates, fat, and protein.

- Carbohydrates are further divided into the simple sugars—small molecules of one or two sugar units each—and complex sugars, also called polysaccharides, which are essentially chains of smaller sugar units linked together. Polysaccharides are commonly called starches, and in the gut, these long carbohydrates and smaller two-unit carbohydrates are chopped into single simple sugar units called monosaccharides for absorption. The main monosaccharide absorbed from food is glucose, and for practical purposes, the terms "blood glucose" and "blood sugar" refer to the same thing.

- Glucose is crucial at many levels of metabolism. It is the essential energy source for many body tissues and can be converted to a variety of forms, including the building blocks of fat, by processes in the liver. The level of blood sugar is tightly controlled by several overlapping homeostatic mechanisms to ensure good health and energy availability.

- The word "**homeostasis**" is a central way that living organisms maintain health. Homeostasis is an active process that regulates the internal environment, keeping essential parameters like pH, temperature, electrolytes, and metabolic substrates all in a normal range. Once homeostasis is disturbed, all sorts of problems ensue.

- Diabetes comes in two types. Type 1 diabetes used to be called juvenile diabetes, and though it usually occurs in children, it can begin in adulthood. In type 1 diabetes, the beta cells of the pancreas are destroyed by the body's own immune system, eliminating the body's ability to secrete insulin. This condition had been uniformly and rapidly fatal prior to the development of insulin injections in the 1920s.

- In contrast to type 1 diabetes, type 2 diabetes more commonly begins in adulthood, usually in people who are overweight. Although the exact mechanisms aren't completely understood, many overweight people will eventually seem to develop resistance to insulin; even though their pancreas can produce plenty of it, the circulating insulin becomes ineffective in driving down blood sugar.

- Eventually, in type 2 diabetes, there is decreased insulin secretion as well (though insulin isn't typically completely gone, as it is in type 1 diabetes). The combination of insulin resistance and relative insulin insufficiency leads to high blood sugar, or hyperglycemia, in type 2 diabetes. And it's the hyperglycemia that causes most of the mischief.

- Although they can be life threatening, acute complications of high blood sugar are not very common in type 2 diabetics. The main goals of therapy are to prevent the very significant, late effects of long-term hyperglycemia. These late effects can affect almost every organ system of the body. Although treatment and good control of blood sugar will prevent or delay most of these complications, even with very good therapy, patients with diabetes remain at risk.

- These complications of diabetes include the following.
  o Heart disease, including an increased risk of heart attack and stiffening of the heart wall, leading to chronic heart failure

  o Other arterial disease, which can cause stroke or a loss of circulation in the extremities that may lead to amputation

  o Kidney disease – in fact diabetes is the most common cause of kidney failure in the developed world;

- o **Neuropathy**, or nerve damage, that can lead to abnormal or decreased sensation or weakness

- o Retinopathy, or eye damage—this can cause severe vision loss or blindness

- There is also an increased risk of dementia, chronic lung disease, frequent infections, and skin ulcers. All of these complications develop after many years of disease, typically 10-20 years, though there's quite a bit of variability. Though better glucose control decreases the likelihood of complications, it is difficult to predict which patients remain at the most risk.

Treatment and Weight Control
- The treatment of diabetes is primarily concerned with achieving euglycemia—that is, a normal blood sugar during, after, and between meals. In type 2 diabetes, first-line therapy is losing weight and improving exercise habits. Sometimes, these steps alone can be sufficient to essentially "cure" diabetes.

- More typically, though, medications are necessary. These include oral medicines—so-called oral hypoglycemics—that increase insulin sensitivity, increase insulin release, or both.

- In many patients with type 2 diabetes, insulin must also be administered, typically by one or more daily injections. Type 1 diabetics, who lack any of their own insulin, must rely on injections. The treatment of diabetes also requires frequent home glucose monitoring with finger sticks.

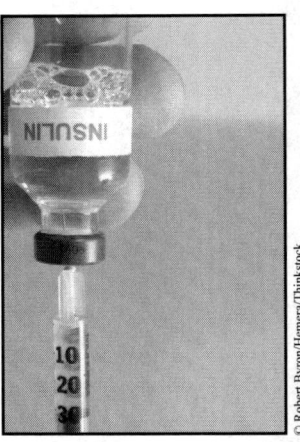

Some diabetics need to be injected with insulin because their pancreases don't secrete it.

- A more advanced treatment strategy, more typically used for type 1 diabetics, is an insulin pump to administer a constant flow of insulin to the body, similar to the way a healthy pancreas secretes insulin. There's also technology available to continuously monitor blood sugar.

- Though tight control—that is, using intensive therapy to keep blood sugar close to normal—has been shown to best prevent the long-term complications of diabetes, it comes at a price. Deciding how tightly to control blood sugar depends on such factors as the life expectancy of the patient, the overall health and other risk factors, and an honest assessment of compliance and a patient's ability to self-medicate.

- With the exception of a few patients with new-onset type 2 diabetes who successfully lose weight and improve their exercise habits, most patients with diabetes require lifelong active management.

- Diabetes is a good example of a disease whose treatment requires not just taking pills and visiting the doctor, but also taking charge of your health and making changes in your life.

- Effective weight control involves primarily changing the diet to consume fewer calories. Many different styles of diet have been proposed and studied, including ones that especially discourage carbohydrates or that stress consuming more foods with lower energy content. The best predictor of success isn't which diet is followed, but whether changes in habits can be sustained for years.

- Although exercise alone is usually ineffective in leading to weight loss, exercise combined with dietary changes works better than diet alone. Medications can sometimes be an additional part of a weight-loss program, but none are really ideal or particularly effective.

- Objectively, the most effective therapy for weight loss for obese patients is surgery. This is a fast-growing field called bariatrics, and it involves a variety of surgical options to lower the stomach volume or bypass some of the digestive and absorptive parts of the intestine—or both.

- Although the results of **bariatric surgery** can be impressive, surgery will not be successful without the patient committing and following through with lifestyle changes as well. Bariatric surgery also entails considerable risks, so it's really only offered to people with severe obesity or who are already suffering from health consequences of their weight.

Important Terms

bariatric surgery: Surgery intended to assist weight loss.

glucosuria: Glucose in the urine.

homeostasis: Physiologic equilibrium, as maintained by mechanisms that control vital processes.

neuropathy: Damage or malfunction of nerves.

white blood cells: The cells in the blood that are part of the immune system.

Suggested Reading

Pollan, *Food Rules*.

American Diabetes Association, http://www.diabetes.org/.

Questions to Consider

1. Who is responsible for making sure that prior records are available and reviewed—the doctor or the patient?

2. What kinds of illnesses can cause unexpected and unhealthy weight loss?

Weight Loss
Lecture 10—Transcript

Have you ever noticed what a weird sense of humor medical students and doctors have? Sometimes their professors do too! A professor is in front of his first-year class, teaching a group of new medical students. He takes out a jar of yellow liquid, holds it up in the light. "This," he explains, "is urine. To be a doctor, you have to be observant. Observe the color, the smell, the sight, and the taste." Then he dips his finger into the jar, puts it into his mouth. The class watches in amazement and disgust. But being dedicated students, as the jar was passed along, one by one, they each dipped their finger into the jar and put it into their mouths to take a taste.

After the last student was done, the lecturer shakes his head. "If any of you had been observant," he says, "you would have noticed that I put my second finger into the jar and my third finger into my mouth." That's an old joke, but there must be a kernel of truth to it. The name of the disease we're going to discuss in depth today does come from, yes, the taste of the urine.

We're in clinic today, general internal medicine, and today's patient is a 46-year-old woman named Charlene. She's coming in for a scheduled checkup. When asked what's on her mind today, she says, "I feel fine." So that's what we have to work with; our chief complaint today is a Beatles song title, "I feel fine."

We take a glance down at the paperwork, the sheet with all of the little check marks for potential symptoms that patients fill out for their yearly checkup. The patient has checked off no, no, no. No concerns here. The only yes box is fatigue, but Charlene wrote in the margin "I have four kids, what do you expect?"

Typically, here in our presentation, before the physical exam, we develop a brief differential diagnosis to help keep us focused, to hopefully help us see what we need to be looking for. Today, our brief differential diagnosis looks like this.: Charlene is either, 1) perfectly healthy or 2) has something wrong with her that she hasn't noticed yet, or at least she hasn't told us about yet. Does a differential like that make you nervous? It should. We have no clues as to what we're looking for, and we don't even know if there is anything to look for. So, on to the physical exam!

Charlene is a well appearing woman, she's 180 pounds, 5 foot 4 inches tall. The remainder of her vital signs are normal, including a normal blood pressure of 108/72, normal pulse of 78, and a normal respiratory rate at 18 per minute. There's nothing notable on the skin exam; HEENT exam is fine; the belly exam is normal; GU exam, including a pap smear, that's normal; rectal exam is normal; her gait and strength and the rest of her exam are all normal. Everything seems fine, right?

Well, maybe not. That weight, that 180, that corresponds to a body mass index at 5'4" of 31, which is in the overweight zone. You bring that up, in order to encourage improved diet and exercise habits. And Charlene responds, she says, "Actually, doc, that's pretty good. I think I've lost a lot of weight this past year." You look back at last year's physical, and sure enough, she's lost 30 pounds. In one year! "How did you do that?" you ask. Charlene responds, "I don't know. Maybe I'm eating better."

You take a brief lifestyle history, then, diet and exercise habits. Charlene gets no regular exercise, though she spends a lot of time with her kids, kind of shuttling them around, doing what moms do. Because of her children's hectic lifestyle and her husband often working late, the family eats out a lot, four, maybe five times a week, often at fast food, and often eating on the run in the car. If anything, it sounds like over the last year, her eating habits have gotten worse, not better.

So, why is Charlene losing weight? A quick observation, Charlene was honest with her doctor. She really hadn't been trying to lose weight. If she had lied and made up some story about her new weight loss program, the entire weight loss concern would have been dropped, which in the long run, could have been disastrous for Charlene. The lesson, be truthful with your doctor. Now, we have an unexplained 30-pound weight loss. That is a problem. For those of you who've struggled with your weight, you know that losing 30 pounds takes work. Significant weight loss without effort means something is wrong. Now, what could it be?

Let's go backwards. We'll get some more history, a few more questions now that know we need to ask. There's been no belly pain, no nausea, no vomiting, no diarrhea; Charlene says her appetite has been fine, and her energy she thinks has been OK. Maybe, she says she's tired sometimes, but not more than she thinks is normal for a mom. She hadn't been trying to lose weight, really, but she was happy to see the weight go.

A detailed, comprehensive differential diagnosis for weight loss would be huge; almost any chronic disease will eventually lead to weight loss. So to help organize our list, let's think of it this way. Weight loss has to be related to energy balance. On one side of the equation is the energy absorbed—what you eat and digest, or what goes into your system. On the other side of the equation is the energy you use for life's activities—staying warm, moving around, exercising, thinking, keeping your heart beating. All of this takes energy. If the net amount of energy you bring into your body exceeds what it needs, you will store the extra energy and gain weight. If the net available energy is insufficient, you will use up the body's stored energy, and will end up losing weight. There is no way around this simple law. At the heart of weight control is energy balance. What goes in versus what you use up.

So, for now, let's come up with a brief differential looking at things that can influence either side of the energy balance equation. We'll start with the input side. Weight loss will occur with conditions that decrease what's eaten. These conditions can include depression, poor food availability, dental disease, abdominal pain, functional disabilities that prevent someone from getting to food, altered taste or smell that might makes food less appealing, social isolation, economic hardship. Even this first idea, decreased intake, can have a whole lot of potential causes.

Once food is eaten, it has to be digested, so gut diseases that interfere with digestion can lead to weight loss. These include conditions like cystic fibrosis, where there are insufficient digestive enzymes, or lactose intolerance, where a lack of a specific enzyme interferes with the digestion of milk sugar. After digestion, food particles have to be absorbed. Gut conditions can interfere with the absorption of nutrients, including some we've met already, like Celiac disease. Also in this category of malabsorption would be diseases of the gut wall, including Crohn disease.

Then, on the other side of the equation, are many diseases that increase the metabolic activity of the body. Even if intake doesn't change, if the metabolic costs of staying alive increase, the body will net not have enough energy, so stored fat will be utilized, leading to weight loss. Conditions like this include chronic infections, heart disease, COPD or any other chronic lung disease, chronic kidney or liver disease, many metabolic or endocrine diseases, and cancer—especially colon, breast, ovarian, lung, or prostate cancers. That is a long list.

There is one other category of illnesses that leads to weight loss, one that's kind of intermediate between two we've mentioned. Let's say our patient Charlene is consuming and absorbing enough calories, and her body is spending the same number of calories that she's taking in. What if she's losing calories somewhere else, maybe by losing excessive protein or other nutrients through her gut, perhaps into her stool, or maybe she's losing calories somewhere else?

One disease we've mentioned, Crohn's Disease, has overlapping mechanisms of weight loss. With Crohn's Disease, a patient may feel bad and have a lot of abdominal pain, decreasing appetite. Because of the gut inflammation that's part of Crohn's Disease, nutrition may not be absorbed efficiently. And, because of chronic inflammation that keeps the immune system churning, patients with Crohn's Disease have increased metabolic needs. It's a triple whammy.

So far, do we have a clue about which of these issues is affecting Charlene? It doesn't really sound like her appetite or intake has decreased; if anything, she seems to be eating more than normal. How about her digestion or absorption of nutrients? Most of the conditions, like Celiac, that affect digestion and absorption will cause other GI symptoms. If food isn't being digested right, you'd expect GI pain, or bloating, or diarrhea; malabsorption syndromes, like lactose intolerance, cause symptoms quickly after eating. Charlene is sure; her gut has been fine, and her stools are normal. Malabsorption or gut disease is still possible, but doesn't seem as likely.

Maybe her metabolic demands are increased. Let's see if she has any signs of chronic, ongoing diseases, especially ones that would burn up calories. She's had no fever, no night sweats, no chronic cough, no chronic aches or pains, or anything else that she can some up with. Changes in the metabolic rate caused by hyperthyroidism often cause diarrhea, a feeling of feeling kind of warm a lot, or thinning of the skin or hair. Charlene denies those symptoms, too. Really, going back to our initial intake forms, all she does report is some fatigue. So we don't yet have much to hang our hat on.

There was that third category. Is our patient somehow losing nutrition from somewhere? Losing nutrition via the gut, into the stool, seems unlikely, since there's no diarrhea. But there's another way to lose nutrition, in the urine. Normally, urine is almost all water, plus some salts and electrolytes, and a little bit of waste products. There should not be much protein, and there should not be any sugar spilled in the urine. But if there were, that could be a source of net energy loss that would affect energy balance.

Labs and tests, What to look for? As is often the case, simple, old favorites are the most useful tests. Markers of inflammation, like a sed rate, are normal, and the CBC, the complete blood count, that's also normal. With no signs of infection or inflammation or anemia on these simple tests, whole categories of disease have become unlikely. There's very little chance of cancer, inflammatory bowel disease, or chronic infection. A chemistry profile shows no liver disease and normal kidney function. That's good.

But the blood glucose from the chem panel is high, at 210. Though the range of normal glucose is wide and depends on when the last meal was eaten, blood glucose level in an adult should almost always be less than 180, and is usually less than 140. How would a high blood glucose cause weight loss? The hint will be in the urine. And no, I won't ask you to taste it.

An ordinary, in-office urinalysis is done using a dipstick—it's a thin strip of plastic with little pads glued onto it. Each pad contains chemicals that change color when they react to different things in the urine. One pad will turn darker if there are red blood cells, another for white cells; one will change color if there are urine chemicals that are produced by bacteria, which can indicate a possible urine infection. On Charlene's urine dipstick, one pad lit up, the one for glucose. Charlene is spilling a lot of sugar into her urine, and may have been doing this all year. Can that cause weight loss? You bet.

Normally, the kidneys filter out glucose, so there is none in the urine at all. But if blood sugar concentration, if those concentrations are high enough, as they are in Charlene, some of the sugar will spill out into the urine. There are no immediate symptoms of this; people can't feel that their blood sugar is high or that they're spilling glucose into their urine. But in time, that lost sugar is equivalent, in a way, to being on a diet, though not a healthy diet, as we will see. People who spill sugar in their urine, may be losing the equivalent of 400 to 500 calories every day. As dieters know, that's a big number, and unless you consistently eat extra to make that up, you will lose weight.

So, the diagnosis. Charlene has increased blood sugar, and sugar in the urine. She has diabetes, specifically diabetes mellitus. Diabetes comes from a Greek word referring to a siphon or something that passes a great deal of water. Mellitus refers to the sweet taste of the urine, as if it is sweetened with honey. It's been known for at least 3,500 years that people with diabetes have sweet-tasting urine. Early sort of proto-physicians in India, they noted that the urine of people who had diabetes would attract ants. In 1776, the glucose concentration of the urine of diabetic patients was first measured, confirming the central role of so-called glucosuria—glucose in the urine—as a defining feature of diabetes.

Understanding diabetes means understanding glucose and carbohydrate metabolism, and how altered-glucose metabolism causes illness. All foods contain one or more of the three so-called macronutrients, the common molecules that we eat and absorb for energy. These three macronutrients are carbohydrates, fat, and protein. Carbohydrates are further divided into simple sugars, those are small molecules of one or two sugar units each; and complex sugars, also called polysaccharides, which are essentially chains of smaller sugar units, linked together. Polysaccharides are commonly called starches, and in the gut, these long carbohydrates and smaller, two-unit carbohydrates, are chopped into single, simple sugar units called monosaccharides for absorption. The main monosaccharide absorbed from food is glucose, and for practical purposes, the terms blood glucose and blood sugar refer to the same thing.

Glucose is crucial at many levels of metabolism. It is the essential energy source for many body tissues and can be converted to a wide variety of forms including the building blocks of fat by processes in the liver. The level of blood sugar is tightly controlled by several overlapping homeostatic mechanisms to ensure good health and energy availability.

That word—homeostasis—we haven't mentioned it before, but it's a central way that living organisms maintain health. Homeostasis is an active process that regulates the internal environment, keeping essential parameters like pH, temperature, electrolytes, and metabolic substrates all in a normal range. Once homeostasis is disturbed, all sorts of problems ensue, which we will see.

Let's use an example of eating a meal to illustrate the tight way that blood glucose concentrations are regulated. You eat an apple, and the natural fruit sugars are digested and absorbed, immediately increasing blood sugar. When that change is detected by beta cells in the pancreas, increased production and secretion of the hormone insulin occurs. Insulin, in turn, drives the blood sugar downwards by encouraging sugar uptake by body tissues, especially muscle cells, and by increasing the liver's activity to store glucose in fat and other molecules. So insulin net decreases blood glucose.

There are also so-called counterregulatory hormones that can increase blood glucose by either suppressing insulin's action or release, or by increasing the liberation of glucose from storage tissues. These hormones, which balance against the actions of insulin, include cortisol, growth hormone, glucagon, and epinephrine; all of these affect each other's actions and metabolism. Rarely, diabetes can be caused by a markedly increased level of one of these hormones, but far more commonly, diabetes is caused by either a deficiency of insulin, or the body becoming resistant to the effects of insulin, or sometimes, a combination of both.

Because of a lack of insulin effect, in diabetes, blood glucose will be high, and it will spike higher and longer than normal after a meal. The blood glucose will be high enough so that some glucose spills into the urine, wasting metabolic energy. This also has the effect of increasing net urine output. So there is excessive urination, often with increased hunger and eating to make up for the loss of sugar. Despite having plenty of sugar in the blood, the lack of insulin prevents many tissues from being able to absorb and utilize the energy of glucose, so the body has to break down excess fat and other tissues, contributing to weight loss, like the kind seen in Charlene. She didn't report excessive appetite or increased urination, as is often the case in adult-onset diabetes.

Diabetes comes in two types. Type I diabetes used to be called juvenile diabetes, and though it usually occurs in children, it can begin in adulthood. In type 1 diabetes, the beta cells of the pancreas are destroyed by the body's own immune system, eliminating the body's ability to secrete insulin. This condition had been uniformly and rapidly fatal prior to the development of insulin injections in the 1920s.

In contrast to type 1 diabetes, type 2 diabetes more commonly begins in adulthood, usually in people who are overweight, like our patient today. Though the exact mechanisms aren't completely understood, many overweight people will develop resistance to insulin. Even though their pancreas can produce plenty of it, the circulating insulin becomes ineffective in driving down blood sugar. Eventually, in type 2 diabetes, there is decreased insulin secretion as well, though insulin isn't typically completely gone, as it is in type 1 diabetes. The combination of insulin resistance and relative insulin insufficiency leads to high blood sugar, or hyperglycemia, in type 2 diabetes. And it's the hyperglycemia that causes most of the mischief.

Though they can be life threatening, acute complications of high blood sugar are not very common in type 2 diabetics. The main goals of therapy are to prevent the very significant, late effects of long-term hyperglycemia. These late effects are bad news, and they can affect almost every organ system of the body. Although treatment and good control of blood sugar will prevent or delay most of these complications, even with very good therapy patients with diabetes remain at risk.

These complications of diabetes include heart disease, including an increased risk of heart attack and stiffening of the heart wall, leading to chronic heart failure; there could be other arterial disease, which can cause strokes or a loss of circulation in the extremities that may lead to amputation. Kidney disease, in fact, diabetes is the most common cause of kidney failure in the developed world; neuropathy, or nerve damage—that can lead to abnormal or decreased sensation or weakness; retinopathy, or eye damage—this can cause severe vision loss or blindness.

There is also an increased risk of dementia, chronic lung disease, frequent infections, and skin ulcers. All of these complications develop after many years of disease, typically 10 or 20 years, although there's quite a bit of variability. Though better glucose control decreases the likelihood of complications, it is difficult to predict which patients remain at the high risk.

The treatment of diabetes is primarily concerned with achieving euglycemia, that is, a normal blood sugar during, after, and between meals. In type 2 diabetes, first-line therapy is losing weight and improving exercise habits, and sometimes, these steps alone can be sufficient to essentially cure diabetes. More typically, though, medications are necessary. These include oral medicines, so called oral hypoglycemics that increase insulin sensitivity, increase insulin resistance, or both. In many patients with type 2 diabetes, insulin must also be administered, typically by one or more daily injections. Type 1 diabetics, who lack any of their own insulin, must rely on injections. The treatment of diabetes also requires frequent home glucose monitoring with finger sticks.

A more advanced treatment strategy, more typically used for type 1 diabetics, is an insulin pump to administer a constant flow of insulin to the body, similar to the way a healthy pancreas secretes insulin. There's also a technology available to continuously monitor blood sugar. And within a few years, it's possible that an entirely self-enclosed electronic instrument will combine these technologies, essentially, creating an artificial pancreas that can, at the same, time monitor blood glucose and adjust its secretion of insulin into the body. You can imagine, if this were small, that the whole thing could be implanted below the skin. We're not quite there yet, but such a device like this ought to be feasible soon.

Though tight control, that is, using intensive therapy to keep blood sugar close to normal, has been shown to best prevent the long-term complications of diabetes, it comes at a price. If you try to control the sugar and keep it low, you increase the risk of occasional episodes of hypoglycemia, or too-low blood glucose. This can cause seizures or coma, so it has to be avoided. Deciding how tightly to control blood sugar depends on factors including the life expectancy of the patient, the overall health and other risk factors, and an honest assessment of compliance and a patient's ability to self medicate. This is sometimes not an easy decision. With the exception of a few patients with new-onset type 2 diabetes who successfully lose weight and improve their exercise habits, most patients with diabetes require life-long active management.

Charlene, in fact, she wasn't surprised at her diagnosis. She had struggled with her weight for years; she had never found the time to exercise regularly or try to improve her diet. Both of her parents, actually, had had diabetes, so she may have known what was going on, even before her appointment. You remember her actual chief complaint? It was "I feel fine." She probably did feel well, at least for now, but perhaps she knew that she was headed in the wrong direction.

Meeting with a dietician and coming up with some weight-loss goals seemed to help Charlene at first, but, as happens so often, lifestyle modification alone was not successful in attaining normal blood glucose. That doesn't mean people with diabetes shouldn't keep up those efforts; improved diet and exercise can help prevent complications by not only helping control diabetes, but also by improving blood lipids, like cholesterol, and keeping blood pressure in a healthy range. It's often the combination of several factors like these that contribute to overall declining health.

In fact, there's a name for this combination of interrelated health problems now so commonly seen in the U.S.A. and in many parts of the developed world. This is the so-called metabolic syndrome, a combination of high blood pressure; abnormal cholesterol and other lipids; high fasting glucose related to diabetes; and obesity, especially central body obesity. Together, these dramatically increase the risk of cardiovascular disease and stroke. Charlene's evaluation did not yet show high blood pressure or an abnormal cholesterol, but it will be very important to continue to take lifestyle steps needed to prevent these problems.

Diabetes is a good example of a disease whose treatment requires not just taking pills and visiting the doctor, but taking charge of your health and making changes in your life. We can instruct and teach and prescribe, but Charlene and patients like her are the people who make the big decisions that end up having the most impact on their health.

The genetics of diabetes, both type 1 and type 2, is complicated. It's not related to a single gene that's transmitted either recessively or dominantly. Instead, there are sets of genes that create varying susceptibility, probably to some other environmental influences. Type 1 and type 2 diabetes, though they share some similar physiology, are not carried on the same genes, so a family history of one kind increases only the risk of that same kind of diabetes. If type 2 diabetes is recognized early, even before there is marked hyperglycemia, it's sometimes referred to as pre-diabetes. It may be that earlier medical therapy, especially when combined with lifestyle improvements, could prevent the progression of full blown diabetes.

Back to our patient, Charlene, the first hint that something was wrong was her weight loss. Yet, I've just said that weight loss can prevent the appearance or progression of type 2 diabetes. It turns out that there is effective, healthy weight loss, there's the weight loss that accompanies disease, and they aren't the same thing. Healthy weight control strategies are not methods that rely on disease mechanisms. You can't get healthy by losing weight because you have a tapeworm, or you make yourself vomit, or you've got sugar spilling into your urine.

Effective weight control involves primarily changing the diet to consume fewer calories. Many different styles of diet have been proposed and studied, including ones that especially discourage carbohydrates, or diets that stress consuming more foods with lower energy content. The best predictor of success isn't which diet is followed, but whether changes in habits can be sustained for years. In fact, the very concept, the word "diet", is probably already a losing proposition. If you say you're going on a diet, it kind of implies that some day you will go off the diet. What people need isn't a diet that lasts weeks or months or years, but a change in eating that lasts the rest of their lives.

Though exercise alone is usually ineffective in leading to weight loss, exercise combined with dietary changes works better than diet alone. Medications can sometimes be an additional part of a weight loss program, but none are really ideal or particularly effective. Objectively, the most effective therapy for weight loss for obese patients is surgery. This is a fast growing field, called bariatrics, and it involves a variety of surgical options to lower the stomach volume or bypass some of the digestive and absorptive parts of the intestine, sometimes both. Though the results of bariatric surgery can be impressive, surgery will not be successful without the patient committing and following through with lifestyle changes as well. Bariatric surgery also entails considerable risks, so it's really only offered to people with severe obesity or who are already suffering from health consequences of their weight. The risks can include potentially catastrophic complications from surgery itself, or later on bowel obstructions, gallstones, malnutrition, or prolonged problems with nausea, vomiting, or diarrhea.

In some ways, we've made great strides against diabetes. We understand far more about the physiology of both type 1 and type 2 diabetes, and we have the tools to aggressively keep blood sugars normal. We've also gotten much better at treating the complications of diabetes, using strategies, like renal transplantation or laser eye surgery to prevent blindness.

But what we really haven't been able to do is to make any strides in preventing diabetes in the first place. In fact, the rates of both type 1, and especially, type 2 diabetes are increasing dramatically, and we're seeing even teenagers now with the early onset of what we used to think of as an adult disease. So though we can better identify and treat diabetes, the vastly increasing quantity of diagnoses has dwarfed these advances. We're net seeing an ever-increasing negative impact of diabetes. We have insulin; now we need something better—a way to prevent diabetes in the first place. Diabetes and its complications are the direct cause of about 70,000 deaths a year in the U.S.A.

Next, we'll talk about a disease that causes about half that many deaths, though, unlike diabetes, it's fairly easily prevented. What's the preventable cause of death of 35,000 Americans each year? We'll see in our next grand rounds.

I Can't Walk
Lecture 11

Influenza is the preventable cause of death of 35,000 Americans each year. It's an old disease that has been thought to be caused by astrological influences or by cold air at various times. Despite some of the myths about flu vaccines, they are safe, and although they are far from perfect, they are one of the best ways we have to fight infection. Yearly influenza vaccination is recommended for everyone over six months of age, and the years it works best are the years when more people get the vaccine.

Subacute Leg Pain

- A 19-year-old man is brought to the emergency department. His name is Christopher, and his chief complaint is: "Doc, I can't walk." He says that for the past two days, his legs have been hurting very badly, and it's getting worse. The pain is mostly in his calves. As long as he doesn't try to move much, it's okay, but if he stands or stretches out his legs or feet, the pain becomes much worse.

- This is an unusual presenting symptom; we need more history. He can't recall exactly when it started but says that he noticed the pain when he awoke two days ago. He's had no recent injury, and he hasn't exercised much lately. He's says he's in great shape, though. He usually exercises a lot, just not in the past two weeks.

- The physical exam confirms that he has tender calf muscles and a lot of pain with stretching. This is some kind of muscle disease that is primarily affecting his calves. A general term for muscle inflammation is **myositis**. Pain and **tenderness** are inflammatory signs.

- Myositis can also occur as part of autoimmune disease, when the body's immune system attacks its own tissues. Rheumatological disease can include myositis among other manifestations.

- Primary infection in muscle itself isn't common, and it would be kind of unusual to have muscles in both legs get infected at the same time. Influenza can cause muscle aches both during and sometimes for several days after the main symptoms of infection.

- Christopher had a recent fever illness and was quite ill. In fact, this case took place in February, during flu season. Influenza is a likely diagnosis that fits the history and physical exam.

- We do a quick test for influenza virus on a nasal swab, which is positive. These rapid tests are widely available in hospitals and doctors' offices and can be done in a few minutes. The current tests are very specific for influenza—meaning that a positive test is quite reliable.

- However, they're not very sensitive. A negative rapid influenza test may be false, missing maybe 20 to 30 percent or more of people who truly have the flu. The exact accuracy depends on what kinds of flu virus are circulating.

- Influenza-associated myositis is common, especially in children, and it occurs toward the end of the fever or a few days later. It most typically affects the calf muscles, though sometimes other muscles hurt, too. They'll hurt to move, and they'll be tender to touch.

- Often, the urine will be dark, and if you do blood tests, you can see the high CPK values. Urine will show the passing of muscle proteins, the myoglobins, by testing positive for blood but negative for red blood cells.

- The treatment is supportive: pain medicine and extra fluids to keep urine flowing. Rarely, this can progress to severe muscle breakdown and resulting kidney damage. Although there are anti-influenza medicines available, myositis usually begins later, beyond the time when these medicines can help. Symptoms of influenza myositis typically last about a week.

Influenza

- Influenza strikes millions of Americans each year and remains a very significant cause of death, directly killing about 35,000 in the United States each year and probably contributing to the ill health and decline of many more, especially elderly adults.

- Influenza is more common in the winter—in the cold months. This may be because people congregate indoors, passing their germs around more efficiently, or perhaps in part because damage to the lining of the nose by cold air makes it easier to catch influenza (and other viruses as well).

- The typical course of influenza begins with exposure to the virus, followed by a brief incubation period of one to four days. People become contagious the day before symptoms begin. Symptoms are typically sudden and include fever and aches and chills, often with some respiratory symptoms, such as cough and runny nose, and sometimes with GI symptoms, including nausea and vomiting. The disease typically lasts about five to seven days.

- Many people mistakenly think that influenza is just a bad cold, but it really is a distinct, different disease, caused by the specific influenza virus. Influenza causes much higher fevers, plus characteristic body aches that aren't seen with ordinary colds.

- The treatment of most cases of influenza is mostly supportive. Medicines like acetaminophen or ibuprofen—more widely known by their brand names, Tylenol or Advil or Motrin—will help reduce fevers and relieve the achy feelings. Extra fluids are also needed during fevers to prevent dehydration. Rest, stay away from other people, and stay in bed until you feel well.

- There are medicines that can be used to specifically fight the flu. The most widely prescribed one is oseltamivir, which is sold as the brand Tamiflu. It can help some, but it's no wonder drug. It works best when started very early in the infection, within 48 hours—or, better yet, within 24. After that, it doesn't help much. It can modestly reduce symptoms and the duration of the infection, but it's not overall very effective in reducing serious complications.

- It is the complications of influenza that we fear. Myositis, like Christopher experienced, can be painful and even debilitating, but with supportive care, full recovery is expected. The most serious complication of influenza, which contributes to most of the deaths, is pneumonia.

- We've talked about pneumonia some before, but it's such a common condition both as a primary infection and as a complication of other illnesses that we ought to cover it more thoroughly. Pneumonia comes from the Greek, meaning inflammation of the lungs; the word is probably related to older root words that refer to fluid or flowing in the chest. Even the ancients knew that fluid in the lungs, leading to a wet cough, wasn't a good thing.

Influenza Pneumonia
- Pneumonia is commonly understood as a bacterial infection in the lungs, but it can be caused by viral or fungal or other kinds of infections, or sometimes by noninfectious things like chemical irritants or an immune-mediated inflammatory reaction.

- In most circumstances, though, pneumonia is caused by infection of the lung tissue—infection that causes an accumulation of fluid and debris that leads to coughing and fever.

- Lung tissue itself is particularly prone to infection, because we're constantly breathing in air and bringing in whatever we breathe. Also, the air sacs in the lungs are normally a little moist, and that warm, moist mucus is a breeding ground for microorganisms.

- Fortunately, we have immune systems to keep infection away. There are also little hair cells that beat up and down to keep mucus moving around and out so that it won't get infected easily. But advancing age, lung damage from mild infections, asthma, and many other conditions can compromise lung integrity, increasing the risk of pneumonia.

- Influenza, the infection itself, causes fever and cough, so how can we tell it has turned into pneumonia? The time course of the symptoms is a crucial clue. Influenza usually includes about five days of fever that gradually decline. Increasing fevers after a few days often indicates a second, superimposed infection like pneumonia. Cough that's getting much worse is another clue.

- On the physical exam, a patient with pneumonia—influenza pneumonia or any pneumonia—will often be breathing rapidly. There may be signs of increased difficulty breathing, such as pulling in the ribs with each breath, and the breath sounds themselves heard through a stethoscope will sound crackly and abnormal.

- Sometimes, a chest X-ray is done to confirm pneumonia. It will show an area of brightness where the X-ray beam is blocked by the accumulated infected fluid. The bigger the area of brightness, the worse the pneumonia (though there isn't a 100 percent correlation).

- X-rays can also be done to monitor therapy for pneumonia to ensure improvement.

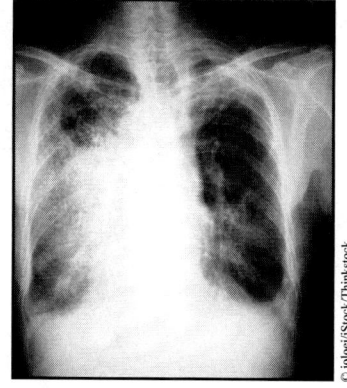

From a chest X-ray, a doctor can diagnose pneumonia, a disease of the lungs.

However, chest X-rays aren't perfect. The findings on the film can lag a day or so behind what's going on with the patient, so very early pneumonias may not be seen yet.

- Although pneumonia in young, healthy patients can usually be treated as an outpatient, in older or ill people, it may require hospitalization and extra support with oxygen. Pneumonia remains a significant cause of death in the developed world, often contributing to illness and decline in people with other health problems but occasionally killing someone who was otherwise well.

- In the case of influenza pneumonia, the secondary pneumonia itself can be caused by the flu virus invading the lung tissue or by secondary bacterial infections by bacteria that happened to be nearby and have taken advantage of the patient's illness to cause another infection.

The Flu: Prevention and Myths

- To prevent influenza, most importantly, stay away from sick people during flu season—typically in the winter, from December to March. If you're sick, especially with fever, stay home. Influenza virus can spray in the air through coughs and sneezes, but it usually gets into your system through your own hands. If you keep your hands away from your face, and wash or sanitize your hands frequently, you'll keep most influenza infections away.

- Immunization is also crucial. The currently available vaccines aren't perfect. The protection varies from year to year; from perhaps 40 to 80 percent protection is expected, depending on circulating strains. But even in poorly matched years, the vaccine provides at least some protection, and the more people get the vaccine, the more protected all of us will be.

- There are some persistent myths about the flu vaccine. First of all, the vaccine cannot give anyone the flu. You can get some achiness and fever, which happens in one to two percent of vaccine recipients, but that is not the flu.

- Some people are under the impression that they "got the flu" from the vaccine, either because of mild side effects or because they indeed got the flu or some other illness right after getting the vaccine. After all, the vaccine is given right during flu season, and it takes about three weeks to work—so if you're exposed to the flu within a few weeks of the vaccine, you're going to get the disease, and it's not the fault of the vaccination.

Important Terms

myositis: Inflammation of muscle.

tenderness: Pain that is increased with palpation.

Suggested Reading

Barry, *The Great Influenza.*

Plotkin, et al, eds, *Vaccines.*

Centers for Disease Control (CDC), http://www.cdc.gov/flu/.

Questions to Consider

1. Why are viral respiratory infections, such as influenza and the common cold, more common in the winter?

2. A good diet can help maintain health. Are there popular diets that contribute to ill health? How?

I Can't Walk
Lecture 11—Transcript

We have an old disease to confront today, and like many old diseases it's gone by different names in the past. It's been called sweating sickness, and at other times it's been called epidemic catarrh. That word itself, catarrh, means "a flowing down," probably referring to a very runny nose. This disease has been thought to be caused by astrological influences, or at other times, by cold air. Is there any truth to that? Let's find out.

A 19-year-old young man is brought to the emergency department, the ED, where we're working tonight. His name is Christopher, and he's brought in by his college roommate. He looks reasonably comfortable, there in the room. You ask, what can we do for you? His answer is our chief complaint, "Doc, I can't walk."

Christopher says that for the past two days his legs have been hurting very badly, and it's getting worse. The pain, he points down, is mostly in his calves. He thought he had just pulled a muscle, but now the pain has gotten so bad that he can't bear to walk. As long as he doesn't try to move much, it's OK, but if he stands or stretches out his legs or feet, the pain becomes much worse.

OK, this is an unusual presenting symptom. What's going on? A good pain differential diagnosis can start with the body part that's hurting. Think, what is there, and why would it hurt? The pain is in the legs, the calf area. Could be bone, could be muscle or tendons, could be perhaps the blood vessels that are running through there. Could even be the skin. And, like any pain, it could be so-called referred pain. He feels it in his legs, but remember that pinched nerves or spinal cord problems higher up in the nervous system can create a sensation of pain further down. As always, an open mind is needed.

We do have one other comment that points us in a certain direction; this pain, he said, is worse when he just stretches his feet out. That doesn't sound like something that could happen because of a spinal cord mass or a problem with the nerves up high. Stretching the feet stretches the muscles, but doesn't really affect the nerves and things up higher. Bone pain? Well, maybe, but just stretching out the feet doesn't really affect bone. Standing, putting weight on the legs, that would put mechanical load and some stress on bones, but he says it hurts badly even when he doesn't do that. Is this sounding kind of muscley to you?

Time for more history; he can't recall exactly when it started, but says he noticed the pain when he awoke two days ago. He's had no recent injury, and he hasn't exercised much lately. He's says he's in great shape, though. He usually exercises a lot, just not in the past two weeks.

There's a good history question for pain complaints. "What were you doing when it started?" Very acute pain, something like a slipped disc in the back, or a broken leg, or a dislocated shoulder, that kind of thing starts suddenly, all at once, and people remember exactly when it started and what they were doing when it started. Christopher has what we'll call subacute pain. It's been brief, just a few days, but it wasn't acute in onset. So it's unlikely to have been any kind of sudden biomechanical or traumatic change.

Christopher denies taking any substances, including no weight gain or muscle building supplements or anything like that. He is on the college wrestling team, and he says, "I keep myself in shape; I'm a vegan." He adamantly denies any sort of recreational drug use. There's no family history of any kind of muscle disease.

On to the physical exam. Christopher, indeed, looks very healthy. He's Caucasian, small and wiry, barely a touch of fat on him, like a typical wrestler. He weighs 155 pounds, is 5'9" tall, and his vital signs include a blood pressure of 130/88, pulse 68, temperature 99.4, and respirations 20 per minute.

What do you think of those vitals? The BP is a little high, as can happen when someone is anxious or in pain. It would be a good idea to repeat that down the line or at a follow-up visit to make sure he really doesn't have high blood pressure. What about that temperature, 99.4? That is entirely normal. It is a myth that 98.6 is the normal temperature; that number is not a normal temperature, it is an accepted average temperature, and measured normal temperatures will sometimes be higher or lower than this 98.6, so 99.4 is well within the normal range, and is not a fever. Most physicians consider a fever above 100.4 or 100.8 degrees.

The rest of the exam next; HEENT exam is fine, and his skin appears normal. He has no swollen lymph nodes, thyroid exam is normal, lungs are clear, his heart is normal, belly is fine. He is very apprehensive about your moving his legs. They look normal; there is no swelling; there's no redness. But he seems very tender when you gently squeeze his calf muscles, and gentle flexion of the ankles, which stretches those calf muscles, causes intense pain on the stretched side.

The exam confirms he's has tender calf muscles and a lot of pain with stretching. This is some kind of muscle disease here, primarily affecting his calves. Now we're focused on what the problem is, and we can better develop our differential diagnosis. A general term for muscle inflammation is myositis. That's myo, for muscle, and our old friend itis, which is used as a suffix meaning inflammation, attached to just about anything. Appendicitis, gastritis, cholecystitis, and now we have myositis. That's not a specific diagnosis, but a descriptive, general term for muscle inflammatory disease.

Do we know it's inflammatory? I think so. Pain and tenderness are inflammatory signs. There are other muscle diseases that are non-inflammatory, like muscular dystrophy; those cause, mainly, weakness. But pain, and especially tenderness with gentle squeezing, that's inflammation. Now, why is there inflammation in our patient's muscles? Trauma is the most common cause of muscle pain and inflammation, but there's no history of that. He was pretty adamant about that. He said he's on the wrestling team, but hasn't been working out for a few weeks.

How about some kind of substance abuse? He denied it, but athletes as we know, aren't always honest about things like steroids that might be taken as performance enhancing drugs. These are meant to build muscle tissue but can sometimes cause muscle damage and inflammation. Some prescription drugs, including the statins used commonly to lower cholesterol, can also trigger muscle damage, inflammation, and pain.

Our patient is a vegan—meaning no animal products, no meat, no dairy, no eggs. Could there be some kind of nutritional deficiency associated with veganism that can cause muscle pain? A careful vegan diet, including supplements, can supply a healthful, complete diet, but do we know he's getting what he needs?

Myositis can also occur as part of autoimmune disease, when the body's immune system attacks our own tissues. Two examples are dermatomyositis, which includes both skin and muscle damage, and polymyositis, which basically affects muscle alone.

How about infectious causes? Primary infection in muscle, that's not very common, but it would be kind of unusual to have muscles in both legs get infected at the same time. Still, some infections, like Lyme disease and Rocky Mountain Spotted fever, do cause a lot of muscle pain. Influenza can cause muscle aches, both during and sometimes for several days after the main symptoms of infection. He didn't say anything about other symptoms of those kinds of illnesses.

We have a good list, but honestly, just a few thin leads this time. What do you think the leading diagnosis ought to be? In most presentations, we'd move on the lab evaluation now to confirm our working diagnosis. But I don't think we have one, yet. Here's a good lesson from today's case; when in doubt, go talk to the patient some more. I think we missed something.

We ask Christopher, in detail, about his diet. He's been a vegan for years, and his parents are vegans, and he knows he needs to take his iron pills and vitamin B12 supplements. His parents actually mail him organic versions of these and other supplements at college. Now, there have been cases of supplements contaminated with substances that cause illness. Keep in mind, in the U.S.A., supplements are not regulated by the FDA or any other authority. Could some kind of toxin from these supplements have led to muscles damaging Christopher? There are a large range of chemicals that could cause muscle breakdown, including tryptophan, ipecac, PCP, many pharmaceutical agents. We'd better keep that in mind.

Then we ask, "Christopher, when, exactly, did you start hurting?" He's sure about that. It was two days ago; he woke up in pain. Again, we ask about trauma. There had been none, and he hadn't been exercising for a few weeks prior to the pain starting anyway. He had been a very fit, working out kind of guy, so why hadn't he been in the gym lately? Good question. Let's ask him. "I was sick," he says.

We ask for details. About 10 days ago he developed a fever, headaches, body aches, and vomiting. The fever was very high, up to 104, and he basically stayed in bed for five days. He thought we already knew about that, see, because he had been seen in this very ED last week with that illness and sent home with a diagnosis of probable influenza. He had been getting better, he says, but hadn't yet felt up to working out.

Another lesson, this time for patients, but a reminder for doctors too, don't assume that the doctor knows the history. This young man was seen in our same ED last week, and it was logical for him to assume that we had those records and we had reviewed them. Logical, yes, but that's often not the way it works. ED records go into a folder and then to the basement where they're picked apart for billing, and sometimes scanned into a computer. In fact, in many cases, the ED doc wouldn't even know those prior records existed.

Even if you're being seen in the same practice, or in the same hospital, or even by the same doctor, it's best to speak up. Say something like, "I saw you three days ago," or "I was here in the ED last week" to ensure that someone knows to look at those old records. The problem, of course, is even worse when patients see multiple doctors at different medical facilities. Should we have easy access to these records? Sure. Do we? Well, probably not.

We need to reorder our differential, I think. This recent illness, that probably makes it far less likely that a toxin has made him sick and less likely that this is some kind of chronic autoimmune disease. Of course, it's possible that the recent illness and these new muscle aches are unrelated, but it's logical to assume that they are related, to see if one illness can explain the whole story. If that doesn't work, we can go back to those other theories.

Christopher had a recent fever illness, and he was quite ill. Remember the infectious causes of muscle pain? One of the most common is influenza. And, in fact, this case took place in February, during flu season. Now we have a likely diagnosis that fits the history, and a physical exam. Let's confirm with a few labs.

A standard chemistry panel is normal. We've seen chem panels before, but to go over what they include, let's have a little bit more detail. A chemistry panel includes the electrolytes—sodium, potassium, and chloride; and a measurement called bicarb that reflects the acid/base balance of the blood. It also includes a few measurements of kidney function, including a creatinine. That value is very, very sensitive. The creatinine creeps up quickly when the kidneys are not functioning properly. There are also measurements of what are called liver enzymes. These become elevated when liver cells or other kinds of tissue are damaged. The exact items in a chem panel vary from lab to lab, so ordering physicians need to know if they're getting all of the components they expect. For Christopher, the most important part of the chem panel to check was that creatinine, which was normal. We'll see why soon.

We also checked a CBC, the complete blood count, and that was normal too. A sed rate, our favorite marker for inflammation, was mildly elevated at 25. Typically, a chronic autoimmune disease would give a much higher number; that 25 fits well with a recent viral illness, like influenza, as we suspect.

There's one other test we did, a CPK, for creatinine phosphokinase. This is a measurement of a muscle protein, and it becomes elevated if there's muscle damage. Sure enough, his was elevated, about three times the upper limit of normal. This could be seen with either chronic or acute muscle injuries, though with his history we're pretty comfortable assuming this is a new, acute problem.

If the CPK is very high, and especially if there is also dehydration or some kind of preexisting kidney disease, the high CPK proteins and other related muscle proteins can themselves damage the kidneys. This condition is a severe form of myositis called rhabdomyolysis—that's muscle damage and breakdown enough to cause organ damage. It can be seen after severe burns or injuries, or very intense exercise, heatstroke, drug exposures, or other conditions that severely damage muscles. It's very uncommon after infections like influenza; that can damage muscle and cause pain, but it would rarely lead to damage to the kidneys.

We did though check a urine, to be sure that the kidneys were OK. His urine looks dark, kind of a dusky-red color—that's from muscle protein. The dipstick is normal, except for one positive for blood. It's negative, though, for red blood cells. That's a good illustration of how labs can be misleading. That urine dipstick for blood—we call it blood, but it's really testing for the presence of the main blood protein, the protein that's in red blood cells, called hemoglobin. Under most circumstances, if there is hemoglobin in the urine, that means there's blood in the urine. Except, not today. Another test on the dipstick is actually for those red blood cells, testing for the cells themselves, and it is negative. So why is the dipstick positive for blood?

The answer is, it's not blood. It turns out that muscles contain a protein called myoglobin that's similar enough to hemoglobin that it fools the dipstick. Christopher's dipstick positive for blood is actually positive because of muscle protein. This is confirmed because the actual red blood cell test on the same urine dipstick was negative. So, be careful with labs; sometimes they'll fool you if you don't know exactly how they're done and what they mean.

We also did a quick test for influenza virus on a nasal swab, which sure enough was positive. These rapid tests are widely available in hospitals and doctors' offices and can be done in a few minutes. The current tests, they're very specific for influenza, meaning that a positive test is very reliable. However, they're not very sensitive. A negative rapid influenza test may be false, missing maybe 20, 30 percent or more of people who truly have flu. The exact accuracy depends on what kinds of flu virus are circulating that year.

Tests were also done to confirm Christopher's nutritional status. His serum ferritin—that's a measurement of iron stores—was normal, as were his vitamin B12 and folate levels. Vitamin B12, in particular, can be difficult for vegans to get from plant sources, and the serum measurement may not accurately reflect whether he was truly getting enough B12 in his diet. Still, he said he was taking supplements, so this is probably OK.

Now, to recap, Christopher had ordinary influenza, which sounds like it hit him pretty hard. He was sick in bed with high fevers for five days and was seen in the ED several days ago; he was sent home; he was starting to feel better until about two days ago when calf pain began, again, caused by the same influenza virus infection. This is actually not such an unusual story.

Influenza-associated myositis is common, especially in children, and it occurs towards the end of the fever or a few days later. It most typically affects the calf muscles, though sometimes other muscles hurt too. They'll hurt to move. The muscles will be tender to touch. Often the urine will be dark, and if you do blood tests you can see that high CPK value. Urine will show the passing of muscle protein, the myoglobins, by testing positive for blood but negative for red blood cells.

The treatment is supportive—pain medicine and extra fluids to keep urine flowing. Rarely, this can progress to severe muscle breakdown and resulting kidney damage. Though there are anti-influenza medicines available, myositis usually begins later, beyond the time when these medications can help. Symptoms of influenza myositis typically last about a week or so. A few other viruses can cause a similar picture of myositis, either during or after the infection. These include coxsackie viruses—those also cause fevers and hand-foot-mouth disease; HIV; hepatitis; several others. Christopher made a full recovery and resumed wrestling a week later.

Today's case was a common illness. Influenza strikes millions of Americans each year and remains a very significant cause of death, directly killing about 35,000 in the U.S.A. each year and probably contributing to the ill health and decline of many more, especially elderly adults. The presentation, though, wasn't very common. Here's a little bit of wisdom. It is more common for a common disease to present in an uncommon way, like influenza presenting with muscle aches, than it is for an uncommon illness to present at all. Another way of putting this: when you hear hoofbeats, think of horses rather than zebras. I actually had a mentor from South Africa who liked to quote that maxim, adding that in his home country, zebras were actually more common than you think! Again, as we've said before, an open mind is more likely to figure something out, whether uncommon or not.

Influenza is of course more common in the winter, in the cold months. This may be because people congregate indoors, passing their germs around more efficiently, or perhaps in part because damage to the lining of the nose by cold air makes it easier to catch influenza, and other viruses as well. An older name for this illness is an Italian phrase—influenza del freddo, meaning "influence of the cold."

The typical course of influenza begins with exposure to the virus, followed by a very brief incubation period of one to four days. People become contagious the day before symptoms begin. Symptoms are typically sudden and include fever and aches and chills, often with some respiratory symptoms, like cough and runny nose, and sometimes GI symptoms, including nausea and vomiting. The disease typically lasts about five to seven days.

Many people mistakenly think influenza is just a bad cold, but it really is distinct; it's a distinct, different disease caused by the specific influenza virus. Once you or a loved one has had full-blown influenza, you'll know it's not just a cold. Influenza causes much higher fevers, plus characteristic body aches that aren't seen with ordinary colds. From my point of view as a practicing physician, patients coming into the office with influenza are often lying on the table, sometimes huddled under a blanket. They look glassy eyed and miserable.

The treatment of most cases of influenza is mostly supportive. Medicines like acetaminophen or ibuprofen—those are more widely known by their brand names Tylenol or Advil or Motrin—those will help reduce fevers and relieve the achy feelings. Extra fluids are also needed during fevers to prevent dehydration. Rest, stay away from other people, stay in bed until you feel well.

There are medicines that can be used to specifically to fight flu. The most widely prescribed one is oseltamivir, sold as the brand Tamiflu. It can help some, but it is no wonder drug. It works best when started very early in the infection, between 24 and 48 hours. After that, it doesn't help very much. It can modestly reduce symptoms and the duration of the infection, but it's not overall very effective in reducing serious complications, and it is the complications of influenza that we fear. Myositis, like Christopher experienced, can be painful and or even debilitating, but with supportive care, full recovery is expected. The most serious complication of influenza, which contributes to most of the deaths, is pneumonia.

We've talked about pneumonia some before, but it's such a common condition, both as a primary infection and as a complication of other illnesses, that we ought to cover it more thoroughly. Pneumonia comes from the Greek, meaning inflammation of the lungs. The word is probably related to older root words that refer to fluid or flowing in the chest. Even the ancients knew that fluid in the lungs, leading to a wet cough, was not a good thing.

Pneumonia is commonly understood as a bacterial infection in the lungs, but keep in mind that it can be caused by viral, or fungal, or other kinds of infections, or sometimes by non-infectious things, like chemical irritants or an immune-mediated inflammatory reaction. In most circumstances, though, pneumonia is caused by infection in the lungs, infection that causes an accumulation of fluid and debris that leads to cough and fever. Lung tissue itself very prone to infection, because we're constantly breathing in air and bringing in whatever we breathe. Also, the air sacs in the lungs are normally a little bit moist, and that warm, moist mucus is a breeding ground for microorganisms. Fortunately, we have immune systems to keep infection away. There are also little hair cells that beat up and down to keep mucus moving around and out so it won't get infected easily. But advancing age, lung damage from mild infections, asthma, smoking, and many other conditions can compromise lung integrity, leading to a risk of pneumonia.

Influenza, the infection itself, causes fever and cough, so how can we tell it's turned into pneumonia? The time course of the symptoms is a crucial clue. Influenza usually includes about five days of fevers that gradually decline. Increasing fevers after a few days, say a patient starts at 103 for two days, then goes to 105 on day three, that often indicates a second, superimposed infection, like pneumonia. Cough that's getting much worse is another clue.

On the physical exam, a patient with pneumonia—here I mean influenza pneumonia, or any pneumonia—will often be breathing rapidly. There may be signs of increased difficulty breathing, like pulling in the ribs with each breath, and the breath sounds themselves heard through a stethoscope will sound crackly and abnormal. Sometimes, a chest X-ray is done to confirm pneumonia. It will show an area of brightness where the X-ray beam is blocked by the accumulated infected fluid. The bigger the area of brightness, the worse the pneumonia, though there isn't a 100 percent correlation there. X-rays can also be done to monitor therapy for pneumonia to ensure improvement. However, chest X-rays aren't perfect; the findings on the film can lag a day or so behind what's going on with the patient, so very early pneumonia may not be seen at all.

Though pneumonia in young, healthy patients can usually be treated as an outpatient, in older or ill people, they may require hospitalization and extra support with oxygen. Pneumonia remains a significant cause of death in the developed world, often contributing to illness and decline in people with other health problems, but occasionally killing someone who was otherwise well. In the case of influenza pneumonia, the secondary pneumonia itself can be caused by the flu virus invading the lung tissue or by secondary bacterial infections by bacteria that happened to be nearby; they've taken advantage of the patient's illness to cause a second infection.

Can influenza be prevented? Yes. Most importantly, stay away from sick people during flu season, typically in the winter from December to March. And if you're sick, especially with fever, stay home. Influenza virus can spray in the air through coughs and sneezes, but it usually gets into your system through your own hands. You touch a contaminated doorknob, for instance, and now flu virus is on your hands. But it can't make you sick though your skin. It's only a few minutes later, when you offhandedly rub your eyes or nose, that the flu virus can get you. That's why hand washing is so important. If you keep your own hands away from your face and wash or sanitize your hands frequently, you'll keep most influenza infections away.

Immunization is also crucial. The currently available vaccines aren't perfect; the protection varies from year to year from perhaps 40 to 80 percent protection is expected, depending on the circulating strains. But even in poorly matched years, the vaccine provides at least some protection, and the more people get the vaccine, the more protected all of us will be. This is the so-called herd effect, which is so important to the way vaccines work. We know the vaccines can't be effective 100 percent of the time, but if most of our community is vaccinated, there will be reduced exposures and transmission for everyone, even in people in whom the vaccine didn't work. Yearly influenza vaccination is recommended for everyone over six months of age, and the years it works best are the years when more people get the vaccine.

There are some persistent myths about the flu vaccine. First of all, the vaccine cannot, ever, give anyone the flu. You can get some achiness and fever, that's going to happen in one or two percent of vaccine recipients, but that is not the flu. Some people are under the impression that they "got the flu" from the vaccine either because of mild side effects or because they indeed got the flu or some other illness right after getting the vaccine. After all, the vaccine is given right during flu season, and it takes about three weeks to work. So if you're exposed to the flu within a few weeks of the vaccine, you're going probably going to get the disease, and it's not the fault of the vaccination. Flu vaccines are safe, and though they're far from perfect, they're one of the best ways we have to fight infection. There should be no hesitation about getting the vaccine.

One of the clues that got lost in this case was the recent medical history, that the patient who couldn't walk actually had the flu a few days earlier. Sometimes these kinds of mistakes can really add up. Patients see multiple doctors, get multiple tests, and a lack of clear coordination of care can make a diagnosis even more difficult to pin down. We'll see a good example of that in the next grand rounds. See you then.

Learning from Failure
Lecture 12

One of the most important goals of discussing cases is to learn from the mistakes of others, so that the mistakes don't have to be made again and again. Poor communication among a patient's doctors can lead to a prolonged diagnostic journey, including multiple doctors, a whole lot of tests, and—most importantly—a significant delay in helping the patient. For good patient care, it is essential for doctors to communicate well with patients, for patients to communicate well with doctors, and for doctors to communicate well with each other.

Persistent Itching
- Leslie, a new patient to the general adult medicine clinic, is a 45-year-old woman with a chief complaint of "I'm tired of the itching." She has brought a voluminous stack of prior medical records that is loaded with lab reports and letters from specialists.

- Leslie says that she had been in good health until about nine months ago, when she started to develop itchy rashes. The rashes appear and disappear quickly, within an hour or so, and they're always itchy. If they pop up at night, they interfere with sleep; if they occur during the day, they interfere with work.

- Leslie says that she's seen doctor after doctor and knows she's allergic to certain foods. She's tired of taking all of the medicines that she's been prescribed, and she's sick of doctors, labs, and tests. She seems very frustrated.

- Having recurrent hives with no identified trigger persisting for a long time, Leslie's diagnosis is chronic **idiopathic** urticaria, a condition that is not uncommon and can lead to significant disruption and very distressing symptoms. In fact, she was diagnosed with chronic idiopathic urticaria by two allergists and a dermatologist, but it was never communicated clearly to Leslie.

- Leslie's story teaches us a number of lessons.
  - When a patient is offering a confusing story, the doctor shouldn't settle for yes/no answers.

  - Insist on clear instructions. When you see a doctor, you need clear instructions on what to do; when you're the doctor, you must make sure that your patient understands you, even if that means writing things down. In fact, it should always mean writing things down, which means including both brand and **generic** names and avoiding using doctor abbreviations that some people might not know.

  - The more doctors involved, the more the patient has to insist on clarity. One of the confusing things with Leslie is that multiple doctors were prescribing multiple things and ordering multiple tests. Everyone was making mistakes, and—more importantly—nobody was learning anything from anyone else's mistakes. When one medicine was tried but didn't work, the next doctor didn't know that and maybe even tried the same medicine again.

  - A medical encounter should always address the primary concerns of the patient. Our patient's concern is a recurring, itchy rash, but she was sent to the endocrinologist because someone thought that she had thyroid disease. There were two main issues that the endocrinologist should have addressed: the rash and the thyroid tests. From our patient's point of view, she didn't get clear feedback about either of these issues.

  - Beware when the diagnosis or plan doesn't make sense. This goes for doctors and patients. As a doctor, if you can't explain the working diagnosis and plan clearly, it's probably because it's not clear in your own mind. You need to think more. From the patient's point of view, if you don't understand the diagnosis and plan, you need to speak up and ask—and ask again.

○ Treating the disease is not the same as treating the patient. Our patient wanted relief from a recurring, itchy rash; she didn't want to have a bunch of blood tests and see a bunch of specialists. All of these tests unfortunately led to doctors focusing on the test, not on the patient herself. In fact, the side effect of all of these tests—the worry and distraction and expense—may have been almost as bad as the itchy rash itself.

○ Whether to do a test depends on both how likely it is that the patient has the disease that you're looking for and on how accurate the test is. Less accurate tests should be done only when absolutely indicated, or they're going to lead to mischief. In any case, tests should only be done if the result of the test will be useful; if the result isn't going to change the plan, then the test shouldn't have been done in the first place.

Allergy Tests

- In general, there are two kinds of allergy tests: blood tests and skin tests. Blood allergy testing is often preferred by **general practitioners** and non-allergists, because anyone can order it and draw blood. These kinds of tests will also not be affected by allergy medicines that patients are often taking.

- The older generation of allergy blood tests were based on **IgG** antibodies and are worthless. These IgG-based tests should never be done, though they're still offered by some less mainstream labs and doctors. The newer tests, based on

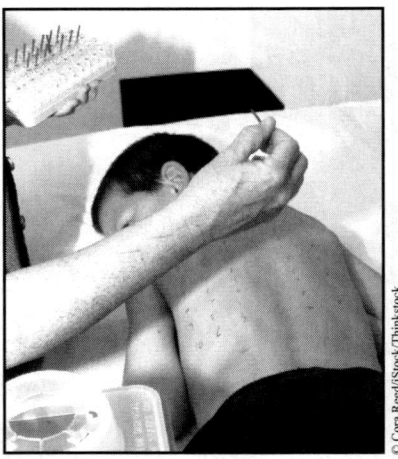

One type of allergy test is a blood test, which can have false positives, so the results should be confirmed.

IgE molecules, are more accurate. But even the best of these blood tests can still be misleading.

- Skin testing is more often performed by allergists, because it can be done in their offices with results available the same day. The results can be affected by certain medications.

- The bottom line for both skin and even the best blood testing is that these tests have many false positives and can have false negatives, too. They can be helpful to get a clue about what exposures could be triggering an allergy but should be confirmed before declaring that a patient is actually allergic.

- Allergies are immune-mediated reactions to exposures to environmental things, including foods, pollen, and dust. Very characteristically, allergic symptoms occur very shortly after exposures, and they're stereotyped—meaning that the reaction is the same every time, after the same exposure. This is especially true for food allergies, which usually trigger reactions within minutes or maybe an hour after ingestion.

- Typical reactions to food allergies include reactions in the skin, such as hives or swelling. It can also include GI symptoms, such as vomiting, diarrhea, or crampy pain; or difficulty breathing or cough. Severe reactions can lead to low blood pressure and loss of consciousness. These usually occur very quickly after the food trigger is eaten.

Urticaria
- There are a few conditions that can kind of mimic chronic idiopathic urticaria, but it's easy enough to tell the difference. Allergic contact dermatitis occurs only where a contact allergen touches the skin, so it's in the same place every time. A so-called fixed drug eruption can be a recurring swollen area, but it's in the same place every time, and as it heals, it leaves a dusky area.

- The only rash that occurs like Leslie's, popping up quickly anywhere on the body and then disappearing quickly, is urticaria.

- At least 30 to 50 percent of chronic idiopathic urticaria is autoimmune—that is, there are antibodies against our own tissues that trigger the reaction. It's likely that perhaps the other 50 percent is autoimmune, too, but we haven't been able to test for the antibodies yet. So perhaps that term "idiopathic," meaning "of unknown cause," is misleading.

- Food allergies can cause acute episodes of urticaria, but it's very unlikely that foods will cause longstanding, chronic urticaria without clear correlation. Some people with chronic urticaria can have hives triggered by physical things, such as pressure on the skin, warmth, or cold. These triggers are usually clear from the history.

- Many patients with chronic urticaria, like Leslie, have thyroid antibodies, but these don't seem to be the actual trigger. Usually, thyroid functioning is normal, and these antibodies require no treatment. Even if thyroid functioning is abnormal, treating the thyroid condition doesn't help resolve the urticaria.

- There is good therapy available for chronic idiopathic urticaria. It's crucial that patients are taught how to use the medicines correctly. Daily use of antihistamines at relatively high doses, every day, can help suppress the rash. It's important that these antihistamines not be stopped on days when the rash is absent—staying on them daily, long term, even on days without rash, helps keep the rash suppressed. Sometimes, multiple antihistamines that work via different receptors are used simultaneously.

- If maximal, regular, scheduled use of antihistamines is ineffective, daily or every-other-day oral steroids can be used, though side effects of this strategy can be significant. To avoid long-term steroids, other immune-modifying medications, such as cyclosporine, can be useful. Even more aggressive strategies can include the administration of intravenous immunoglobulin or

plasmapheresis, a method of filtering out immune molecules from the blood.

- Ironically, Leslie was prescribed the correct medications, but because multiple doctors had given her different instructions, she didn't understand how to use these medications correctly. In our clinic, no further tests were done, and written instructions were provided for the use of two simultaneous antihistamines.

- Leslie, as is typical for most people with chronic urticaria, did not have any food allergies, but food allergies are a significant problem for many people, and they're often misunderstood. It's important to make a distinction between an adverse reaction to food—something like the bloating and diarrhea that goes with lactose intolerance—and a true food allergy, because only real food allergies can progress to life-threatening reactions.

- Most food allergies cause only mild symptoms. The best predictor of who is at risk for serious food reactions is what has happened with that food exposure in the past. Anyone who has had a life-threatening or severe reaction to a specific food is at risk for that happening again.

- Also, some foods, especially peanuts and tree nuts, are more likely to cause more severe reactions than other food allergens. In addition, any person who has a history of asthma or recurrent **wheezing** who also has food allergies is more likely to experience a severe reaction to foods. These are generalities. If you have food allergies or a suspicion of food allergies, work with your own doctor for specific recommendations.

Important Terms

general practitioner: A physician who treats general conditions; this title does not require a residency or board certification.

generic: Referring to medications, "generic" means manufactured by a company that does not own the patent.

idiopathic: Of unknown cause.

IgE: Immunoglobulin E, a specific subtype of antibody that's often associated with allergic disease.

IgG: Immunoglobulin G, the most common subtype of antibody circulating in blood.

plasmapheresis: A medical procedure that separates out the plasma from the whole blood and then filters out certain elements, typically proteins, before returning the blood to the body.

wheezing: A physical exam finding of the lungs, heard best with a stethoscope. Wheezing sounds like air rushing through small tubes and is most typically heard in expiration.

Suggested Reading

Montgomery, *How Doctors Think*.

Wanderer, *Hives*.

Questions to Consider

1. Do you think doctors learn more from their successes or their mistakes?

2. What is the difference between treating a disease and treating a patient?

Learning from Failure
Lecture 12—Transcript

Welcome back! Let me start today's grand rounds with a quote from the literature. "Smart people learn from their mistakes. But the real sharp ones learn from the mistakes of others." That's a quote from *Fablehaven*, by Brandon Mull. Because I'm a pediatrician, I can get away with quoting young adult literature like that. For those of you with pre-teens, or those of you with a taste for children's fantasy, Fablehaven is a wonderful series.

Now, all of the cases we're discussing during these grand rounds are fictionalized. I'm deliberately changing some details to protect patient privacy. However, every single one of the patients discussed is based on a real case, including the one today. Not all of them, I'll admit, make the doctors look very good. Our cases leave in the real mistakes that doctors and patients make. I will tell you I've learned a lot from my own mistakes, as have all doctors.

One of the most important goals of discussing cases like these is to learn from the mistakes of others, so all of these mistakes don't have to be made again and again. One more quote to help us get started, this, from a slightly more adult book, from Bram Stoker's Dracula: "We learn from failure, not from success."

A day in clinic; we're doing general adult medicine. It's a nice day out, and I think we'd probably rather be walking in the park than meeting our next patient, who is a new patient to the clinic. She has brought a voluminous stack of prior medical records, about six inches high, and we can tell it's loaded with lab reports and letters from specialists. A past medical record like this can be helpful, in a way, but it can also be like taking a drink from a fire hose. I'd rather talk with the patient first, before diving into a big stack of paper.

Leslie is a 45-year-old woman with a chief complaint of "I'm tired of the itching." She says she had been in good health until about nine months ago, when she started to develop these itchy rashes. The rashes appear and disappear quickly, within an hour or so, and they're always itchy. If they pop up at night, they interfere with sleep; if they occur during the day, they interfere with work.

Leslie says she's been seeing doctor after doctor, and she knows she's allergic to certain foods, and none of it has helped. And she's tired of the testing; and she's tired of all the medicines; and she's sick of doctors, and labs, and tests, and she's ready to … "What?" you say. "You're ready to what?" Leslie answers, "I'm just going crazy with this, OK?" and she starts to cry. You sit down, and hand her a box of tissues, and you start to sort of idly flip though the stack of old records to give your patient a few moments to recover.

There's a letter from an allergist, and a letter from another allergist, and a letter from a dermatologist. Here's another letter from maybe an endocrinologist, and a letter from a rheumatologist, and then page after page of labs. Many look normal, though some are flagged in the abnormal column as well. There are all sorts of scribbles and notes on them. Looking at this stack, you may want to cry, too, but we'll be professional and we'll hold it together.

After a little while, you say, "I want to try to help you. It's going to be hard to go through this entire record. Can you walk me through it; what happened; what have you been told?" Leslie answers, "I'm only here because my insurance changed, and I have to get referrals from you to see the specialists." Did I mention, this is a real case? Well, anyway, you say, "I'd like to get to know what's been going on. I'd like to see if I can help, too." Leslie sighs. Then she tells us more.

The itchy rash was diagnosed as hives by her first doctor, who told her it was probably from some kind of allergy and prescribed allergy medicines. That seemed to work at first, but the rash just kept coming back, so he changed medicines a bunch of times, and then it seemed like the medicine itself, maybe a new medicine, was actually triggering more of those hives.

So Leslie saw an allergist who did a bunch of tests, and she was told she was allergic to eggs and wheat, which she's pretty much avoided ever since. They also told her she was allergic to Timothy grass and two different indoor molds. She tried some different medicines from that allergist that didn't seem work and had some more blood tests, and was then told that she had a problem with her thyroid. But the endocrinologist said that her thyroid was OK.

And then there were more tests, and she saw a rheumatologist, and she doesn't remember what he said. And then she saw a dermatologist, or maybe, I think, two dermatologists, and more tests were done, and it turns out that she's also allergic to milk and corn and cinnamon, and avoiding these, maybe, has helped some, but she still gets the rash several times a week. And it itches. And it drives her crazy. Sometimes medicine seems to help the rash go away, but other times it seems to make it worse.

Our differential here, it's not long at all. There's really only one rash that comes and goes this quickly, and it's characteristically very itchy—hives, or what doctors call urticaria. I'm not sure why we have a different name for hives, but as you've already learned, that's typical. Doctors like to have different words for things. Anyway, our patient has been having recurrent hives for almost a year. Why?

More history. There seems to have been a lot of suspicion of allergies as a trigger, so we might as well start there. We ask, is there a certain food that triggers the hives? Leslie says, yes, eggs, wheat, and she thinks dairy, and cinnamon. So have four yes answers. Today's lesson one: when you have a confusing story, don't settle for yes/no answers.

You ask Leslie, how do you know? What happens when you eat those things? Well, it's different, she says. With eggs, she thinks she gets her rash about two days later, or maybe three days, depending on the amount of eggs. It's more quick if she eats more eggs, or if eggs are baked into a cookie or bread. Or with cinnamon, Leslie thinks the rash begins later that same day, or especially at night; the night rash, she says, that's often from cinnamon, or even from something cooked in the same bakery where they use a lot of cinnamon. With milk, it's OK if she drinks organic milk, but ordinary milk will start the hives, though sometimes that can start even a week later. With chicken, she can eat processed chicken, like chicken strips, but not plain baked chicken.

"Wait," you ask, "You're allergic to chicken, too?" "Yeah, that was on the last set of tests done by the new allergist. I don't think I brought those with me. Do you want to see them?" You say, "Maybe later." OK, so there's a lot of itchy rash, and it seems maybe related to different kinds of food. Taking further history along these lines is likely to get maybe even more confusing, so let's try a different tactic. Let's see if we can figure out what sort of workup has been done and what the specialists have concluded.

"So," you ask, "what did the allergists say?" OK, I'm not going to go through the blow by blow. But she's probably seen three different allergists, from two different allergy groups, and it sounds like at least three sets of blood tests and skin-prick allergy tests have been done. You're trying to pin this down, here, and you ask, "So bottom line, did they tell you this was an allergy? What did they tell you to do?" "I'm supposed to take these medicines," Leslie says. "And these allergy tests came up positive." "What medicines?" you ask.

Leslie brings out a brown lunch sack filled with bottles of pills, and dumps them out on the table. "Do you take these every day? Which ones? How do you take these?" you ask. It's clear that she just doesn't know. She starts pawing through them and holding them up, and she can't remember which ones are which. You look at the labels, the instructions that the pharmacist puts on each bottle, and they don't make sense to you either. Some say "for hives," and some say the initials P.R.N., which is doctor abbreviation for "as needed."

Another added confusion is that doctors often refer to medications by their common brand names, like Motrin or Atarax. However, when prescriptions are filled, the pharmacy label may only have the generic name. So, for Motrin, that would be ibuprofen, which many people know, but for an allergy medicine, like Atarax, the label may just say "hydroxyzine." Sometimes, there are even multiple brands or generic names for the exact same medicine. This really is unfortunate, and it makes communication about medications unnecessarily complicated.

Today's lesson number two: Insist on clear instructions. When you see a doctor, you need clear instructions on what to do; when you're the doctor, you must make sure that your patient understands you, even if that means writing things down. In fact, really, it should always mean writing things down. And writing things down means including both brand and generic names, and avoiding using doctor abbreviations like P.R.N. that ordinary people might not know.

And, let's just jump to today's lesson number three: The more doctors involved, the more the patient has to insist on clarity. One of the confusing things here is that multiple doctors were prescribing multiple things and ordering multiple tests. Everyone was making mistakes here, and, more importantly, I don't think anyone was learning anything from each other's mistakes. One medicine was tried; it didn't work, but the next doctor didn't know that, and maybe even tried the same medicine again.

OK, so you ask, Leslie, what did that endocrinologist say? "Well, I went to see him because of the thyroid test. Did I bring that with me? Anyway, the dermatologist said I had low thyroid, so I went to see the endocrine, but he just sent me away." "Did he say your thyroid was normal?" you ask. She kind of looked at the stack of paperwork. "I guess so," she says.

Today's lesson four: A medical encounter should always address the primary concerns of the patient. Our patient's concern is a recurring itchy rash, but she was sent to the endocrinologist because someone thought she had thyroid disease. So there were really two main issues that the endocrinologist should have addressed, the rash and the thyroid tests. It sounds like from our patient's point of view, she didn't get clear feedback about either of those issues.

I think we're all getting a feel here that Leslie's adventure is what should be called, in the common medical jargon, a train wreck. This is not, really, an atypical case. People have confusing histories and see multiple doctors, and we do not do a good job with communicating clearly. It's a huge waste of money, but even more distressing is that situations like these often create worry and anxiety and make health problems worse. You almost regret having to ask your next question, "So, why did the rheumatologist get involved, and what did he say?" Leslie answers, "I just don't know."

Lesson five: Beware when the diagnosis or plan doesn't make sense. This goes for doctors and patients. As a doctor, if you can't explain the working diagnosis and plan clearly, it's probably because it's not clear in your own mind. You need to think more. From the patient's point of view, if you don't understand the diagnosis and plan, you need to speak up. You need to ask and ask again.

OK, I'm exhausted, and we have a lot more to cover today. So let's just say that there isn't any more helpful history and that the physical exam is absolutely, completely normal. Leslie is a well-appearing woman of Asian ancestry who has no rash right now. But our patient did bring a photo, on her cell phone, and it looks like large, raised, pink-red areas with surrounding pink skin. She says when the rash pops up it feels warm, and then it always goes away in an hour or so. By the way, the cell phone is a great diagnostic tool, both for photos of rashes and for videos of funny movements, or recordings of peculiar sounds. In this case, the photo looks exactly like we expected it's a photo of hives, also known as urticaria.

Let's go though that stack of labs, at least briefly. There are a bunch of CBCs, all of them look OK; there are sed rates and CRPs, those are normal, too. So, there's no anemia, there's no inflammation; it doesn't look like there's much of chance of chronic or serious infections, or of anything terrible, like cancer, with these labs.

There are a few sets of thyroid tests. Let's see what those are all about. Thyroid testing has changed a lot in the last 20 years. Older tests had been often inaccurate or misleading, but the current testing is very reliable, using only two measurements—the TSH and the free T4. TSH is thyroid stimulating hormone. It's produced by the pituitary gland in the brain to rev up the thyroid gland to work harder, kind of like stepping on the gas. The free T4, the other test, is the best measurement of the hormone made by the thyroid gland.

Our patient's measurements of TSH and free T4 were all normal at every test, so Leslie does not have thyroid disease. What was abnormal was a different kind of test, a test for anti-thyroid antibodies. However, even when that's positive, most people who have this never develop any thyroid disease.

It's a marker for a slightly increased risk of late thyroid disease. Tests like this don't help management in most cases, and as in this case, just kind of muddy the water. The test was done, it was positive, but it was irrelevant.

By the way, Leslie had another "abnormal test," called an ANA; that's why she was referred to a rheumatologist. The ANA is another test, kind of like the antithyroid antibodies, that is very often falsely positive or positive in a way that's irrelevant and doesn't help the patient. With no other evidence on the history, or physical exam, or on any of those other screening labs of rheumatologic disease, the positive ANA is meaningless, and the test really should not have even been done in the first place. Yet, there it is, worrying the patient and driving more visits to more doctors.

Today's lesson number six: Treating the disease is not the same as treating the patient. Our patient wanted relief from a recurring, itchy rash; she didn't want to have a bunch of blood tests and see a bunch of specialists. All of these tests unfortunately led to doctors focusing on the test, not on the patient herself. In fact, I would say that the side effect of all of these tests—the worry, the distraction, and the expense—may have been almost as bad as the itchy rash itself.

Another blood test was done, celiac antibodies, which were negative. This wasn't a bad idea, because celiac disease can cause, among many other things, recurrent itchy rashes, including hives. The current celiac antibody test is actually quite good and rarely has false results, unlike that ANA and the thyroid antibodies. So adding Celiac testing to the initial screen was reasonable, which leads us to lesson number seven: whether to do a test depends on both how likely it is that the patient has the disease you're looking for, but also on how accurate the test is. Less-accurate tests should only be done when absolutely indicated, or they're going to lead to mischief. In any case, tests should only be done if the result of the test will be useful. If the result isn't going to change the plan, the test shouldn't have been done in the first place.

Speaking of less-accurate tests, we need to address all of those allergy tests that our patient endured. In general, there are two kinds of allergy tests, skin testing and blood testing. Blood allergy testing is often preferred by general practitioners and non-allergists, because anyone can order it and draw blood. These kinds of tests will also not be affected by allergy medicines that many patients are taking. The older generation of allergy blood tests were based on IgG antibodies. Those are worthless. Those IgG based tests should never be done, though they're still offered by some less-mainstream labs and doctors. You should just stay away from them. The newer tests, based on IgE molecules, are more accurate. But even the best of these current blood tests can still be misleading. Skin testing is more often performed by allergists, because it can be done in their offices with results available the same day. Those results can be affected by certain medications.

But the bottom line for both skin and even the best blood testing is that these tests have many false positives and can have false negatives too. They can be helpful to get a clue about what exposures could be triggering allergy but should be confirmed before declaring that a patient is actually allergic. So, how do you really tell if a patient is allergic to something? As is so often is true in medicine, it's not the test. It's the history.

Allergies are immune-mediated reactions to exposures to environmental things, including foods, or pollen, dust, things like that. Very characteristically, allergic symptoms occur very shortly after exposures, and they're stereotyped; that's a good word. It means that the reaction is the same every time after the same exposure. This is especially true for food allergy, which usually triggers reactions within minutes or maybe an hour after ingestion. Typical reactions to food allergies include reactions in the skin, like hives or swelling. It can also include GI symptoms, like vomiting, or diarrhea, or crampy pain, or difficulty breathing, or coughing. Severe reactions can lead to low blood pressure and a loss of consciousness. Again, these usually occur very quickly after the food trigger is eaten.

Let's think back to our patient, Leslie. When we asked her about foods that could be triggers, her answers were, well, they were kind of all over the place. Eggs caused a reaction, sometimes; as did chicken, but it depended on how it was cooked. And a lot of her reactions seemed to be a day or more later. Does this sound like real food allergies? No, it doesn't. Real food allergies happen quickly, and in general, don't depend on how much is eaten or how things are cooked or combined. If you're allergic to milk, it doesn't matter whether it's organic milk or not. What's going on is that Leslie had this inexplicable rash that kept coming and going, and she understandably thought about what could have been the trigger.

Plus, she had all of these allergy tests that supposedly were positive. Foods like eggs and wheat are in many things, and if you start to consider foods cooked in the same facility, or reactions that start three days later, I suppose any of her rashes could seem to have been triggered by some kind of food exposure. But when you dig deeper, there's no consistent, quick stereotyped reaction. Chances are, despite the testing, that there is no food allergy at all that's contributing to Leslie's hives. All of these food tests and restrictions, based on our history, were a waste of time.

What about this thought that medicines could have made the hives worse? Well, maybe yes, some medicines can trigger hives. But her hives started before any of these medications and continued to reappear sporadically, so how do we know if a medicine is really a trigger? It turns out that though hives are possible with any medicine, they're really only likely after certain medications, like antibiotics or seizure medicines. Allergy medicines themselves would very rarely cause hives, though since they're often prescribed in people who are already having hives that come and go on their own, they might seem to make things worse because of the coincidence of timing.

In fact, many people who think they are allergic to medicines, including antibiotics, are not in fact allergic and could take that medicine safely. Rashes after medications are not usually caused by allergy. However, if you've been told you are allergic to a medicine, don't start taking it again on the basis of this lecture. Talk with your own doctor about the circumstances and whether trying that medication would be OK for you.

Pollens, dust mites, mold, and other airborne allergens can cause itchy noses and congestion and sniffles, but they would only rarely cause skin reactions like hives. Leslie tested positive for some of these, but honestly, there's no reason to think that this would have contributed to her hives, and again, there was no reason to have done that testing.

So, recurrent hives with no identified trigger, persisting for a long time, Leslie's diagnosis is Chronic Idiopathic Urticaria. This is a condition that's not uncommon and can lead to significant disruption and very distressing symptoms. That's what Leslie has, and in fact, it was diagnosed by two allergists and the dermatologist, based on their letters. We found that diagnosis; it was typed right there in the notes. But it was never communicated clearly to Leslie.

There are just a few conditions that can kind of mimic chronic idiopathic urticaria, but it's easy enough to tell the difference. Allergic contact dermatitis occurs only where there was contact to allergen where it touches the skin, so it's in the same place every time, like where a nickel belt buckle or a necklace touches the skin. A so-called fixed drug eruption can be a recurring swollen area, but it's in the same place every time, and as it heals, it leaves a dusky area. Honestly, the only rash that occurs like Leslie's, popping up quickly anywhere on the body and then disappearing quickly, is urticarial, or hives.

Is there likely a specific cause of Leslie's urticaria? As we've seen, food allergies can cause acute episodes of urticaria, but it's very unlikely that foods will cause longstanding, chronic urticaria without clear correlation. Some people with chronic urticaria can have hives triggered by physical things, like pressure on the skin, or warmth, or cold. But again, these triggers are usually clear from the history.

Many patients with chronic urticaria, like Leslie, have thyroid antibodies, but these don't seem to be the actual trigger. Usually, thyroid functioning is normal, and these antibodies require no treatment. Even if thyroid functioning is abnormal, treating the thyroid condition does not help resolve the urticaria.

So, to the treatment. That really is what Leslie is interested in. What can she do to stop these rashes and become more comfortable? There is good therapy available for chronic idiopathic urticaria. It's crucial that patients are taught how to use those medicines correctly. Daily use of antihistamines at relatively high doses, every single day, can help suppress the rash. It's important that these antihistamines not be stopped on days when the rash is absent; staying on them daily, long term, even on days without rash, helps keep the rash suppressed. Sometimes multiple antihistamines that work via different receptors are used simultaneously.

If maximal, regular scheduled use of antihistamines is ineffective, daily or every-other-day oral steroids can be used, though side effects of this strategy can be significant. To avoid long-term steroids, other immune-modifying medications like cyclosporine, can be useful. Even more aggressive therapies can include the administration of intravenous immunoglobulin or plasmapheresis, a method of filtering out immune molecules from the blood. Ironically, Leslie actually had the correct medications in her brown paper bag, but because multiple doctors had given her different instructions, she didn't understand how to use these medicines correctly.

In our clinic, no further tests were done, and written instructions were provided for the use of two simultaneous antihistamines. Over the next few weeks, Leslie had fewer flares of hives, and within three months, she was no longer having any rash. She stopped her medications and the rash did return, so the regimen was restarted, and she continues to do well with those medicines about six months later. For the very rare, mild flare up that Leslie does see, she has a backup added medicine to take, as needed, in addition to her usual routine medications.

Leslie, as is typical for most people with chronic urticaria, did not have any food allergies; but food allergies are a significant problem for many people, and they're often misunderstood. It's important to make a distinction between an adverse reaction to food—something like the bloating and diarrhea that goes with lactose intolerance—and a true food allergy, because only real food allergies can progress to life-threatening reactions. Having said that, most food allergies cause only mild symptoms. So who's at risk for serious food reactions?

The best predictor is what has happened with that food exposure in the past. Anyone who has had a life-threatening or severe reaction to a specific food is at risk for that happening again. Also, some foods, especially peanuts and tree nuts, are more likely to cause more-severe reactions than other food allergens. And any person who has a history of asthma or recurrent wheezing who has also food allergies, they're more likely to experience a severe reaction to foods. Now, these are generalities. If you have food allergies or a suspicion of food allergies, work with your own doctor for specific recommendations.

In Leslie's case, there were misunderstandings about the role of food, her actual diagnosis, and the best way to treat her recurring rash. This, unfortunately, led to a prolonged diagnostic journey, including multiple doctors, a whole lot of tests, and most importantly, a significant delay in helping Leslie. Mistakes were made by both the doctors and the patient, and most of them had to do with a single problem—communication. For good patient care, it is essential for doctors to communicate well with patients, and for patients to communicate well with doctors, and for doctors to communicate well with each other.

We have a good case lined up for next time, a mystery with a much younger patient—a baby who's pale and weak. We'll hear more about that next time.

The Children Who Come and Go
Lecture 13

Sickle-cell anemia is an ancient illness. Although it was "discovered" about 100 years ago, it's clear that this disease has afflicted people since ancient times. Although we will probably never know for sure, it's quite possible that this disease caused the death of the king of Egypt, King Tutankhamen, at age 19, about 1300 years before the Common Era. The case presented in this lecture teaches you why patients with sickle-cell anemia become ill and what kinds of therapies can be used to keep them well.

A Pale, Weak Baby

- A 7-month-old boy named Marcus has been brought by his parents to the pediatric clinic. In their words, "He looks weak." They say that Marcus is a happy baby, but he has never been as active as his sister. Lately, though, he seems more fussy at times and isn't interested in sitting up or playing much. In addition, Marcus was anemic last month.

- From the physical exam, we find that Marcus is pale and listless. His eyes are yellow, and his heart rate is fast. He also has a **murmur** and a large spleen. We've already been told that he was anemic one month ago, and he was started on extra iron. Anemia can cause a high heart rate, and when severe, it can cause low energy or listlessness.

- From the history and physical, Marcus seems to have a chronic, ongoing, anemia caused by hemolysis, or the destruction of red blood cells in the blood. Under a microscope, we can examine Marcus's cells. Normal red blood cells are round and flat, sort of like fat pancakes with dimples on both sides. Marcus's red blood cells look very different from each other. Some look normal; some look very small and bent; and many of them have an elongated, crescent shape. Marcus has sickle-cell anemia.

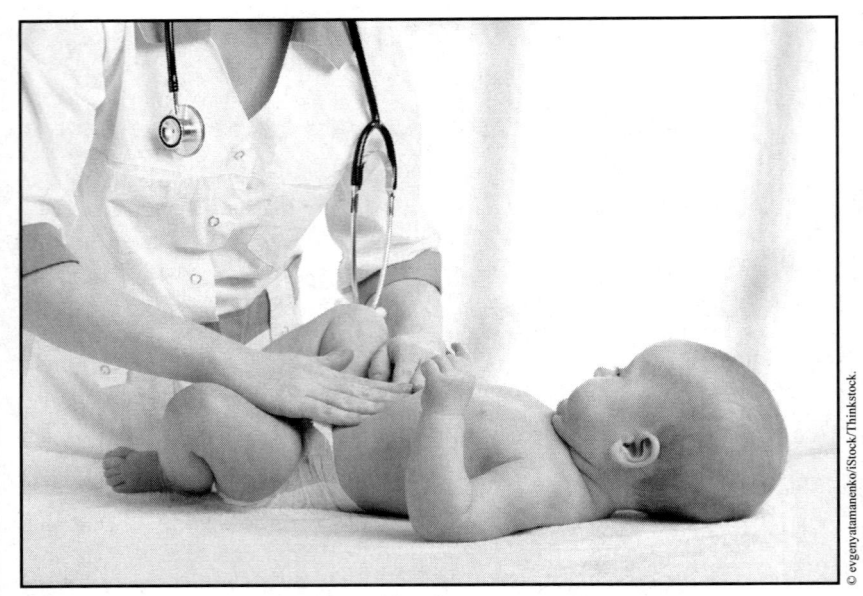

Sickle-cell anemia is a blood disorder that can cause tissue damage.

- Marcus's diagnosis of sickle-cell anemia is confirmed by a test called a hemoglobin electrophoresis, which can confirm the kind of protein that makes up his **hemoglobin**. It's likely that his anemia had been worsened to some degree because he had never had folate supplements but also because he had a mild viral infection that suppressed his marrow.

- After stabilization with several small blood transfusions, Marcus perked up well. There was no evidence of any neurological or cardiac damage. After extensive education for his family, he was sent home on oral folate supplements and oral penicillin to take every day. He will continue follow-up with the sickle-cell center, a multidisciplinary clinic for patients of all ages with sickle-cell anemia and related chronic anemias, as well as with his pediatrician for routine care.

Sickle-Cell Anemia

- Sickle-cell anemia, which is also called sickle-cell disease, had several earlier names that remain quite telling. Hospitalizations for this disease were sometimes called "muscular rheumatism," referring to the intense pain that can occur, or "bilious attacks," referring to both the pain and the **jaundice** (which was also known to be caused by disorders of the bile).

- In 1949, Linus Pauling demonstrated that sickle-cell disease was caused by an abnormality in the hemoglobin molecule; this was actually the first time a genetic disease was linked to abnormalities in the production of a specific protein. Since then, we've been able to map the exact gene, find the exact incorrect instruction, and see how that leads to the production of a protein that doesn't work the way it should. This really was a milestone in the field that was to become molecular biology.

- The genetics of sickle-cell anemia, and they way the genes affect the proteins, is a wonderful lesson to teach both medical genetics and the practical impact of evolution on health.

- Each of us has two copies of each gene (except that men have only one X chromosome and one Y chromosome—all of the other chromosomes come in pairs). One gene comes from our mother and one from our father. Each gene is a string of DNA that gives instructions for making a protein.

- The normal hemoglobin in adults is called hemoglobin A, and most of us have two copies of the gene that makes that normal hemoglobin. In sickle-cell anemia, both copies of this gene are broken; one of the base pairs of the DNA instructions is wrong, so the cell making the hemoglobin molecule substitutes one incorrect amino acid into the chain that makes the protein. That one substitution—just one wrong amino acid—causes the hemoglobin to form rigid polymers that get stuck in a sickle shape, deforming red cells and making them stiff.

- Sickle-cell disease is a classic so-called recessive condition—to have the disease, you have to inherit both abnormal genes from both of your parents. If you only inherit one abnormal gene and one normal gene, you are what's called a sickle-cell carrier, which causes minimal if any health effects.

- In fact, carriers of sickle cell—people with one abnormal gene and one normal hemoglobin gene—have a genetic advantage. Their red blood cells are relatively resistant to infection with malaria.

- People who are most likely to have sickle-cell disease are from areas of the world with the most malaria, especially Africa. In those communities, malaria was and continues to be a huge health problem; malaria continues to cause about a million deaths, worldwide, each year.

- A genetic mutation that confers some protection from this very common infection would confer increased survival, which allows people who carry the trait an increased chance of having more children to pass on this trait. As evolutionary theory predicts, a genetic mutation that confers a survival advantage will spread and become more common in a community, which is exactly what has happened.

- All of the various manifestations of sickle-cell anemia are caused by a single genetic change that leads to a substitution of one amino acid unit in the hemoglobin molecule. This one substitution creates a hemoglobin that can become sticky and stiff, and that one change leads to infections, strokes, pain crises, anemia, chronic jaundice, gallbladder disease, impotence, leg ulcers, heart damage, and eye problems.

Treatment
- The treatment of sickle-cell anemia starts, most importantly, with the early identification of affected babies. Every state in the United States screens for sickle-cell anemia in all newborns.

- As soon as sickle-cell anemia is diagnosed, these babies are started on an extra folate supplement as well as a daily antibiotic to prevent overwhelming infection. These early interventions have dramatically reduced the early mortality of the disease. Thirty years ago, prior to these recommendations, fewer than half of people with sickle-cell anemia lived to reach adulthood.

- It's also crucial that routine vaccines are received because those can prevent some of these bacterial infections, and families also need to be taught how to recognize early symptoms of infection and get immediate care.

- Families need to learn how to prevent crises and complications and when to seek immediate care. For example, dehydration and situations with low oxygen need to be avoided.

- Depending on the severity of the disease, other treatments may be needed. Patients who are having strokes, frequent pain, or chest crises can be given routine transfusions to keep their anemia under control; by diluting the sickling cells with donated, normal cells, vasoocclusion can be at least partially prevented. Frequent transfusions carry their own risks, but in certain patients, it can be lifesaving.

- Pain crises need to be immediately treated with pain medication, oxygen, and fluids to treat dehydration if present. Sometimes, transfusions are also needed during these and other crises.

- There are also medications that can be used, and more are under development, to suppress the sickle kind of hemoglobin and encourage the marrow to produce a different variety called fetal hemoglobin that would otherwise only be produced in the marrow before birth.

- The most aggressive therapy available for sickle-cell anemia is bone-marrow transplantation, which involves essentially killing off a patient's entire marrow and replacing it with donor marrow from someone else. This is curative, but it entails a lot of risk and tremendous expense.

- Bone-marrow transplantation will prevent the development of new or further complications of sickle-cell anemia, but it will not be able to reverse the damage from previous strokes or other preexisting complications. Currently, excluding bone-marrow transplantation, sickle-cell anemia cannot be cured. But it can be treated and managed to prevent and mitigate complications.

- Blood transfusions are an important part of therapy for sickle-cell anemia and many other conditions, and the development of modern blood banking has been a huge contributor to extending healthy lives. Good blood banking requires careful, sterile technique for collection and transfer, plus very specific storage systems with tightly controlled temperatures.

- It's also crucial that blood for transfusion be matched, or the recipient can experience a catastrophic immune reaction to the foreign proteins on the red blood cells. Even with careful matching, there is still a risk of blood transfusion reactions, and these can be severe. About 1 in 20,000 to 50,000 transfusions will cause a life-threatening reaction.

- There is also a risk of transmission of disease. Although blood banks screen both donors and blood for many infections, there may be some infections that we do not know how to test for yet, and no test is 100 percent accurate.

- It's estimated that about 1 in 1.5 million transfusions will transmit HIV virus, and 1 in about 300,000 transfusions may transmit hepatitis B. The risk of infection or serious reactions is small enough to be acceptable only if a patient is truly in need of a transfusion.

- For patients with chronic anemias (including sickle-cell anemia, thalassemias, and other conditions), the frequent transfusions become more likely to cause either infections or reactions. In addition, a risk eventually develops for iron overload, because each transfusion puts extra iron into the body. Hopefully, future therapies will replace the need for blood transfusions for these patients.

Important Terms

hemoglobin: The molecule in red blood cells that binds oxygen. "Hemoglobin" often refers to a quantitative lab measurement of the concentration of this molecule in a blood sample.

jaundice: A yellow color to the eyes and skin caused by excessive bilirubin in the blood.

murmur: A noise heard over the chest with a stethoscope caused by turbulent blood flow through the heart.

Suggested Reading

Hillman, et al, eds, *Hematology in Clinical Practice*.

Centers for Disease Control (CDC), http://www.cdc.gov/ncbddd/sicklecell/index.html.

Questions to Consider

1. What sorts of problems make a person look pale?

2. Are there special health considerations to think about for the children of military families?

The Children Who Come and Go
Lecture 13—Transcript

Today's case is an ancient illness. Though it was "discovered" about 100 years ago, it's clear that this disease has afflicted people since ancient times. Although we will probably never know for sure, it's quite possible that this disease caused the death of the pharaoh of Egypt, King Tutankhamun, at age 19, about 1,300 years before the common era.

We're in pediatric clinic today, and our next patient is a seven-month-old boy named Marcus. His parents have brought him in for evaluation because, in their words "He looks weak." Marcus's father is in the military, and though his parents are American, he was born overseas, at a military base in Central America. He has just moved back to the U.S., and his family is now transferring routine care to your clinic.

Now, with young babies, a traditional medical history starts with pregnancy and birth. Marcus was born after a full term, uneventful pregnancy. It was a routine delivery, and he went home with his mom after a typical two-day hospital stay. Since then, he has been home with mom and an older sister and has been in generally good health. He's been to routine well-child visits and has received all of his recommended vaccinations.

At his six-month-old checkup, a routine finger stick to measure blood hemoglobin was low, and mom was told to begin an iron supplement. She had been nursing exclusively at that time. At that visit, the physician had also thought that Marcus' heart rate was fast and that he seemed kind of listless. They were supposed to follow up for a recheck, but Dad was transferred back to the United States, and they haven't seen a doctor since that visit one month ago. Mom has been giving the iron drop supplement as directed. Marcus takes no other medicines and is nursing and taking complementary foods twice a day. His sister and parents are healthy.

His parents say that Marcus is a happy baby, but he has never been as active as his sister. Lately, he seems more fussy at times and isn't interested in sitting up or playing much. His grandmother, who hadn't seen him until he moved back to the U.S. last month, says he looks kind of weak and tired, and she's worried about his color, so she encouraged his parents to bring him to us right away.

A few quick comments before our differential, pediatricians know to always listen to grandparents! They might not have the specific medical knowledge to make a diagnosis, but they have a very good sense of when something isn't right. Do not disregard grandma's concerns!

So, for now, what we have is a little vague, a baby who's kind of weak or tired, he's listless, and we've been told that last month he was anemic. What could it be? Well, just about anything. In a broad sense, we'll keep in mind that this could be brain or neurologic disease, or a condition affecting the strength of his muscles, or a problem with his blood or bone marrow. Heart failure, malnutrition, chronic kidney disease are all among the possibilities, too. We need more information to move ahead here.

On to our physical exam. Marcus' weight and length are both a little on the small side, at about the 10th percentile; his head circumference is right at 50th percentile, which, by definition, is average. Pediatricians love percentiles, because it allows us to express these growth numbers in comparison to other children of the same age. A height percentile of 10 percent means that if you line up 100 babies of the exact same age and sex in height order, Marcus would be number 10 in line, with 90 babies longer and 9 babies shorter. Percentiles are especially useful to track as a child grows; in general, after growth stabilizes by age two or so, most children will track upwards along their own stable percentile.

Marcus's numbers today show that his weight and length are a little small, which itself isn't concerning. Though, actually, when we looked back at the records from his last well check, we did find that those percentiles had dropped some. This kind of relatively poor weight and height gain could fit with almost any kind of chronic disease. The diagnostic clue from this growth chart is that whatever is going on, it's unlikely to be something acute, but rather something that's been happening for a while.

Vital signs include a heart rate of 160, that's high for a seven month old; respirations are 40, that's probably normal for this age. Marcus also had a normal temperature and blood pressure. He has an African-American complexion, and is noticeably pale. A good trick with darker skinned children is to compare the color of the palms of their hands to that of their parents, who probably have a similar complexion. When compared to mom and dad, Marcus's palms were definitely pale. His eyes, the whites of his eyes, I mean, looked yellow. The remainder of the HEENT exam was OK; lungs are clear; he has a heart murmur, not a loud one; and his spleen feels enlarged when we palpate his belly. The skin exam is normal; there's no bruising. Neurologically, Marcus doesn't really respond very much to the exam. He just kind of lies there, and he doesn't want to sit up.

OK, that's a lot of information. I think we're in agreement with grandma, something here is not right. Let's review the most pertinent physical exam findings to focus our thoughts. Marcus is pale, he's listless, his eyes are yellow, his heart rate is fast; he also has a murmur and a large spleen. We'll get all of this explained soon enough, but for the sake of thinking through the case and putting this all together, we'll focus on his paleness, or pallor. We've already been told he was anemic one month ago, and he was started on extra iron. And we know that anemia can cause a high heart rate, and when severe, it can cause low energy or listlessness. So this anemia can explain a lot and seems central to what's going on.

Why would Marcus be anemic? Anemic means that there are fewer red blood cells than expected. The red cells, of course, carry oxygen to body tissues, so they're essential for health and energy. Normally, red blood cells live for about 120 days, after which, they disintegrate. The bone marrow constantly makes new red cells to replenish the supply. So anemia could occur either if the marrow isn't working right—if it isn't making enough new red cells to replace the old ones—or, if too many red cells are being lost too early. Those red cells could be lost in two ways, either from bleeding, say from a wound or perhaps from oozing in the gut, or if the red cells themselves are dying in the blood too early.

We need a quick red blood cell physiology lesson here. These are simple cells, really. Circulating red cells don't have a nucleus; they're really just floating little bags of hemoglobin, that's the molecule that carries oxygen. There are a few enzymes and other things in there, but that's about it. When they die, they pop open, releasing the hemoglobin molecules directly into the blood. These molecules are processed and recycled by the liver, but if there is too much hemoglobin released, the liver can't keep up with it. In that case, molecules related to the breakdown of the hemoglobin make their way into the blood, including the molecule bilirubin, which is yellow in color.

Wait, yellow, yellow; where did we hear yellow before? Marcus has yellow eyes. That's a physical finding called jaundice, meaning a yellow color to the eyes or skin. And in this case, with a patient who's suspected of being anemic, it probably means that something is destroying a lot of red blood cells, releasing their hemoglobin directly into the blood.

OK, we're making progress. Just from the history and physical, we're thinking that Marcus has a chronic, ongoing, anemia caused by—here's another new word—hemolysis, or the destruction of red blood cells within the blood itself. Let's confirm our suspicions with some lab work.

First, of course, a CBC, a complete blood count. We'll see just how anemic Marcus might be, and we'll also be sure to check if the other kinds of blood cells, the white cells and platelets, are those normal. Marcus's CBC shows a hemoglobin of five; normal at this age would be over eleven, with a normal white count and platelets. By the way, if those other cell lines, the platelets and white cells, if those were also down, it would increase the worry about some very serious problems indeed, like aplastic anemia, or cancer, or overwhelming infection. But they are normal. Only his red cells are affected. Chemistry studies confirm a high bilirubin, which is causing Marcus's yellow eyes.

Will a hemoglobin of five cause listlessness and a fast heart rate? You bet it will. In fact, we might have expected someone with a hemoglobin that low to seem even sicker. But Marcus's illness probably developed gradually, and in that case, people tolerate anemia better. Someone whose hemoglobin dropped from normal to five after, say, sudden blood loss from a car accident, they are going to be much, much sicker than someone whose hemoglobin drifted down slowly, as we suspect Marcus's has.

We don't yet have a definite diagnosis, but even so, it's time to move ahead quickly. We call the blood bank and warn them that this baby will almost certainly need one or more transfusions; and we draw a test called a type and cross match so the blood bank can get matched blood ready for him. We also make arrangements to admit Marcus to the hospital for further evaluation and management. Then we wander over to the lab where they did that CBC—it's just down the hall—to do something kind of old fashioned, but it's critically useful in a case like this. Let's go look at the blood smear under a microscope.

On the way, we'll think about the causes of hemolytic anemia in a baby. One cause is an infection, like malaria, which is a parasite transmitted by mosquitoes that's rarely seen in the U.S.A. But, wait, Marcus was living in Central America until just a few weeks ago! There is plenty of malaria in Central America, in South America, Africa, the Far East, so remember, a travel and exposure history can be very important.

Other causes of hemolytic anemia can be classified as intrinsic or extrinsic, meaning, is there something intrinsic to the red cell that shortens its life, or is there something extrinsic outside of the cell that's destroying it? Extrinsic causes of hemolytic anemia can include artificial heart valves that chew up the cells, or immune mechanisms that trick the body into destroying its own red blood cells. Alternatively, intrinsic problems with the red cells themselves can be a defect in the way the cell membrane is made or a problem with the hemoglobin that fills up the cell.

We're at the hematology lab, so let's look at those cells from Marcus. On the slide, we can see a few platelets and white cells; they look ok. We also do not see any malaria parasites. The red cells themselves, though, now, normal red cells are round and flat, sort of like fat pancakes with dimples on both sides. A collection of red cells under the microscope all pretty much look alike, but when we look at Marcus' red cells on the blood smear, it doesn't look like that at all. His red cells look very different from each other. Some look normal, some look very small and bent, and many of them have an elongated, crescent shape.

Cells like this were first noted under a microscope by an intern named Ernest Irons in 1910, who described the cells of a patient with chronic anemia as "peculiar, elongated, and sickle shaped." That's a good description, and it became the name of the disease in 1922. Marcus has sickle-cell anemia.

Sickle cell anemia, which is also called sickle cell disease, had several earlier names that remain quite telling. Hospitalizations for sickle cell were sometimes called muscular rheumatism, referring to the intense pain that can occur, or bilious attacks, referring to both the pain and the jaundice, which was also known to be caused by disorders of the bile. One other name, ogbanjes, comes from Africa. This means children who come and go, because of the very high infant mortality rate that's caused by untreated sickle cell disease.

In 1949, Linus Pauling demonstrated that sickle cell disease was caused by an abnormality in the hemoglobin molecule; this was actually the very first time a genetic disease was linked to abnormalities in the production of a specific protein. Since then, we've been able to map the exact gene, find the exact incorrect instruction, and see how that leads to the production of a protein that doesn't work the way it should. This really was a milestone in the field that was to become molecular biology.

The genetics of sickle cell, and the way the genes affect the proteins, is a wonderful lesson to teach both medical genetics and the practical impact of evolution on health. Each of us as two copies of each gene, except men, who have only one X chromosome and one Y chromosome; all of the other chromosomes come in pairs. One gene comes from mom and one from dad. Each gene is a string of DNA that gives instructions for making a protein. The normal hemoglobin in adults is called hemoglobin A, and most of us have two copies of the gene that makes that normal hemoglobin molecule. In sickle cell anemia, both copies of this gene are broken; one of the base pairs of the DNA instructions is wrong, so the cell making the hemoglobin molecule substitutes one incorrect amino acid into the chain that makes this protein. That one substitution—just one wrong amino acid—causes the hemoglobin to form rigid polymers that get stuck in a sickle shape, deforming red cells and making them stiff.

Sickle cell disease is a classic so-called recessive condition; to have the disease, you have to inherit both abnormal genes from both of your parents. If you only inherit one abnormal gene and one normal gene, you are what's called a sickle cell carrier, which causes minimal, if any, health effects. In fact, carriers of sickle cell, those are people who have one abnormal gene, and one normal hemoglobin gene, they have a genetic advantage. Their red blood cells are relatively resistant to infection with malaria.

So where are the people who are most likely to have sickle cell disease? They're from areas of the world with the most malaria, especially Africa. In those communities, malaria was and continues to be a huge health problem. Malaria continues to cause about a million deaths, worldwide, each year. So a genetic mutation that confers some protection from this very common infection would confer increased survival, which allows people who carry the trait an increased chance of having more children to pass on that gene. As evolutionary theory predicts, a genetic mutation that confers a survival advantage will spread and become more common in a community, which is exactly what has happened. The mutations conferring sickle cell anemia probably arose about 100,000 years ago in human populations in Africa and India. Today, about 1 in 25 black Americans is a carrier of sickle cell trait.

When two people who are sickle cell carriers have children, each child has a 50 percent chance of getting the sickle gene from mom, and a 50 percent chance of getting the sickle gene from dad. Multiplying those together, each child of these families has a 25 percent chance of getting both sickle genes, meaning having sickle cell anemia; the children also have a 50 percent chance of getting one of the genes, that is, becoming a carrier, and a 25 percent chance of getting neither of the genes.

How does sickle cell make people like Marcus sick? It's the rigid, inflexible, and sticky red blood cells that cause the problems. Blood cells flowing through capillaries have to squeeze through, bending and deforming at branches and through thin capillary spaces. When the hemoglobin sickles, it makes the red cell rigid, and the cell gets stuck. That's called vasoocclusion—cells stuck in blood vessels. Sometimes the cells pop, getting destroyed; or sometimes they just glom there, getting stuck and preventing blood flow. There are also other molecular factors at work that contribute to vasoocclusion. For example, the sickled cells kind of partially turn inside out, exposing internal red cell proteins that themselves stick to the lining of the blood vessels.

The abnormal hemoglobin of sickle cell anemia isn't sickled all the time. It gets sticky and makes those rigid chains especially when there is less oxygen nearby. So tissues with relatively little oxygen tend to be affected most severely by the sickling and vasoocclusion. And unfortunately, once vasoocclusion begins, it reduces local blood flow and reduces the amount of oxygen nearby, which can worsen sickling.

The clinical manifestations of sickle cell disease are caused by several overlapping mechanisms. There's the anemia itself, the red cells in sickle cell anemia last probably 20 or 30 days, compared to the 120 day lifespan of ordinary red cells. So patients with sickle cell are chronically anemic, and their marrow has to continuously pump out a huge number of red cells to keep up with their shortened lifespan. Iron deficiency isn't typical, because the iron released by destroyed red cells can be recycled, but to continue to produce so many red cells, patients need extra amounts of a B vitamin called folic acid.

There can also be short term crises, where a patient's baseline anemia drops much further, leading to complications. These can be caused by infections or other stresses and sometimes require blood transfusions. A crisis might be caused by a spike in hemolysis or destruction of red cells; or a crisis might be caused by a temporary slow down in red cell production; that's called an aplastic crisis.

The vasoocclusion of sickle cell leads to many problems. There can be pain crises involving areas of bone that get insufficient blood and then infarct, kind of like a heart attack, but of bone. These can be very painful. Infarction and vasoocccclusion can also happen in the lungs, leading to a pneumonia-like acute chest syndrome with pain and fever, and that can lower the oxygen absorbed through the lungs, causing more sickling. People with sickle cell usually have damaged kidneys from vasoocclusion, so they cannot concentrate their urine properly; this leads to an increased risk of dehydration, which itself can also worsen sickling. Finally, and perhaps most of all, vasoocclusion can lead to blockage in the blood vessels of the brain, causing strokes. These can be large, devastating events, or can be a series of kind of mini strokes that slowly lead to cognitive problems.

There's more. Vasoocclusion in the spleen inevitably leads to permanent damage to that organ. In babies and young children with sickle cell, the spleen is enlarged and can easily be felt poking down into the abdomen from the left side on the physical exam. In healthy children, the spleen is small; you cannot feel it on the exam. Later in life, the spleen in sickle cell disease will scar down and atrophy, disappearing entirely. This damage to the spleen interferes with the normal development of the immune system and leaves children like Marcus vulnerable to overwhelming bacterial infections and death. Recognition of this risk has led to several recommendations that have dramatically helped extend lives. These steps include teaching families to quickly seek medical care when there are signs of infection, using daily antibiotics to prevent infection, and making sure that children with sickle cell are fully immunized.

Now, think about this. All of these manifestations of sickle cell, all of this, is caused by a single genetic change that leads to a substitution of one amino acid in the hemoglobin molecule. This one substitution creates a hemoglobin that can become sticky and stiff, and that one change leads to infections, strokes, pain crises, anemia, chronic jaundice, and some other complications I didn't even list yet, like gall bladder disease, impotence, leg ulcers, heart damage, and eye problems.

So, I think we've explained all of the findings on that complex physical exam. Marcus is jaundiced from hemolysis; he's pale from anemia; he has an enlarged spleen from vasoocclusion; he's listless because of the degree of severe anemia. Marcus also has a fast heart rate; that can be a subtle finding, and it's easy to overlook on a panel of vital signs. But they're called vital signs for a reason. Those numbers really are important, and they can tell you when a patient might be genuinely in danger.

A fast heart rate can be caused by many things, including pain, anxiety, fever, dehydration, any condition that weakens the strength of the heart muscle, many medications, at times, when the respiratory system isn't bringing in enough oxygen or when the blood isn't carrying the oxygen. There's quite a list of causes of a fast heart rate. In Marcus's case, the low red cell count means that there are fewer cells to carry oxygen, so the blood has to be pumped faster to make up the difference.

There's also a heart murmur, which is a noise made by flowing blood. In children, murmurs are often heard when the blood is being pumped quickly. This can occur with a fever, or when a child is anemic. Many children have murmurs as a completely normal finding on their physical exams.

OK, back to Marcus and his sickle cell anemia. The treatment of sickle cell anemia starts, most importantly, with the early identification of affected babies. Every state in the U.S.A. screens for sickle cell in all newborns. This patient may have been missed because he was born at a military hospital out of the country. In any case, a physician did pick up on the anemia at a previous visit but assumed it was ordinary iron deficiency, perhaps because she thought that sickle cell should have been picked up on the newborn screen.

As soon as sickle cell is diagnosed, these babies are started on an extra folate supplement, as well as a daily antibiotic to prevent infection. These early interventions have dramatically reduced the early mortality of the disease. Thirty years ago, prior to these recommendations, fewer than half of people with sickle cell disease lived to reach adulthood. It's also crucial that routine vaccines are received, because those can prevent, at least, some of these bacterial infections. Families also need to be taught how to recognize early symptoms of infections to get immediate care and how to prevent crises and complications. For instance, dehydration and situations with low oxygen need to be avoided.

Depending on the severity of the disease, other treatments may be needed. Patients who are having strokes, or frequent pain, or chest crises can be given routine transfusions to keep their anemia under control by diluting the sickling cells with donated, normal cells. Vasocclusion can be at least partially prevented this way. Frequent transfusions carry their own risks, but in certain patients, this can be lifesaving.

Pain crises need to be immediately treated with pain medication, oxygen, and fluids to treat dehydration. Sometimes, transfusions are also needed during these and other crises. There are also medications that can be used, and more are under development, to suppress the sickle kind of hemoglobin and encourage the marrow to produce a different variety called fetal hemoglobin that would otherwise only be produced in the marrow before birth.

The most aggressive therapy available for sickle cell disease is bone marrow transplantation, essentially killing off a patient's entire marrow and replacing it with donor marrow from someone else. This is curative, but entails considerable risk and tremendous expense. Bone marrow transplantation will prevent the development of new or further complications of sickle cell, but will not be able to reverse the damage from previous strokes or other preexisting complications. Currently, excluding bone marrow transplantation, sickle cell disease cannot be cured. But it can be treated and managed to prevent and mitigate complications.

Our patient, Marcus, he did well. His diagnosis of sickle cell anemia was confirmed by a test called a hemoglobin electrophoresis, which can confirm the kind of protein that makes up his hemoglobin. It's likely that his anemia had been worsened to some degree because he had never had folate supplements, but also because he had had a mild viral infection that suppressed his marrow. After stabilization with several small blood transfusions, he perked up well. There was no evidence of any neurologic or cardiac damage. After extensive education for the family, he was sent home on an oral folate supplement and oral penicillin to take every single day. He will continue follow up with the sickle cell center, a multidisciplinary clinic for patients of all ages with sickle cell and related chronic anemias, as well as with his pediatrician for routine care.

Blood transfusions are an important part of therapy for sickle cell and many other conditions, and the development of modern blood banking has been a huge contributor to extending healthy lives. Good blood banking requires careful, sterile technique for collection and transfer, plus very specific storage systems with tightly controlled temperatures. It's also crucial that blood for transfusion be matched, or the recipient can experience a catastrophic immune reaction to the foreign proteins on the donated red blood cells.

Even with careful matching, there is still a risk of blood transfusion reactions, and these can be severe; about one in 20,000 to 50,000 transfusions will cause a life-threatening reaction. There is also a risk of transmission of disease. Though blood banks screen donors and screen blood for many infections, there may be some infections that we do not know how to test for yet, and no test is 100 percent accurate. It's estimated that about 1 in 1.5 million transfusions will transmit HIV, and 1 in about 300,000 transfusions may transmit hepatitis B. The risk of infection or serious reactions is acceptable only if a patient is truly in need of a transfusion.

For patients with chronic anemias, including sickle cell, thalassemias, and other conditions, the frequent transfusions become more likely to cause either infections or reactions. And, a risk eventually develops for iron overload, because each transfusion puts extra iron into the body. Hopefully, future therapies will replace the need for blood transfusions for these patients.

Today's case has been an especially good science lesson. It took us from how genes encode for proteins, to how a small change in structure can lead to a huge impact in the functioning of an essential protein, then to the pathophysiology of disease caused by that single change. Understanding why patients with sickle cell become ill leads directly to what kinds of therapies can be used to keep them well.

Next time, we're going to step back from the science a bit and sink our teeth into a new medical mystery. It's a disease we've all heard of, we've read about it, it's affected most all of our lives in one way or another. Think you can figure it out? Join us next time.

Guardians' Day
Lecture 14

Prescription drug abuse is a disease that has affected almost all of our lives in one way or another. It has become a common cause of disrupted lives, lost jobs, and death—striking every age, from teens through elderly adults. We are not, as a whole, doing a particularly good job of tracking prescriptions to identify those at risk, and we're doing a terrible job of getting people who are addicted the addiction treatment they need.

Constipation

- Our next patient in the general medicine clinic, Sandra, is a 35-year-old woman who we have not met before. Her chief complaint, as listed on the intake form, is "constipation." According to her, it's been going on for about a year, maybe longer, but it's just getting worse and worse. She has brought some of her medicines with her so that you could see what she's tried.

- Constipation is very, very common, and most of the time, it's related to lifestyle factors and diet. But it can be part of some important health problems, too. Constipation is often related to several overlapping factors: Basically, anything that either slows down the movement of the gut or leads to dry, hard, firm stools is going to contribute to constipation.

- Normally, as food is digested and absorbed and travels through the gut, water is absorbed through the walls of the large intestine. If gut transit is slowed, more water will be absorbed, leading to firmer, hard, bulky stools—which themselves become more difficult to push through, so they sit even longer, getting even more dry and hard. So anything that either slows the gut or leads to less moisture in the stool is going to be constipating.

- Sandra says that she gets a lot of bellyaches and really has to strain. She says that she's been trying to eat better and drink water and prune juice, but she can't really exercise much because of her back, which she injured about six months ago. She's seen an orthopedist who did X-rays and thinks she had a slipped disk. She takes pain medicine and now uses a cane to walk.

- Her past medical history is unremarkable. Upon physical examination, we learn that Sandra vital signs and reflexes are normal. Her labs come back normal. An MRI is done, and the results show that she does have two discs with a small amount of **herniation**, but neither is pressing on any nerves. Discs like that could possibly be causing some pain, though they're seen incidentally in many people and probably don't cause any symptoms most of the time. There's no problem with the spinal cord itself.

- After talking to Sandra for a while and seeing her in the clinic a few more times, it seems like she is doing some doctor shopping; it's not clear why she changed to our clinic. Eventually, we find out that she was also seeing other doctors at the same time. There were reports of stolen drugs or prescriptions, and she may have been using multiple pharmacies. Any of these can have an innocent explanation, but the pattern of behavior, at least in retrospect, seems suggestive.

- Also, it's unclear exactly how Sandra's original back injury led to such significant pain. Her back injury history was kind of vague, and her sustained discomfort was out of proportion to the injury.

- Our patient's apparent addiction to pain medications also caused her to stop working and led to her no longer living with her daughter. Somehow, her daughter had gone to live with another family member—supposedly just because of Sandra's hurt back. These kinds of negative life consequences are typical of true addiction.

- In addition to addiction, there are other side effects of the use of **narcotics**. One of them is constipation—which is what drove Sandra to our clinic in the first place. They can also cause itching, vomiting and nausea, and dry mouth; they can also cause confusion, sleepiness, or dizziness, and it is not safe to drive while taking these medications.

- However, the most severe symptom, the worst side effect, is respiratory depression. Taking higher doses of any narcotic starts to blunt the automatic drive to breathe. The higher the dose, the slower the breathing, and at a high enough dose, breathing will stop. That is the cause of death in narcotic overdose.

- People seek higher and higher doses to satisfy their cravings, and eventually, the dose is high enough to kill. At this point in the United States, there are more deaths from prescription **opioids** than from cocaine and heroin combined.

Prescription Drug Abuse
- Painkillers are the most often abused prescriptions. It turns out that there are really only three medications that are commonly used to treat pain—or at least three groups of medications, and within each group, they're all similar.

- The first group only contains one medicine: acetaminophen, or Tylenol. It's an effective medicine for mild to moderate pain, with minimal side effects when used correctly. It is not addictive.

- The second group, which also has many brands available over the counter, is the nonsteroidal anti-inflammatory drugs (NSAIDs). The most common ones are ibuprofen and aspirin; there are many others available by prescription. They all work in a very similar way. They are also effective for mild to moderate pain and have no addiction potential, and they're pretty safe. Occasionally, and more often with regular use, they can cause GI upset.

- The problem is that neither of these kinds of medicine, alone, is effective for the most severe pain. For the worst pains, the only effective medicines in general use are narcotics and narcotic derivates. They're all essentially based on an extract of the poppy plant, the precursor to opium.

- These medications range from morphine to codeine with many in between; the group also includes heroin, which is another opium

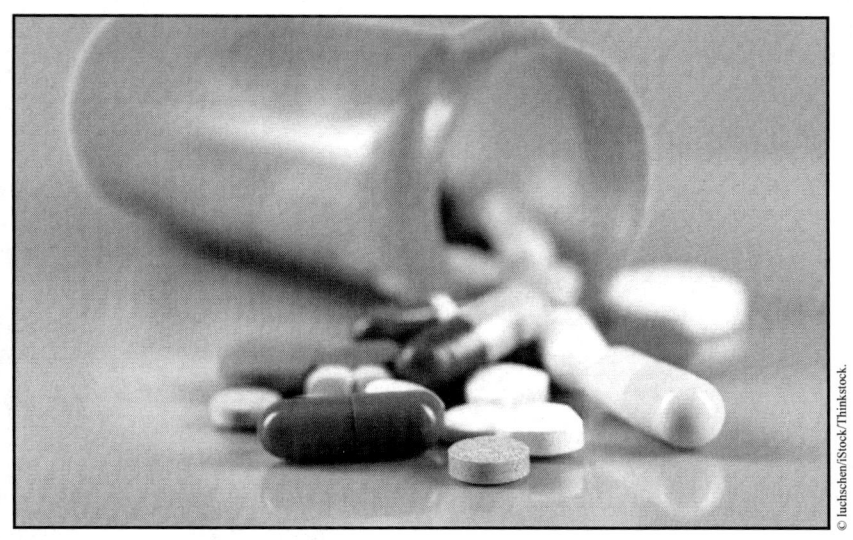

The abuse of prescription drugs is a serious concern in our overmedicated society.

derivative. They can all be used to effectively treat even the most severe pain, but all of them are potentially addictive when used inappropriately. When abused, they not only relieve pain, but they also get the user high.

- Still, for the many people who suffer from pain, especially chronic pain, narcotics are essential for providing relief. One of the biggest obstacles for these patients is misunderstanding the nature of drug tolerance, dependence, and addiction. This leads to the frequent undertreatment of pain, which itself, ironically, can actually contribute to the development of addictive behavior.

- To prevent, recognize, and treat addiction, we first have to make sure we understand what's happening physically and psychologically. Tolerance is a normal physiological change, when the body adapts to, or seems to "get used to," a certain dose of a medication, such as an opioid.

- When tolerance develops, the drug becomes less effective at a given dose, and to get the desired effect, the dose will have to be increased. Tolerance is an inevitable, predictable phenomenon that will occur in anyone who regularly uses certain medications.

- Dependence is different. In modern medical contexts, dependence refers to physical changes in the body as we adapt to regularly taking certain drugs. Biochemical changes take place mainly in the brain, as the body gets used to regular doses of these medications—and if the medication is stopped or reduced quickly, physical symptoms of withdrawal will take place.

- Symptoms of opiate or narcotic withdrawal can include sweatiness, agitation, aches, insomnia, cramping, diarrhea, nausea, and vomiting. These can be very unpleasant or severe, but they are not life threatening.

- Other kinds of medication can cause dependence and withdrawal symptoms, including steroids, antidepressants, anxiety medication, and some heart medicines (such as beta-blockers).

- Addiction, the way that doctors use the term, means psychological symptoms like compulsive drug use and craving for drugs. People who are addicted to drugs will continue to seek and use the drug despite worsening physical, social, and mental harm.

- In a sense, while the term "dependence" refers to the physical symptoms of withdrawal, the term "addiction" refers to a maladaptive psychological need to consume a drug. This definition of addiction is also used in other contexts, such as people addicted to gambling, sex, or Internet use.

- People with addiction may or may not have physical dependencies and may or may not suffer from physical withdrawal symptoms, but they will crave and seek the addiction even at the expense of their jobs or relationships, risking arrest and social isolation to satisfy their cravings.

- Another term that's sometimes used is "pseudoaddiction," which is seen only in people with chronic pain that is inadequately treated. These patients are desperate for effective pain relief and very fearful of worsening pains, so they watch the clock closely and may take steps that could be considered to be drug-seeking behaviors, such as filling prescriptions early or hoarding pills.

- The behaviors associated with pseudoaddiction stop completely when the pain itself is adequately treated. The key to treating pseudoaddiction (and preventing it from developing into true addiction) is in treating pain correctly.

- Not all chronic pain patients become addicted to opioids. In fact, the vast majority will never have addictive symptoms. Most, if not all, patients who use narcotics regularly will develop tolerance, physical dependence, and the potential for withdrawal, but that's different from the craving and compulsive drug-seeking behavior seen with addiction.

- Although it is possible, addiction is not a common problem among those treated for pain, and a fear of encouraging addiction should not prevent doctors from treating pain and relieving suffering.

- Although we don't know the exact contribution of genetics, it's definitely true that some people seem to have a higher built-in risk for addiction than others. Beyond that, the most important factor in predicting addiction is the reason the drug is taken. People who take drugs to get high or avoid life (as opposed to people who take medication to treat pain or other medical problems) are much more likely to develop addiction.

Prescribing Pain Medication
- Ironically, doctors are sometimes criticized from both sides of this issue. Doctor and hospital ratings stress how important it is for doctors to treat pain quickly and effectively; at the same time, federal and state agencies monitor doctors' prescribing habits and investigate those who seem to prescribe too many narcotics.

- Judging whether pain is real or exaggerated is very difficult; we don't have any kind of objective "pain meter." Add to that the complexities of the modern American medical system, the multiple doctors and pharmacies, and it's very difficult to identify patients at risk for addiction, especially when they deliberately cover their tracks to hide drug-seeking behavior.

- This is not a good situation, and it's contributing to the suffering of both pain patients who need effective pain treatment and to patients, families, and communities struggling with addiction.

Important Terms

hernia: A condition where an organ protrudes through the wall of the area surrounding it.

narcotic: A class of pain relievers derived from opium or morphine.

opioid: An opium-like compound, informally synonymous with "narcotic."

Suggested Reading

Fletcher, *Inside Rehab*.

Sheff, *Beautiful Boy*.

Questions to Consider

1. What are the best ways to judge how much pain a patient is experiencing?

2. Why do some people who are prescribed painkillers develop addiction while others do not?

Guardians' Day
Lecture 14—Transcript

Eastern Kentucky, rolling hills, bluegrass music, small towns you'd think maybe isolated and protected from modern worry. But there's an epidemic there that's not getting a lot of attention. Rockcastle County, a county of about 16,000 people, is seeing one death a week; in Knott County, next door, more than half of the children don't live with their parents because of death or abandonment or an inability of parents to take care of their own children. These kids are being raised by grandparents, and aunts, and uncles, many of whom later succumb to the same illness. In Johnson County nearby, school administrators have changed the name of Parents' Day to Guardians' Day because so many kids have lost their parents.

We're back in general medicine clinic today, picking up some extra shifts for a colleague who's out on maternity leave. Our next patient, Sandra, is a 35-year-old woman who we've not met before. Her chief complaint listed on the intake form is constipation. We head into the exam room, and we meet Sandra. She's a well-appearing woman, a little thin, and she's sitting on the edge of her chair with a cane propped against one leg. She has a few bottles of medicines lined up on the desk there, and she reaches out to shake your hand as you walk in. She says, "Sorry, it's hard for me to stand up." You say, no problem, and you shake her hand, and you sit down across from her. She asks a few questions about you, a little chit chat, because she's never met you before. It's nice, when you're not rushed, to spend a little time getting to know patients, even before diving into the medical information. Honestly, it's nice even when you are rushed, but today we have a little extra time. She says her usual doctor is on leave, so she decided to see you because you're new to the area, and she figured you'd be easy to get an appointment with, and she's heard you're very nice.

Sandra is an unemployed teacher, She says she used to work as a substitute teacher, but she hurt her back setting up the background for a school play, and has been on disability for several months. "So what can I do for you today?" you ask. The big problem, she says, is constipation. It's been going on for about a year, and maybe longer, and it's just getting worse and worse. She's brought some of her medicines with her so you could see what she's tried. OK, constipation is our main concern, so let's think about that. It's very, very common, of course, and most of the time, it's related to lifestyle factors and diet. But it can be part of some significant health problems too. Let's put together a brief differential diagnosis so we know what to ask next.

Constipation is often related to several overlapping factors, basically, anything that either slows down the movement of the gut or leads to dry, hard, firm stools is going to contribute to constipation. Normally, as food is digested and absorbed and travels through the gut, water is absorbed through the walls of the large intestine. If gut transit is slowed, more water will be absorbed, leading to firmer, hard, bulky stools, which themselves become more difficult to push through, so they sit even longer, getting even more dry and more hard. So anything that either slows the gut or leads to less moisture in the stool is going to be constipating.

Stool moisture has a lot to do with diet. People who don't drink enough water can be chronically constipated. Food itself is also important, especially fiber, which helps trap moisture in the stool. Fruits and vegetables are especially important to keep the bacteria in your gut active and happy, helping protect the normal structure and function of the gut.

Apart from issues with stool moisture, conditions that slow the muscular contractions of the gut wall can lead to constipation. This includes, most commonly, an overall lack of exercise, but also life habits that include ignoring the urge to have a bowel movement. Holding stool is not good, and delaying BMs does not make for a happy colon. Any changes in routine, including travel, or pregnancy, or life stress, can cause constipation, as can normal aging, when the muscles of the gut and abdominal wall start to lose their ability to squeeze well.

There are some important medical causes of constipation that shouldn't be overlooked. Many teens and adults have irritable bowel syndrome, which can cause constipation or diarrhea, or sometimes, alternating periods of both. Diabetes can affect the nerves in the gut, leading to disturbed gut motility. Neurologic disorders like stroke or Parkinson Disease can also interfere with normal control of the muscular contractions of the gut wall, as can problems and injuries that affect the spinal cord. Hormonal issues, especially hypothyroidism, can cause constipation, as can many prescription and over-the-counter medications.

There can also be an important psychological component to constipation. Anxious people—and that includes people anxious about having large or painful bowel movements, or people who are reluctant to have a BM at work or at school—they may put off normal bowel function, contributing to worsening constipation. So, this is a big differential, with problems ranging from common and trivial to rare and life threatening. We'd better pay attention to the rest of the history and physical.

Sandra says she's had some constipation, on and off, maybe even for years, but it's getting worse. She gets a lot of belly aches now and really has to strain. She says she's been trying to eat better and drink water and prune juice, but she can't really exercise much because of her back. She's tried over-the-counter medications, including stool softeners and laxatives, which haven't helped very much.

There's been no weight loss, no fevers, no blood in the stool; she's had no vomiting; she's had no diarrhea. There's no family history of gut illnesses or Celiac disease. By the way, Celiac can cause diarrhea or constipation. She says she's overall felt OK, but she's not working any more because of her back injury.

"What happened with that?" you ask. About six months ago, Sandra says, she was helping move some backdrops, basically, these are big, wooden painted sheets, to set up for a school play, and she kind of wrenched her back somehow. She's seen an orthopedist who did X-rays and thinks she had a slipped disk. She takes pain medicine, and says it's not that terrible, but she can't move around quickly and now uses a cane to walk. Otherwise, her past medical history is unremarkable. She's had some hay fever allergies and takes over-the-counter medicine for that sometimes. Her last menstrual period was a few weeks ago. Sandra now lives alone. She has one daughter, she's 10, and she's staying with an aunt for the past few months while mom's back gets better. Her husband, Sandra says, ran off years ago.

On to the physical exam. Sandra's vital signs are normal; she has no goiter or swelling of her thyroid gland; heart and lung exams are OK; and her abdominal exam is normal too. Her muscle strength seems normal in all extremities, and her so-called deep tendon reflexes are normal too. Basically, it's a normal and reassuring exam.

Those reflexes—doctors often call those by the abbreviation DTRs for deep tendon reflexes—that's when we give a little rap over a tendon, often right at the knee. That triggers a reflex arc that makes the muscles at the top of the thigh tense up, kicking the leg upwards. Tap, kick, it's pretty much instantaneous. What this tests is a reflex loop. The tap quickly stretches the quadriceps muscle of the thigh, and there's a nerve that detects the stretch of the muscle. That information, the feedback that the quad was stretched quickly, that's transmitted to the spinal cord. There, in the spine, the reflex arc sends a signal back to that muscle to quickly contract; that counterbalances the stretch. If there is a problem anywhere in that pathway, from the muscle to the nerves back and forth, or a problem in the spinal cord itself, the reflex will be abnormal. We're especially careful to compare the kick in either side; they look right about the same.

So, why are we so hung up on these reflexes in Sandra? Remember, we have that history of a back injury. Could something affect the back, the spinal cord specifically, causing constipation? Yes. Nerves from the spine go to the distal colon, and they're necessary to trigger relaxation of the pelvic muscles to allow a bowel movement. Damage to the spinal cord or nerves can cause what can look like ordinary constipation, so the reflexes are important here as a way to see if there has been an injury to the nerves or the spinal cord.

Sandra's reflexes are normal. We also observe that her gait, the way she walks, is pretty much normal too, though she leans on a cane. A spinal injury leading to constipation really ought to have caused other issues, like problems walking, changes in those reflexes, or perhaps numbness in the extremities. For now, we'll say that a spinal problem is unlikely.

Did we learn anything else from the exam? Not really. Overall Sandra looks good. So we discuss with Sandra some strategies to address the constipation, including drinking more water, trying to get some more exercise, improving her diet, and taking appropriate doses of the stool softeners that she brought along. We suggest she make a follow-up appointment in two weeks. Sandra seems happy with the advice; she's written some notes down, and she gets up to leave. On the way out she asks for refills of her back-pain medicines, so we take care of that and we send her on her way.

OK, there, case over, right? Well, no. It's two weeks later, and you head back into an exam room to see how Sandra is doing. "Not any better, doc," she says. She's got her cane, and she's got her little bottles lined up on the desk again. Not much has changed, Sandra says. She'd tried what you said; she's still constipated, and she thinks it's even making her back feel worse now, because she has to sit kind of funny and push a lot. You double check doses on the medicines; they're OK, and repeat the exam, which is unchanged.

OK, it's time to get more aggressive. You ask her to set up an appointment later that day with your dietician to review her food and fiber intake in detail, and to order some labs, and you have her increase the doses of her stool softeners and add a second medication as a laxative to increase the squeezing force of her gut wall. Recheck, two weeks. Sandra walks out, with her scripts for medication refills.

A quick phone call, now. Remember, as I've said before, the telephone is a crucial diagnostic instrument! This time, you call the orthopedist who had evaluated Sandra's back. He comes to the phone; he looks though his notes. He says, a pretty ordinary injury, with minimal changes on the X-ray that could mean a slipped disk, though honestly, many people have those, and it's hard to know if that's really causing her pain. He says her exam was OK, that he doesn't think there was any chance of a serious spine injury, but that he had planned to do an MRI if she didn't improve.

Flipping through, he says Sandra's been back to clinic a few times, and there's been a few phone calls, nothing serious, just med refills. And last time she said she thought she was starting to feel better. So he wasn't going to do any more imaging, and he figured everything was OK. The labs come back the next day; everything looked good. We checked her thyroid, we checked celiac antibodies, we checked a CBC and chemistries, all of that was normal.

Two more weeks go by, and Sandra has returned for follow up. This time, her face looks swollen, and she's talking oddly. It turns out she had been to the dentist and needed some cavities filled, or something,. So she has wadding in her cheek and her face is still half-numb. She says, "I love my dentist, but there's always something there he's got to do." Anyway, Sandra reports no change, no improvement. If anything, she says, her constipation is worse than ever. She saw the dietician. She says she's even eating bran muffins now, and she's trying to exercise, and she's taking her medicines and everything. There's her usual bottles, lined up. It looks like she's done everything she was supposed to do.

Today's exam remains normal, except she's talking kind of funny from the dental procedure. We do an especially careful exam of her back and reflexes and gait, and she seems fine, though she says her back is actually hurting more now. Her pain medicine bottles are mostly empty. She mentions that she lost the last prescription we had written, and she needed more pain medication because of the dental procedure, so that's why she's out of meds, so write for more refills.

Thinking about the worsening back pain and the constipation, we've really made zero progress with that. So we go ahead and order an MRI of her spine. Follow up, two weeks. One week later we get a call from the pharmacist; he just wanted to check. He's a little worried because the dentist had written for pain medicine, too, and you've written for a refill, and so has an orthopedist. And her rheumatologist, too.

What rheumatologist? You ask. It turns out there's a rheumatologist Sandra's been seeing. You ask the pharmacist to go through the medication refills that he's done. It's a lot of refills. They include your prescriptions for laxatives, as well as many refills for pain medicines from her multiple doctors and her dentist. You're starting to get a bit of a creepy feeling, now. A single prescription that should have lasted a month was filled from multiple doctors, and it looks like she's been taking four times the expected amount of painkillers. Well, at least four times; you only have information from this one pharmacy.

The MRI is done, and the results come back. She does have two discs with a small amount of herniation, but neither is pressing on any nerves. Discs like that could possibly be causing some pain, though they're seen incidentally in many people and probably don't cause any symptoms most of the time. There's no problem with the spinal cord itself. Sandra comes back for her two week recheck. She seems well. As usual, she has bottles lined up. She says the constipation is OK now; it's not better, but she says, "I guess it's just something I have to live with."

You ask about her back. She says it's the same-old, same-old, and you tell her about the normal lab work that came back. She thanks you for your kindness in trying to help. Then she asks for a refill on the pain medications. "Since your back is getting better," you say, "it's getting time to get off of these medicines. I think you're using too much of them." Well, the discussion goes on from there. Sandra's apologetic. She says she knows she shouldn't take them much, and she'll try to cut down, but she needs to have them for the bad times, especially at night.

You say, Sandra, look, I think all of these pain medicines are what's causing your constipation. I think we ought to have you seen by one of the addiction counselors at the pain center of the local hospital, and that so you can be safely weaned slowly down from these medicines. "Remember your daughter?" you say. "She's living with her aunt. If we can get you better, off of all these medicines, she can move back in with you, that would be great, right?"

Sandra is crying now; she's really bawling, and she's agreeing with everything you say. She needs to go to the hospital and get off the medicines, and thank you so much, doctor, and I'm going to do that as soon as I can. You give her one last, small refill of the pain medicine and make sure she knows how to get to the pain clinic, and you call over there to make sure they can take her, and you have everything set up for Sandra.

She says goodbye. She leaves, and you never see Sandra again. She doesn't keep her pain clinic appointment. You call the pharmacist, and he says that she just doesn't come there any more. "Of course," says the pharmacist, "she could just be going to a different pharmacy now. "And maybe," he says, "she's just got herself a new doctor."

This is a sad story, and unfortunately, it's the kind of thing that is happening all over the country, not only in Kentucky. Prescription drug abuse, or misuse, has become a common cause of disrupted lives, lost jobs, and death, striking every age, from teens through elderly adults. We are not, as a whole, doing a particularly good job in tracking prescriptions to identify those at risk, and we're doing a terrible job getting those people the addiction treatment they need.

There were all sorts of clues in Sandra's case. She came to see you in the first place because you were young and inexperienced. Remember, the first time you met, she even said that. Her back injury history was kind of vague, and her sustained discomfort was out of proportion to the injury, and really, was never clearly correlated with any imaging study. Somehow, her daughter had gone to live with another family member; I don't think that's typical, for a mom to send her own daughter away just because of a hurt back. And what had actually happened to Sandra's husband, the one that she said ran off years ago? It turns out, we learned later, that he was serving time in prison for buying and selling prescription painkillers.

And it's painkillers that are the most often abused prescriptions. It turns out that there are really only three medications that are commonly used to treat pain, or at least three groups of medications, and within each group they're all similar. The first group only contains one medicine, acetaminophen, or Tylenol. It's an effective pain medicine for mild to moderate pain, with minimal side effects when used correctly. It is not addictive.

The second group has many brands available over the counter too; it's the NSAIDs, or non-steroidal anti-inflammatory drugs. The most common ones in here are ibuprofen and aspirin. And there are many others that are available by prescription. They all work in a very similar way. They're also effective for mild-to-moderate pain and have no addiction potential. They're pretty safe. Occasionally, and more often with regular use, these kinds of drugs can cause GI upset.

The problem is that neither of these kinds of medicine, alone, is effective for the most severe pain. For the worst pains, the only effective medicines in general use are narcotics and narcotic derivatives. They're all essentially based on an extract of the poppy plant, the precursor to opium. These medications range from morphine to codeine, with many in between. The group also includes heroin, which is another opium derivative. They can all be used to effectively treat even the most severe pain, but all of them are potentially addictive when used inappropriately. When abused, they not only relieve pain, but they also get the user high.

So, for the many people who suffer from pain, especially chronic pain, narcotics are an essential tool for providing relief. One of the biggest obstacles for these patients are misunderstandings about the nature of drug tolerance, dependence, and addiction. This leads to the frequent under treatment of pain, which itself, ironically, can actually contribute to the development of addictive behaviors.

To help patients like Sandra, that is, to prevent, recognize, and treat addiction, we first have to make sure we understand what's happening physically and psychologically. Tolerance is a normal physiologic change, when the body adapts or seems to "get used to" a certain dose of a medication such as an opioid. By the way, many classes of drugs can induce tolerance, but many others do not. When tolerance develops, the drug becomes less effective at a given dose, and to get the desired effect, the dose will have to be increased. Tolerance is an inevitable, predictable phenomenon that will occur in anyone who regularly uses certain medications.

Dependence is different. In modern medical contexts, dependence refers to physical changes in the body as we adapt to regularly taking certain drugs. Biochemical changes take place, especially in the brain, as the body gets used to regular doses of these medications. And if the medication is stopped or reduced quickly, physical symptoms of withdrawal will take place. Symptoms of opiate or narcotic withdrawal can include sweatiness, agitation, aches, insomnia, cramping, diarrhea, nausea, and vomiting. These can be very unpleasant or severe, but are not life threatening.

Other kinds of medication can cause dependence and withdrawal symptoms, including steroids, antidepressants, anxiety medication, and some heart medicines, like beta blockers. So tolerance is one thing, the physical adaptation that makes medicines less effective at the same dose if they're taken long term. Dependence is different. That's defined by the occurrence of physical symptoms, or withdrawal, when a drug is stopped. But neither is the same as drug addiction.

Addiction, the way that doctors use the term, means psychological symptoms, including compulsive drug use and craving for drugs. People who are addicted to drugs will continue to seek and use the drug despite worsening physical, social, and mental harm. In a sense, while dependence refers to the physical symptoms of withdrawal, addiction refers to a maladaptive psychological need to consume a drug. This definition of addiction is also used in other contexts, such as people addicted to gambling, or sex, or internet use. People with addiction may or may not have physical dependencies and may or may not suffer from physical withdrawal symptoms, but they will crave and seek the addiction even at the expense of their own jobs or relationships, risking arrest and social isolation to satisfy their cravings.

Another term that's sometimes used is pseudoaddiction. This is seen only in people with chronic pain that is inadequately treated. These patients are desperate for effective pain relief and very fearful of worsening pain, so they watch the clock closely and may take steps that could be considered drug-seeking behaviors, like filling prescriptions early, or hoarding pills. The behaviors associated with pseudoaddiction stop completely when the pain itself is adequately treated. The key to treating pseudoaddiction and preventing it from developing into true addiction is in treating pain correctly. By the way, these terms—addiction and dependence—I've been stressing their medical definitions. In the common literature and lay press, the terms are often used interchangeably, which is unfortunate. There is an important difference.

So, do all chronic pain patients become addicted to opioids? No. In fact, most patients treated with narcotic painkillers will never have addictive symptoms. Now, most, if not all patients who use narcotics regularly will develop tolerance, physical dependence, and the potential for withdrawal, but that's different from the craving and compulsive drug-seeking seen with addiction. In one study of 24,000 patients with chronic pain treated with opioids, only seven developed addiction. Though it is possible, addiction is not a common problem among those treated for pain, and a fear of encouraging addiction should not prevent doctors from treating pain and relieving suffering.

If it's not common in chronic pain patients, who are the people who get addicted to opiates or who get addicted to other medications or other things? There certainly seems to be a genetic predisposition, though we don't know the exact contribution of genetics, it's true that some people seem to have a higher built-in risk for addiction than others. Beyond that, the most important factor in predicting addiction is the reason the drug is taken. People who take drugs to get high or avoid life, as opposed to people who take medication to treat pain or other medical problems, are much more likely to develop addiction.

Looking back at Sandra's case, there were some warning signs. She seemed to be doing some doctor shopping. It's not clear at all why she changed to our clinic in the first place, and we found out later that she was also seeing other doctors at the same time. There were reports of lost prescriptions, and she may have been using multiple pharmacies. Any of these could have had an innocent explanation, but the pattern of behavior, at least in retrospect, seems suggestive. Also, it's unclear exactly how that original back injury led to such significant pain. Her apparent addiction also caused her to stop working and led to her no longer living with her daughter. These kinds of negative life consequences are typical of true addiction.

Ironically, doctors are sometimes criticized from both sides of the issue. Doctor and hospital ratings stress how important it is for us to treat pain quickly and effectively, while at the same time, federal and state agencies monitor our prescribing habits and investigate doctors who seem to prescribe too many narcotics. Judging whether pain is real or exaggerated is very difficult. We don't have any kind of objective pain meter. Add to that the complexities of the modern American medical system, the multiple doctors and pharmacies, and it's very difficult to identify patients at risk for addiction, especially when they deliberately cover their tracks to hide drug-seeking behavior. This is not a good situation, and it's contributing to the suffering of both pain patients who need effective pain treatment, and to patients, families, and communities struggling with addiction.

Back to Sandra again. We've been focusing on addiction, but there are other side effects of the use of narcotics. One of them is constipation, which is what drove her to our clinic in the first place. Narcotics can also cause itching, vomiting and nausea, and dry mouth; they can also cause confusion, sleepiness, or dizziness, and it is not safe to drive while taking these medications. However, the most severe symptom, the worst side effect, is respiratory depression. Taking higher doses of any narcotic starts to blunt the automatic drive to breathe. The higher the dose, the slower the breathing, and at a high enough dose, breathing will stop. This is the cause of death in narcotic overdose. People seek higher and higher doses to satisfy their cravings, and eventually the dose is high enough to kill. At this point in the United States, there are more deaths from prescription opioids than from cocaine and heroin combined.

OK, ready for our next Grand Rounds? Coming up is the story of Joe, who is tired all the time. What the Dickens could be going on? We'll see if you can figure it out.

Dickens's Diagnosis
Lecture 15

Obesity contributes to more ill health, poor quality of life, and early death than smoking—yet we still don't have a good handle on the best ways to prevent or treat it. Obesity results when someone regularly takes in more calories than needed, but there is far more to the modern obesity epidemic than that. There seem to be neurohormonal and psychological factors, genetic influences, and changes in gut function related to bacterial colonization. Disentangling these factors to come up with comprehensive, workable, and effective ways to prevent and treat obesity is emerging as the health challenge of the 21st century.

Constantly Falling Asleep
- Joe is 55 years old, and he comes to our general medicine clinic with his wife. His chief complaint is: "I fall asleep all the time." Joe says he's not sure how it happens; he just kind of nods off, and someone has to wake him up.

- There are primary sleep disorders, such as narcolepsy, where control of sleep cycling is disrupted and sudden sleep can occur—especially right after an emotional outburst, such as crying or laughing.

- Or perhaps Joe is just tired; he's not getting enough sleep or enough quality sleep. His sleep could be interrupted by something like sleep **apnea** or restless legs syndrome, both of which can interfere with sleep quality.

- Or maybe he's on some kind of medicine that makes him drowsy. This could be a prescribed medicine, something over the counter, street drugs, or maybe he's consuming too much alcohol. Depression is also a possibility; it can present with excessive sleeping.

- Joe says that he has problems with feeling tired, headaches, shortness of breath with exercise, weight gain, and impotence. He also says that he has swollen feet. He denies smoking or drinking or any substance use; it looks like he hasn't taken any prescriptions or seen any doctors in years.

- On the physical exam, we've found that his resting heart rate is fast (a finding called **tachycardia**), his blood pressure is mildly elevated, and his heart is heaving against his chest. He also has pitting **edema** of his lower extremities, which means that he has puffy skin that you can press into pits.

- The finding of edema means that there is excessive fluid in the spaces between the cells—fluid that is essentially seeped out of the circulation and is just sitting there. This kind of fluid buildup usually occurs from disease of the kidneys, liver, or heart.

- Joe has several indications of heart disease, including edema (with no other explanation), and some kind of issue seems apparent with his lungs or breathing—his blood oxygen is low, and his blood carbon dioxide is high.

- We need more information about lungs and heart. A good test of both is a chest X-ray. On Joe's film, his lungs look fine, but his heart is enlarged. We've found that there is something going on with his heart, and his body isn't getting enough oxygen, and he's not effectively blowing off his carbon dioxide. Heart disease can make you tired, but falling asleep all the time is odd.

- Joe said that he gets enough hours of sleep, though he wakes up still tired. His wife says that he snores, gasps, mutters, snaps awake, and rolls over. In addition, Joe is overweight. His blood oxygen is low, and his blood carbon dioxide is high. Our diagnosis is that Joe has obstructive sleep apnea. And worse, he's now developed complications from that: **congestive heart failure** caused by chronic **hypoventilation**.

Obesity Hypoventilation Syndrome

- The modern name for the whole package of what Joe has is obesity hypoventilation syndrome, which was first described in the medical literature in 1956 in a case report that named it "Pickwickian syndrome."

- During sleep, Joe's upper airway flops closed, causing the snoring and gasping. During these events, blood oxygen falls and blood carbon dioxide rises—because, essentially, Joe stops breathing. He struggles, wakes, and gasps to normalize ventilation, but this is happening so often that his body has trouble compensating and normalizing his ventilation.

- Worse, over time, exposure to high CO_2 actually blunts the body's response to the CO_2; essentially, Joe has gotten somewhat used to these ventilatory pauses. In part, this may be from sleep disruption and exhaustion, though there are hormonal changes that occur, too.

- When lung tissue is underoxygenated, the blood flow to those parts of the lungs shuts down. That's normal physiology, and it makes sense: The body sort of shunts blood to areas of the lungs with more oxygen, and it does this by constricting blood flow to areas with less oxygen.

- If all of the lungs are underoxygenated, the blood vessels throughout both lungs constrict. But the blood has to get through, so the heart has to pump harder and harder. Like any muscle, the heart, when it exercises more, will hypertrophy, or grow larger. This actually diminishes the efficiency of how the heart muscle contracts, forcing the heart muscle itself to need more oxygen, which is becoming less available.

- Joe's tiredness is from sleep apnea, from frequent interruptions in sleep that are preventing him from getting good rest. His tiredness is compounded by chronic low oxygen and high CO_2, which have led to heart failure from what is called pulmonary hypertension—a high resistance to blood flow through the lungs, a physiological

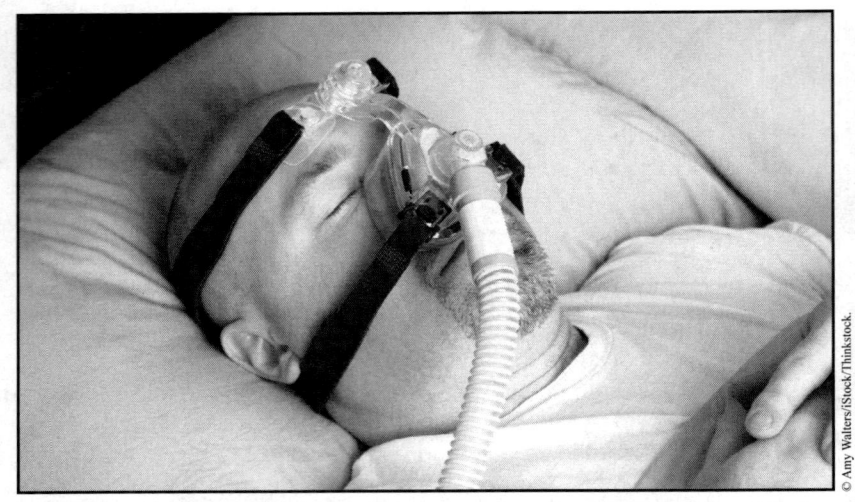

A sleep study, which involves hooking a patient up to several monitors while he or she sleeps, can be conducted to determine whether the patient experiences sleep apnea.

effect of chronic underventilation. The correct medical term is "hypoventilation," meaning basically breathing less than one should.

- There were a few other things on the review of systems that are also part of the obesity hypoventilation syndrome. These patients have frequent headaches, especially in the morning, perhaps related to poor sleep, poor ventilation, or both.

- Joe also reported a poor ability to exercise, because his heart is already working as hard as it can; if he tries to exercise, there is no cardiac reserve left to pick up the pace. His heart is beating rapidly, and his blood pressure is high—these are part of the neurohormonal response to heart failure, the body trying to get as much blood flow as possible out of a failing heart.

- Erectile dysfunction is also a common complaint of those with sleep apnea and sleep hypoventilation syndrome (as well as other men with heart failure from other reasons).

- The phrase "heart failure" does not mean that the heart has stopped working entirely; instead, it means that the heart's pumping power is decreased and that it is not delivering enough blood to the body tissues.

- Heart failure can be caused by coronary artery disease that leads to a heart attack, which kills some of the heart muscle; or it can be caused by a problem with a heart valve, so the blood doesn't flow efficiently in the direction it's supposed to; or it can be caused by problems with the working of the heart muscle itself, which can occur with severe thyroid disease or muscular dystrophy. Heart failure can also occur because of a problem with the heart rhythm.

- Whatever the cause of heart failure, some of the symptoms that result are the same. These include exercise intolerance—an inability to stay physically active—plus fluid and water retention. That's the edema in Joe's legs.

- The water retention can also occur in the abdomen and lungs— what's called congestive heart failure. There is often also a rapid or irregular heartbeat, dizziness, fatigue, and weakness. Congestive heart failure is the leading cause of hospitalization in the United States among patients older than 65 and is one of the most common causes of death.

- To confirm Joe's diagnosis, a sleep study can be done; although in this case, the history and physical are so clear that it might not be necessary. A sleep study entails having a patient sleep while hooked up to several monitors that can detect via brain waves what part of the sleep cycle a person is in.

- Simultaneously, monitors check blood oxygen levels; plus, monitors on the chest wall can detect if a person is making a respiratory effort. Another sensor can detect airflow through the nose or mouth, and if necessary, yet another sensor can even measure the carbon dioxide in the breath.

- Joe's sleep study confirmed that he has many, many complete apneas at night, during which his blood oxygen falls dramatically. During some of the apneas, he struggles to breathe; during others, he doesn't even try.

- Joe he has a mixed picture of both obstructive apnea (when the airway closes up) and what's called central apnea, where the brain isn't even driving breaths. This is typical of Pickwickian syndrome. The sleep study also confirmed that he does not have narcolepsy.

Treatment: Weight Loss
- The treatment of obesity hypoventilation syndrome starts with weight loss. This is not easy to do, and often patients are not successful in losing weight. However, if weight can be lost, sometimes even a small percentage, there can be a big improvement in sleep quality and ventilation.

- For a patient like Joe, who is already in heart failure, weight loss is still a goal, but more aggressive therapy would be started right away. This would include ventilatory assistance during sleep, using a mask device that can provide positive pressure—a sort of push on the air to keep the airway open and make sure that there is airflow both in and out. The device also makes sure that enough breaths are taken each minute to ensure adequate ventilation.

- Joe also needs treatment for his heart failure. This may include diuretic medications to increase urine output and decrease retained fluid; it may also include medicines to get the heart to pump harder or more efficiently, plus medication to control Joe's blood pressure.

- If treatment of his obesity hypoventilation syndrome itself is successful, his heart can recover, and he may not continue to need these heart medicines, but for now, there isn't time to wait and see.

- The most aggressive therapy to help patients like Joe lose weight is bariatric surgery, which includes methods like stomach stapling or intestinal bypass to decrease the amount of food he can eat or decrease the number of calories that he can absorb.

- In Joe's condition, with heart failure, this kind of surgery is too risky, but perhaps with some improvement he may be able to tolerate a bariatric procedure. Improvements in bariatric techniques are making the surgery less risky, but they're still not suitable for patients like Joe.

- Obesity can lead to heart failure. Obesity also contributes to orthopedic problems like bad knees and hips, high blood pressure, coronary artery disease, some cancers, cholesterol disorders, stroke, liver and gallbladder disease, etc.

Important Terms

apnea: Cessation of breathing.

congestive heart failure: Insufficient output of blood from the heart, leading to fluid accumulation.

edema: Swelling, typically of an extremity.

hypoventilation: Insufficient breathing, resulting specifically in increased carbon dioxide in the blood.

tachycardia: Fast heart rate.

Suggested Reading

Chokroverty, *Questions and Answers about Sleep Apnea*.

Dickens, *The Pickwick Papers*.

Questions to Consider

1. What are the health consequences of poor or inadequate sleep?

2. The biggest historical health challenges have been poor nutrition, sanitation, and infectious diseases. What are the new challenges for the 21st century?

Dickens's Diagnosis
Lecture 15—Transcript

We've talked about doctors and writers, both being keen observers of human nature. Here's a case where a writer beat the doctors to a diagnosis by over a hundred years! Charles Dickens had little formal education in literature, writing, or medicine. His first novel, The Pickwick Papers, was published in 1837. It included a supporting character, Joe, who is described as greatly overweight, continuously consuming vast quantities of food. Joe falls asleep many times throughout the day, in any situation. Over 100 years later, in 1956, a medical report of a similar case was published. These medical authors suggested a literary name for their "new" condition, acknowledging that Dickens had described it a century earlier.

So Joe is our patient today, a modern Joe, but one based on Dickens's character. He's 55 years old, and he comes to our general medicine clinic with his wife. His chief complaint is: "I fall asleep all the time." Joe explains that his wife made him come in, because she says it's not normal. He falls asleep too much. Sometimes, Joe says, he's kind of laughing now, he even falls asleep while his wife is talking! That never goes over well. He's fallen asleep at work more than once, and his coworkers kind of cover for him and wake him up quickly so he doesn't get in trouble. But his wife is concerned that he might fall asleep while driving or he might lose his job, so she made him come in.

"What do you mean," you ask, "you fall asleep? Just suddenly?" Joe says he's not sure how it happens, he just kind of nods off, and someone has to wake him up. OK, let's step back and think about this problem. We have some kind of sudden falling asleep, or at least some kind of sudden loss of consciousness. What could it be?

My first thought, is this really sleep? I mean, could Joe be having some kind of seizure or faint, or some other kind of phenomenon that causes a sudden loss of consciousness? You know, at first blush, probably not. Seizures are a brain phenomenon, a sudden electrical storm of sorts. They're like a hard reset on a computer. Seizures that affect enough of the brain to cause a loss of consciousness will usually be more dramatic than this, and certainly, a wife or coworker wouldn't be able to kind of wake him up quickly from a seizure. Likewise, a loss of consciousness from a faint, you couldn't instantly wake someone up from that. We'll want to ask some clarifying questions, but really, so far Joe's case really is sounding like someone who just falls asleep a lot.

So, if it is sleep, where do we go from here? There are primary sleep disorders, like narcolepsy, where control of sleep cycling is disrupted, and sudden sleep can occur, especially right after an emotional outburst, crying or laughing, or something like that. Or, perhaps Joe is just tired; he's not getting enough sleep or enough quality sleep. His sleep could be interrupted by something like sleep apnea, or restless legs syndrome, both of which can interfere with sleep quality. Or maybe Joe's on some kind of medicine that makes him drowsy. This could be prescribed medicine or something over the counter, or street drugs, or maybe he's consuming too much alcohol. Depression is also a possibility; we've run across that diagnosis before, and we know depression can present with excessive sleeping.

That's enough to get started. Let's hear more of Joe's story. We glance up at Joe, over the paper chart. We see that he's leaned back in his chair, and it looks like he's fast asleep! Joe, Joe, you ask. Then a little louder. Joe! Then his wife swats his arm. He wakes up quickly, with a bit of a start, and says, "Sorry doc." He rubs his eyes, and Joe continues his story.

He says, as far back as he can remember, he has felt tired a lot. He doesn't have a lot of energy for exercising, and actually, he thinks when he does try to exercise he quickly gets out of breath. And Joe says, he knows he should exercise more; he's patting his big belly, but you know, it's hard to do that. You ask about sleep habits in detail. Joe goes to bed at 10, he says he quickly falls asleep, and he sleeps through until the morning at 6:00; that's eight hours, which should be enough. He says he think he sleeps well, but his wife complains that he snores.

Joe says, even when he wakes up in the morning, he doesn't feel rested, but it's always been like that. He often wakes up with a headache, too. He denies any other symptoms or any change in these symptoms lately. Really, this tiredness, this falling asleep thing, he thinks it's been going on for years.

You ask a few specific questions about narcolepsy, and it doesn't look like that's likely. Many people with narcolepsy have cataplexy—a sudden onset of sleep with emotional outbursts, And many have so-called sleep paralysis, with a prolonged feeling of being unable to move upon first awakening. Joes says, no, he doesn't have these kinds of symptoms. However, some people with narcolepsy really only complain of excessive sleepiness and napping, so we may need to investigate further to make sure Joe definitely doesn't have narcolepsy, that would require a sleep study.

You look down through the printed list he completed in the waiting room; that's his review of symptoms, with the little check boxes, and there are a lot of positives. Let me take a moment for a quick medical lingo explanation. That word, positive, in the medical discussion, that means that a symptom or finding is present. Negative means absent. So, in medical parlance, positive doesn't always mean good. A positive test for cancer is not good news.

So, back to Joe. He's checked off as positive that he has problems with feeling tired, with headaches, with shortness of breath with exercise, with weight gain, and with impotence; he also says that he sometimes has swollen feet. Joe denies smoking or drinking or any substance abuse, It looks like he hasn't taken any prescriptions or seen any doctors in years. The family history isn't helpful. Joe lives with his wife, and they have two children who have moved away to college. He works in an office as a customer sales rep, mostly desk work and answering phone calls.

Time for the physical exam. Joe is a big guy, 6' 2", 280 pounds. He's Caucasian, though he looks kind of ruddy, with a reddish kind of complexion. He's joking; he's engaged, and that makes you think that depression really is unlikely. His heart rate is 92; blood pressure 134/88; respirations 22; and temperature normal. HEENT exam is normal. His chest wall, when you go to listen to his heart, you can feel it beating very strongly against his chest; that's called a ventricular heave, and it can be a sign of an enlarged, overly muscular heart. Joe has no murmurs.

His lungs are clear, and abdominal exam is normal. You cannot feel a liver or a spleen, though you think to yourself, in an individual who is overweight like this, it can be difficult to palpate these organs even if they were enlarged.

His pulses are strong. When you get down to examine his legs and his feet, you notice that, as he said, his feet are kind of swollen, with puffy skin over his feet and up towards his ankles. You can push the skin down in a pit with your finger. This finding is called pitting edema. The neurologic exam is normal; Joe seems alert, well, and comfortable during the exam.

OK, we have a lot going on here, and probably more than first meets the eye. Let's review a problem list, the main issues that have come to our attention. We have excessive sleepiness, a decreased ability to exercise, fatigue; plus, on the physical exam, we've found that his resting heart rate is fast, that's a finding called tachycardia. His blood pressure is mildly elevated, and his heart is heaving against his chest. He also has pitting edema of his lower extremities. So that's a long list to juggle all in your head at once.

One strategy to tackle a list like this is to start with one of the problems that's simpler, maybe one that doesn't have a long list of possible causes. You think about just one problem; think about what could be causing it, and then see if any of those explanations could fit some of the other issues on the longer problem list.

Let me give you an example. Joe has a fast heart rate, but that's not a good starting point. The list of causes of fast heart rate is huge, from genuine heart disease, to anemia, anxiety, dehydration, thyroid disease, fever, infections, all sorts of things. So instead of starting with a fast heart rate, let's think about that pitting edema. What could cause puffy skin that you can press into pit shapes? As you'll see, the differential diagnosis of edema is smaller and more manageable to think through. So starting with causes of edema, I'll bet we'll be able to work our way back to an explanation that covers everything.

So, edema. The finding of edema means that there is excessive fluid in the spaces between the cells—fluid that's kind of seeped out of the circulation, and it's just sitting there. Without belaboring the physiology too much, this kind of fluid buildup usually occurs from disease of the kidneys, liver, or heart. Let's see which one seems most likely in our patient.

Is it kidney disease? The way kidney disease causes edema is when the kidneys start spilling out protein into the urine. Normally, blood proteins are filtered out of the urine, and kept in the body; but some kidney diseases affect this function, leading to excessive protein loss in the urine. Once that occurs, blood protein levels drop. And it is the blood proteins that effectively hold water in the blood through a process called osmotic pressure. You can think of the protein as a sponge, holding on to water; with less protein in the blood, more water will spill out between the cells, causing edema. Could Joe have kidney disease? Maybe, and kidney disease can cause high blood pressure. So let's keep that in mind.

Liver disease can also cause edema. Those blood proteins that hold the water, they are made in the liver, so once that liver protein synthetic function is affected, there will be less blood proteins to do many jobs, one of which is to hold water in the circulation. Patients with liver disease can develop edema of the extremities, like Joe has. But there are no other findings to suggest liver disease; there's no jaundice, no abdominal swelling or pain, and there's really nothing in the histories to suggest a cause of liver disease, such as excessive alcohol consumption. Still, we'll be looking for any evidence of liver problems in our further evaluation.

Finally, the heart. Heart disease, and in particular, a kind of heart disease called congestive heart failure, will cause edema. In heart failure, the heart does not deliver enough blood to the body tissues. The kidneys, sensing decreased blood flow, will hold onto water and salts, thinking that the body is in effect dehydrated—that there is insufficient blood. In fact, there is plenty of blood, but in heart failure the kidneys are fooled because blood is not flowing effectively. So the kidney holds on to our water and salt, mistakenly trying to fight the apparent decrease in body fluid. The net effect is excessive retention of water and salt, and that extra fluid becomes edema, not only edema in the legs, but often extra fluid in the lungs, causing shortness of breath and exercise intolerance, and extra fluid in the abdominal cavity as well; that's called ascites. We might not be able to appreciate ascites because of Joe's obesity. But he did complain of shortness of breath and an inability to exercise. These symptoms, like the edema, could be caused by congestive heart failure.

So does Joe have heart disease? There were some other clues. He has a fast heart rate and hypertension, and he has that ventricular heave, that big lift feeling over his chest with each heart beat. Heart disease, and congestive heart failure in particular, could explain many of Joe's findings. Can we fit that in with the bigger picture here, the falling asleep all the time? That's the concern that brought him to the doctor? I think we can, but first, let's check on our lab and other data to make sure we're headed down the right road. We need to close the door on some of these other mentioned diagnoses that are still possibilities.

Let's start with blood tests. A CBC, complete blood count, has a normal white cell count and platelets, but the measurement of his red cells is actually elevated above normal. We've seen anemia, that's a low red cell count, before, but this is kind of the opposite thing, a high red cell count; that's, called polycythemia. Remember the physical exam, when I mentioned that Joe's complexion was kind of red or ruddy looking. Now we know why. He has a high red blood cell count. Can this fit into what we already know?

There aren't a lot of causes of a high red cell count. One of them is a disease like polycythemia vera, which is, in a way, similar to cancer, where there is poor regulation of the proliferation of red cells. The marrow churns out too many of them. Also, any condition that causes chronic low oxygen will trigger the body to increase the red cell count to compensate. This takes place via a hormone called erythropoetin, produced in the kidneys. Examples of this include people who smoke, or people who live at high altitudes, or lung or heart conditions that decrease the amount of oxygen in the blood. There's that mention of heart disease, again. Are we getting closer to a diagnosis?

Let's check blood chemistries. The tests of kidney function and liver tests are completely normal. Remember, we had said edema can be caused by liver, kidney, or heart disease, though it's now looking like we can forget about the liver and kidneys. The urinalysis is also normal; there's more evidence that Joe's kidneys are healthy. But there was one result from the chemistries that stood out, a measurement of serum bicarbonate was high. OK, understanding that, I promise, will go a long way towards understanding what's going on with our patient.

Normally, there is a balance between acid and base in our bodies, and mechanisms are in place to keep your blood pH at pretty much exactly 7.4.

Sure enough, we do another test called an arterial blood gas; a sample of arterial blood is taken to quantify pH, oxygen, and carbon dioxide. The blood pH is normal, 7.4. But the blood CO_2, the carbon dioxide, is very high. That blood carbon dioxide acts as an acid. So to compensate and to make sure that the pH stays normal, the body is holding onto extra bicarb; that's a base. The blood bicarb is high to compensate for high CO_2. By the way, the blood oxygen level was a little bit lower than expected, too. Low blood oxygen, the body compensates for that by making more red cells, and Joe's doing that. High blood carbon dioxide, the body compensates by retaining bicarb to keep the pH normal.

OK, I know we have a lot of diagnostic plates spinning in the air, a lot is going on here. Joe has several indications of heart disease, including edema, with, really, no other explanation, and now some kind of issue seems apparent with his lungs or breathing. His blood oxygen is low, and his blood carbon dioxide is high. Keep those facts in mind; that's what to focus on.

How to proceed? We need more information about lungs and heart. A good test of both is a chest X-ray. On Joe's film, his lungs look fine. There's no pneumonia; there's no collapsed lung or anything like that. As far as we can see, his lung tissue itself seems fine. But his heart on the X-ray, it's enlarged. The silhouette we see of his heart on the film, it's too big.

Let's think back to the history, the physical. Let's think back to what we already know. And especially, and you knew I was going to bring this up again, the chief complaint. Why did Joe come here today? We've found there is something going on with his heart, and his body isn't getting enough oxygen, and he's not effectively blowing off his carbon dioxide, but really, why Joe came to see us was his chief complaint, "I fall asleep all the time." Now, heart disease can make you tired, sure, but falling asleep all the time, Joe even fell asleep during our interview. That's kind of odd, isn't it?

Joe said he gets enough hours of sleep, though he wakes up still tired. But what was that his wife said; he snores. You head back into the exam room to talk to Joe and his wife. What do you mean, you ask, he snores? How much snoring? Oh, his wife, Mrs. Joe, she says, you wouldn't believe it. He snores and gasps and mutters and snaps awake, and he rolls over, and it's a huge amount of noise over there on his side of the bed.

Joe is a big guy, remember, quite overweight. And now we know there are gasps and pauses in his breathing, all night long. And his blood oxygen is low, and his blood carbon dioxide is high. We have our diagnosis. Joe has obstructive sleep apnea. And worse, he's now developed complications from that—congestive heart failure caused by chronic hypoventilation. The modern name for this, the whole package, is the obesity hypoventilation syndrome. It was first described in the medical literature in 1956 in a case report, which named it Pickwickian syndrome, after the character Joe in Dickens's *The Posthumous Papers of the Pickwick Club*, or *The Pickwick Papers*.

Let's go back through the physiology. During sleep, Joe's upper airway flops closed. That causes the snoring and gasping. During these events, blood oxygen falls and blood carbon dioxide rises, because, essentially, Joe just stops breathing. He struggles, he wakes, and he gasps to normalize ventilation, but this is happening so often, that his body has trouble compensating and normalizing his ventilation. Worse, over time, exposure to high CO_2 actually blunts the body's response to that CO_2. Essentially, Joe has gotten somewhat used to these ventilatory pauses. In part, this may be from sleep disruption and exhaustion, though there are hormonal changes that occur too. So he has these events when he stops breathing, and his body is kind of getting used to them, and his body is kind of getting used to high CO_2. Compensatory mechanisms, like holding onto bicarb and making more red cells are kicking in.

But there's more physiology here that starts to go wrong, and it concerns the heart and the lungs. When lung tissue is under oxygenated, the blood flow to those parts of the lungs shuts down. That's normal physiology, and it makes sense. The body sort of shunts blood to area of the lungs with more oxygen, and it does this by constricting blood flow to areas with less oxygen. But what happens if all of the lungs are under oxygenated? The blood vessels throughout both lungs constrict. But the blood has to get through, so the heart has to pump harder and harder. Like any muscle, the heart, when it exercises more, will hypertrophy, or grow larger. This actually diminishes the efficiency of how the heart muscle contracts, forcing the heart muscle itself to need more oxygen, which is becoming less available. You can see, we're heading into trouble here.

Joe's tiredness is from sleep apnea, from frequent interruptions in sleep that are preventing him from getting good rest. His tiredness is compounded by chronic low oxygen and high CO_2, which have led to heart failure from what is called pulmonary hypertension, that high resistance to blood flow through the lungs; that's a physiologic effect of chronic under ventilation. The correct medical term, we've used that word before, is hypoventilation, meaning basically breathing less than one should.

There were a few other things on the review of systems which are also part of the obesity hypoventilation, or Pickwickian, syndrome. These patients have frequent headaches, especially in the morning, perhaps related to poor sleep, poor ventilation, or maybe both. Joe also reported a poor ability to exercise, because his heart is already working as hard as it can. If he tries to exercise, there is no cardiac reserve left to pick up the pace. His heart is beating rapidly; his blood pressure is high. These are part of the neurohormonal response to heart failure. The body trying to get as much blood flow as possible out of a failing heart. Erectile dysfunction is also a common complaint of those with sleep apnea and sleep hypoventilation syndrome, as well as other men who have heart failure for other reasons.

Let's go back to that phrase—heart failure. It's a term that doctors use that might not mean what people think it means. It does not mean that the heart has stopped working entirely. It means that the heart's pumping power is decreased and that it is not delivering enough blood to the tissues. It can be caused by coronary artery disease that leads to a heart attack that kills some of the heart muscle. Or, it can be caused by a problem with a heart valve, so the blood doesn't flow efficiently in the direction it's supposed to; or heart failure can be caused by problems with the working of the heart muscle itself. This can occur with severe thyroid disease or muscular dystrophy. Heart failure can also occur because of a problem with the heart rhythm.

In any case, whatever the cause of heart failure, some of the symptoms that result are the same. These include exercise intolerance, that's an inability to stay physically active, plus fluid and water retention. That's the edema we saw in Joe's legs. The water retention can also occur in the abdomen and lungs, and that's what's called congestive heart failure. There is often also a rapid or irregular heartbeat, dizziness, fatigue, and weakness. Congestive heart failure, abbreviated CHF, is the leading cause of hospitalization in the U.S. among patients older than 65, and it's one of the most common causes of death.

To confirm Joe's diagnosis, a sleep study can be done. Though, honestly, in this case, the history and physical are so clear that I'm not entirely sure it's necessary. A sleep study entails having a patient sleep while hooked up to several monitors. These can detect via brain waves what part of the sleep cycle a person is in. Simultaneously, monitors check blood oxygen levels, plus monitors on the chest wall can detect if a person is making an effort to breathe. Another sensor can detect airflow through the nose or the mouth, and if necessary, yet another sensor can even measure the carbon dioxide in the exhaled breath.

Joe's sleep study confirmed that he has many, many complete apneas at night, during which his blood oxygen falls dramatically. During some of the apneas, he struggles to breathe; during others, Joe doesn't even try. So he has a mixed picture of both obstructive apnea, when the airway closes up, and what's called central apnea, where the brain isn't even driving breaths. This is typical of Pickwickian syndrome. By the way, the sleep study also confirmed that Joe does not have narcolepsy.

The treatment of the obesity hypoventilation syndrome starts with weight loss. This is not easy to do, and often patients are not successful in losing the weight. But, if weight can be lost, sometimes even a small percentage, there can be a big improvement in sleep quality and ventilation. For a patient like Joe, who is already in heart failure, weight loss is still a goal, but we'll start more aggressive therapy right away. This will include ventilatory assistance during sleep, using a mask device that can provide positive pressure; that's a sort of push on the air to keep the airway open and to make sure there is airflow both in and out. The device also makes sure that enough breaths are taken each minute to ensure adequate ventilation.

Joe also needs treatment for his heart failure. This may include diuretic medicines to increase urine output and decrease retained fluid; it may also include medicines to get the heart to pump harder or more efficiently, plus, medication to control Joe's blood pressure. If treatment of his obesity hypoventilation syndrome itself is successful, his heart can recover, and he may not continue to need these heart medicines, but for now, I don't think there is time to wait and see.

The most aggressive therapy to help patients like Joe lose weight is bariatric surgery, which includes methods like stomach stapling or intestinal bypass to decrease the amount of food he can eat, or, decrease the amount of calories that he can absorb. In Joe's condition, now, with heart failure, this kind of surgery is just too risky, but perhaps with some improvement he may be able to tolerate a bariatric procedure later. Improvements in bariatric techniques are making the surgery less risky, but they're still not suitable for patients like Joe.

We've discussed obesity before, while talking about type II diabetes. Now we know it can also lead to heart failure. Obesity also contributes to orthopedic problems, like bad knees and hips, high blood pressure, coronary artery disease, some cancers, cholesterol disorders, stroke, liver and gall bladder disease; the list goes on and on. At this point, obesity contributes to more ill health, poor quality of life, and early death than smoking.

Yet we still don't have a good handle on the best ways to prevent or treat obesity. Certainly, overeating plays some role, as does decreased physical activity. We know that obesity results when someone regularly takes in more calories than needed. But there is far more to the modern obesity epidemic than that. There seem to be neurohormonal and psychologic factors, genetic influences, and changes in gut function, perhaps related to bacterial colonization. We know that factors in early life, even influences on the developing fetus before we're born, contribute to obesity risk. Something as simple as a lack of sleep seems to be another risk factor, though we don't understand why. Disentangling these factors to come up with a comprehensive, workable, and effective way to prevent and treat obesity is emerging as the health challenge of the 21st century.

Our next case is a much younger patient, a four month old. We're in the ED; the parents are scared, and we're pretty scared too. See you next time.

Shaking Sammi
Lecture 16

The case in this lecture illustrates one way that medical cases proceed: A logical chain develops from a chief complaint, step by step, to a diagnosis and treatment plan. One question, correctly answered, leads to another, and eventually, the last question gives us our final answer. But that's not always the way it works. Real medical cases sometimes have blind alleys and distractions and, frankly, misleading clues that lead to a twisted medical journey. And, sometimes, real patients have multiple diagnoses—sometimes related, sometimes unrelated—that contribute to their symptoms. Remember to keep an open mind, and pay attention to details.

A Shaking Infant

- On a snowy winter night in Boston, a four-month-old African American girl named Samantha is brought to the emergency department, and the chief complaint, as written on a form by the parents, is: "She's shaking; is something wrong?"

- Samantha, or Sammi, has been healthy. She's been nursing well and growing well. But over the last three days, she's having periods of time when she seems to either go stiff or kind of shake. They saw their family physician earlier today, but she didn't see an episode and thought maybe the baby was having some reflux. Worried, the parents brought her to the emergency department.

- This could be a seizure. Babies are actually a high-risk group for seizures, because there can be brain malformations or metabolic problems that could just be coming to light. Babies are also the highest-risk group for brain infections like meningitis.

- Or maybe it's not really a seizure. There are several neurological symptoms that can kind of mimic seizures, at least at first. For example, sleep myoclonus is the name for those few jerking movements that many people have as they fall asleep. Another common benign, normal movement is a shuddering spell, which looks like a quick sort of trembling movement.

- Or this could be something not neurological at all, such as reflux. All babies spit up, but some find it painful. Occasionally, we will see a baby with reflux from the stomach up into the throat who arches and stiffens, looking in many ways like a seizure. This is called Sandifer's syndrome.

- Or, maybe, this will turn out to be nothing at all—or nothing that has a name. Babies will sometimes move in kind of weird ways. Odd movements, including some trembling or shaking or jerking, are just something that babies sometimes do.

- Sammi's parents agree that the shaking or funny movement she does sort of comes out of nowhere. It can happen at any time. The shaking lasts about three or four minutes, and then it stops.

- The family history doesn't add much. There are no health problems reported in the parents; there's no family history of **epilepsy** or seizures or movement disorders. Her vital signs are normal, including temperature, pulse, respirations, and blood pressure.

- While examining her, you notice that both of her hands start rhythmically trembling or jerking upward. To determine whether this is a seizure, we'll reassess how she looks overall. Her color is good, and she's not having any trouble breathing—but when we try to engage her eyes, they have kind of rolled up and aren't looking at anything. Her attention is no longer engaged with her environment.

- If you think a baby, or anyone else, may be having a seizure, gently hold or touch the extremity that's shaking. Normal baby trembling stops with a gentle touch. Sammi's shaking does not stop when you touch and hold her hands. This is a seizure. We'll have to figure out why, and what we ought to do about it, but first, it's time for first aid and stabilization.

- When someone—anyone—is having a seizure, first let them lie down so that the head is at the same level as the heart. This is the same thing you do when someone faints or collapses, to maximize blood flow to the brain. Loosen any tight clothing. Glance at your watch so that you know how long this might go on.

- Don't put things in people's mouths. There is a myth that people might swallow their tongue during a seizure and that somehow you need to prevent that with a spoon or something. That's just false; it doesn't even make anatomic sense. Putting a spoon or anything in someone's mouth may cause gagging and vomiting, which would be very bad during a seizure.

- In babies especially, seizures are often caused by metabolic conditions, including low blood sugar, low calcium, or low sodium or high sodium. Also, any kind of brain injury or problem can cause seizures. Fevers of any cause can sometimes trigger seizures in young children. Another cause is trauma. Furthermore, a large proportion of seizures remain unexplained, probably 25 to 30 percent in babies.

- The results of Sammi's blood tests show that her blood calcium is very, very low; normal would be from about 9 to 11, and Sammi's is 6.5. Such a low level can cause seizures.

Low Vitamin D

- Calcium is essential for life and for growth, and there are elaborate and interconnected mechanisms for ensuring that the right amount of calcium is absorbed and maintained in the body.

- Ingested calcium is actively taken up by cells in the small intestine and transported within these cells by a specific calcium-binding protein. That protein acts as a little carrier, and the more of these proteins there are in each absorptive cell, the more calcium will make its way from the gut into the body.

- The amount of these carrier proteins produced in each cell is regulated by vitamin D. Even if there is plenty of calcium in the diet, if there is not enough activated vitamin D, the gut will not efficiently absorb calcium.

- Vitamin D itself comes from two sources: It can be ingested as part of the diet, or the human body can essentially manufacture it in skin cells when exposed to sunlight. Natural sources of vitamin D are actually very, very scarce; vitamin D can be found naturally in fish and fish liver, some in beef liver, and perhaps a small amount in eggs and mushrooms.

- Many foods are fortified with vitamin D—that is, vitamin D has been added—including milk, commercial baby formulas, some juices, and some breakfast cereals. Dairy products other than milk are not typically fortified with vitamin D.

- Babies don't get much liver in their diets, and Sammi was relying on mother's milk, which, like unfortified cow's milk, has almost zero natural vitamin D. In this case, Sammi probably can't get enough vitamin D from sunlight exposure. Children with darker skin need longer sunlight exposures to make the same amount of vitamin D as Caucasian children.

- Sammi had all of the pieces in place to put her at risk for low vitamin D: She has dark skin; it is winter (so there is less daylight and less time spent outside); and she is fed exclusively on breast milk, which has no vitamin D. She is also four months old, and by then, babies have often used up their stored vitamin D from birth.

- To confirm our diagnosis, we draw a vitamin D level (it's actually measured as 25-hydroxy vitamin D, which is a marker for the most active form). We expect a level of 30 to 35 to be sufficient. Hers is 3.

- Over the next few days, Sammi is continued on first IV then an oral calcium supplement, plus a big oral dose of vitamin D. She has no further seizures, and she is sent home to continue

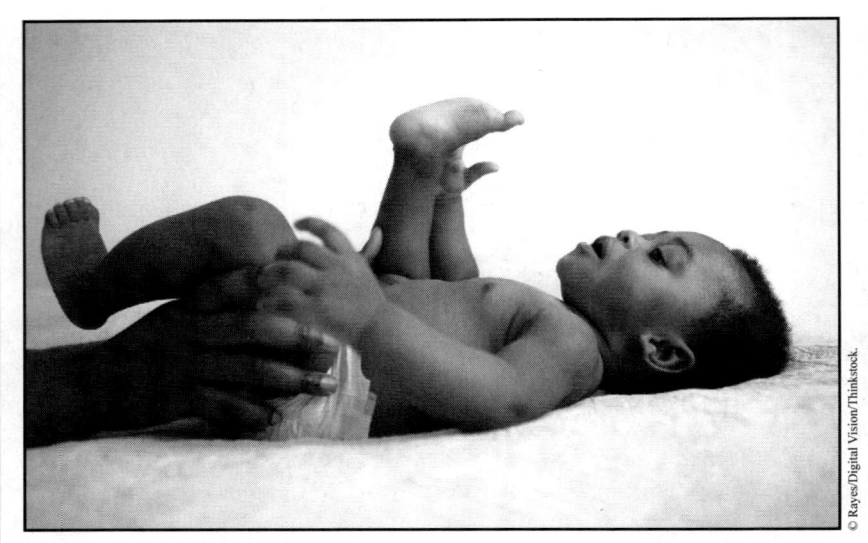

Breast milk does not contain vitamin D, so babies who are breast-fed are at a higher risk for having low levels of vitamin D.

nursing, with supplemental vitamin D. She was actually a little low in iron on other lab studies, so it was suggested that she start some complementary foods, including iron-rich meats and fortified cereals.

- Sammi will probably not suffer any long-term effects from this. Her seizures were brief, and she probably only had them a few days. Short and infrequent seizures do not cause brain damage (though any seizures should be investigated and prevented when possible). Keeping Sammi on a diet with adequate vitamin D and calcium should ensure that there are no further seizures and that her bones develop normally.

- Just about every pediatrician recommends nursing as the best nutrition for most babies, unless there is a medical or other reason for choosing formula. Human milk is a great source of nutrition: It's easy to digest, it's cheap, and it provides unique immune benefits.

- However, human milk isn't perfect; it is not a sufficient source of vitamin D. That's why it's recommended that exclusively nursing babies begin an oral vitamin D supplement at birth and continue it until they're consuming vitamin D–enriched foods, milk, or formula.

- This recommendation is especially important for babies with the following risk factors: dark skin, wintertime, not spending much time outside, and living in cooler climates. It's also crucial for babies born preterm, because they've had less chance to absorb calcium and vitamin D from their mother.

- Calcium is an interesting molecule, and it's essential for many life functions. Along with phosphorus, it makes up the mineral matrix of bones, so prolonged vitamin D deficiency can cause rickets in children. The symptoms of rickets can include delayed growth, bone pain, and muscle weakness along with skeletal deformities like bowed legs.

- Adults don't develop rickets because their bones aren't growing, but if they are deficient in vitamin D or calcium, they can have decreased mineral density, leading to osteoporosis and fractures. Calcium is also essential for normal muscle functioning, clotting of the blood, normal heart contraction and rhythms, and normal functioning of nerve cells and the brain.

- The control of calcium levels is actually fairly complicated. Vitamin D has to be activated by metabolism in the kidney and liver, and that step of activation itself is regulated by hormones from the parathyroid gland. Parathyroid hormone along with vitamin D and another hormone, calcitonin, regulate the uptake of calcium from cells that both build and repair bone; they also influence the amount of calcium excreted into the urine. There are multiple overlapping feedback loops that are all in place to keep calcium levels controlled in a very narrow range.

- The role of vitamin D goes far beyond calcium metabolism and bone health. Vitamin D modulates cell growth, regulates neuromuscular and immune function, and helps control inflammation. The exact functioning of vitamin D, and optimal levels of intake for health, are active areas of current research.

Important Term

epilepsy: A neurologic disorder characterized by recurrent seizures.

Suggested Reading

Hochberg, *Vitamin D and Rickets*.

Pediatrics, http://pediatrics.aappublications.org/content/122/5/1142.full.

Questions to Consider

1. What are the advantages—and disadvantages—of breastfeeding?

2. What sorts of things does a baby do that tells a doctor that his or her brain is normal?

Shaking Sammi
Lecture 16—Transcript

Today's presentation isn't common—this will be a bit of a brain stretch. But we've made it this far, and you've learned a lot, so let's see how you do. Here's your hint. Risk factors for what's about to happen to our patient include being born in the winter and growing up far from the equator.

We're working an ED shift tonight, which means, well, anything can happen. It's a snowy night in Boston, and we're hoping the weather keeps some of the less severe emergencies away. Our next patient is ready to be seen in the walk-in side—that's where those less severe emergency patients end up, at least as judged by the triage nurse. That's one drawback to seeking care at an ED. It is not first come, first served. The sickest, most-likely-to-die patients go to the front of the line, and patients judged to be less sick will have to wait longer. Unfortunately, sometimes that means initial triage misses something important.

Anyway, here we go. Let's take a look at the intake form. We have a four-month-old little African-American girl named Samantha, and the form here has the chief complaint posed as a question written by the parents, They've written, "She's shaking. Is something wrong?" We head in, and there's a little girl sitting in mom's lap, kind of half propped up. You introduce yourself, shake hands, and dad says, "She seems OK now, but she's really had us scared."

The parents tell the story. Samantha—they call her Sammi—she's been healthy. She's their first child, and she's been nursing well and growing well. But over the last three days, she's having periods of time when she seems to either go stiff or kind of shake. They thought Sammi was just startling at first. They saw their family physician earlier today, but she didn't see an episode and thought maybe the baby was having some reflux. But the parents are still worried, so they came to the ED to get her checked out again.

By the way, for some clarification, a family medicine physician has done a three-year residency and kept up specific requirements for specific board certification in family practice. This specialty focuses on primary care of people of all ages, from birth to geriatrics. And many family practice doctors also perform minor surgery and obstetrics. Family practice is not the same as GP, or general practice; those are people who typically have not completed a specific residency and do not hold any board certification.

OK, you take a quick look-see, a once-over at this little baby. She's a cute little thing, smiling back at you, her color is good, she looks fine. So, whatever's going on, we can at least think about it for a few minutes. What do you think about this story? It's one of these chief complaints, it could be nothing, or it could be something kind of big and scary. On the one hand, Sammi may just be shaking a bit because of a startle or a shudder, or could there be a serious neurologic or other problem going on here?

Let's put together our brief differential. This could be a seizure; that's the scary thing that we worry about with shaking. Little babies are actually a high risk group for seizures, because there can be brain malformations or metabolic problems that could just be coming to light. Babies are also the highest risk group for brain infections, like meningitis.

Or, maybe it's not really a seizure. There are several neurologic symptoms that can kind of mimic seizures, at least at first. Some examples: Sleep myoclonus is the name for those few jerking movements that many people have as they fall asleep. Another common, benign, normal movement is a shuddering spell, which looks like a quick sort of trembling movement.

Or, could this be something not neurologic at all, like reflux. Now, all babies spit up, but some find it painful. And occasionally, we will see a baby with reflux from the stomach up into the throat who arches and stiffens, looking in many ways like a seizure. This even has a name. It's called Sandifer Syndrome. So reflux may indeed be the culprit here. Or, maybe, this will turn out to be nothing at all, or nothing that even has a name. Babies will sometimes move in kind of weird ways. Sometimes odd movements, including some trembling or shaking or jerking. It's just something normal babies do.

Let's get more history, then our exam. Sammi had a routine pregnancy, with no history of abnormal prenatal ultrasounds or problems. The delivery was at term, and there were no known problems that could have affected or damaged Sammi's brain. She went home after an ordinary two-day hospital stay, she lives with her parents. She's had only a few doctor visits for routine care and routine immunizations. No medical concerns have really been raised previously. Her growth, including measurements of height and weight and head circumference, have all been normal.

You ask for a little more detail, this shaking or funny movement she does, when does it occur? Her parents agree, it sort of comes out of nowhere. It can happen any time. Once it was during nursing, once it was just while playing, and they think it happened once while she was napping. The shaking lasts maybe three, maybe four, minutes, and then it stops.

I'm just going to interject here; that history, that it happens pretty much any time, that does fit with seizures. Funny movements that only occur at a certain time, let's say, a baby who shakes his fist during a diaper change, or turns his head only when he's fed with a spoon, or a child who gets red in the face and trembles only when he's mad, maybe when he gets hurt, those movements are much less likely to be seizures. Seizures really should occur just out of the blue, not under only specific circumstances. One exception—there's always an exception—is that there are some kinds of seizures that are more common during sleep, or more common when a baby is just falling asleep or waking up. Sammi's history of funny movements at random times is not particularly reassuring.

So, back to the history, Sammi is fed exclusively breast milk, and she nurses well. Her parents are planning to add some complementary foods soon, though they haven't yet. She takes no medicines and no vitamins or anything else. The family and social history don't add much else. This is the family's first baby; there are no health problems reported in the parents, and there's no family history of epilepsy or seizures or movement disorders.

A good history on a little baby includes at least a brief developmental assessment, especially when we're potentially thinking about a neurologic issue, like a seizure. Sammi is said to be bright and engaged, she babbles, she will turn to look when she hears her name. She is just starting to roll over and grab for toys. Overall, that sounds like pretty normal developmental for a four-month-old baby, and we'll make our own observations about her development and the way she interacts during the exam. Normal brain development is very reassuring, that makes it much less likely that there is a serious brain malformation and much less likely that these could be frequent or severe seizures, or that they've been going on a long time.

Vital signs are normal, including temperature, pulse, respirations, and blood pressure. Often, blood pressure isn't checked in babies, but electronic devices have made this more practical. In an emergency department we'd probably be able to get a measurement. You measure her head circumference to check brain growth, and it plots normally on the chart.

Sammi, overall, looks great. Four month olds, they're really a pleasure to see as a doctor, they're happy; they're smiling, and sometimes you can even get them to laugh or giggle. She's an adorable girl, She's sitting in mom's lap; she's holding her head up just fine. Her color is good; her pulses are strong; she's moving all extremities equally. Her "soft spot"—that's also called the anterior fontanel, it's the open area on the front of the skull that usually doesn't close until 18 months of life; that's normal; it's flat; it's not bulging. Again, we're concerned about a possible brain event or seizure, so our exam is going to concentrate on clues about how her brain is doing. A bulging fontanel would have indicated increased pressure in the cranium, and that's not a good thing.

Her eyes—here's another way to test her brain function—they look normal, they follow your face as you move, and they move together. Both pupils constrict normally with light. Her neck seems to move normally in all directions. The remainder of the exam seems to be entirely normal, , except something odd starts to happen as you're counting her toes. Wait, quick aside here, as a pediatrician, it is important to count up toes when you first meet a baby, especially in a newborn. It doesn't matter how good a doctor you are, if you miss that sixth toe, the parents will never trust you again. OK, back to Sammi. You're examining her, counting those toes, and dad says, Look, look what she's doing with her hands. You look up, and they're kind of trembling, or jerking upwards a bit, rhythmically, both hands. That's what she does, dad says. That's the thing. What is that? OK, now it's crunch time. Here's the baby, here's the thing she's doing. Is it a seizure or not?

First, we'll re-assess how she looks overall. Her color is good, she's not having any trouble breathing, but when we try to engage her eyes, she's not really interested in looking at us now. Her eyes have kind of rolled up and aren't looking at anything. "Sammi," we say. She doesn't turn to look at us. Her attention is no longer engaged with her environment. And that shaking, itself, a good trick if you think a baby or anyone else may be having a seizure is to gently hold or touch the extremity that's shaking. Normal baby trembling stops with a gentle touch. This shaking of Sammi's, it does not stop when you touch and hold her hands. She's still jerking—up, up, up. This is a seizure. We'll have to figure out why and what we ought to do about it, but first it's time for first aid and stabilization.

When someone, anyone, is having a seizure, first let them lie down so the head is at the same level as the heart. This is the same thing you do when someone faints or collapses to maximize blood flow to the brain. Loosen any tight clothing. Glance at your watch so you know how long this might go on. We'll gently lift Sammi up onto the exam table from Mom's lap. Since she's shaking some, we'll stay very close so she can't possibly fall off the table. With an older child or adult with big body shaking during a more-dramatic seizure, it may be best to leave the patient on the floor if you can't be sure you can prevent a fall.

Do not, ever, put something in someone's mouth during a seizure. There is a myth, an old wives tale, that people might swallow their tongue during a seizure and that somehow you need to prevent that with a spoon or with something in the mouth. That's just false; it doesn't even make anatomic sense. Putting a spoon or anything in someone's mouth can cause gagging or vomiting, which would be very bad during a seizure.

Right now, it doesn't look like Sammi is having trouble breathing, Her color is good. It never hurts to start oxygen if you're not sure if a patient is breathing well during a seizure. Sometimes there can be gasping or ineffective breathing during seizures. When in doubt, get some extra oxygen on. Since we're in the ED, we can call for a little extra help too. We get some monitors on, a pulse ox, a cardiorespiratory monitor with little electrodes on her chest; those can count breathing and pulse.

By now, a few minutes have gone by. Sammi's still jerking her hands, and now her arms are also getting involved in the movement, up to her shoulders. Seizures can be very scary, especially in babies, so we'll keep our cool to reassure mom and dad, even while inside we're thinking, OK, now, it's time for this seizure to stop. But it doesn't stop. It's been almost 10 minutes; we've had a nurse working on getting an IV started. Ideally, with an IV, we'd be able to give some seizure-stopping medicine, but we don't have that access yet. Fortunately studies have looked at several other options for medicine delivery, including rectal administration, there's a version that parents can use at home, or spraying certain medicines into the nose or into the inside of the cheeks. That's what we do, at nine minutes, a dose of midazolam is given inside the cheek, and a few minutes later the shaking stops. Sammi looks well. Her parents look frazzled.

Our IV is started, so we can give more medicine if needed. The nurse also drew some blood for tests, because she's experienced and she knows we're about to ask for those. Let's catch our breath and think about a more focused differential. This isn't reflux; this isn't some normal trembling. This was a real seizure. Why would a baby like Sammi do that?

The brain is an electrical organ. Each nerve cell, those are called neurons, conducts electric impulses between parts of the brain and interconnects with hundreds or thousands of other neurons. In babies and children, these interconnections are actually even more dense and numerous than in adults. Normally, the flow of signals between neurons is very tightly regulated, so neurons fire in a synchronous, or organized, pattern. A seizure is like an electrical storm—a group of neurons just fires, uncontrollably sending out signals to adjacent neurons. Because children have more interconnections, they're actually more prone to seizures than adults. About four to eight percent of children will experience at least one seizure during childhood.

The manifestations of seizures, the symptoms you see, depend on what area of the brain is affected and how much of the brain is affected. A seizure in a small area of, say, the motor part of the cortex, may only cause one shaking limb, without a loss of consciousness. A wider seizure that affects more of the brain can cause whole body shaking, a loss of consciousness, and a loss of bladder control. Some kinds of seizures can cause only a change in sensory perception, or a dramatic change in behavior, or just a sudden drop to unconsciousness.

So what sorts of things trigger seizures? In little babies especially, they're often caused by metabolic conditions. Low blood sugar, low calcium, low sodium, or high sodium. These small molecules are essential to the normal functioning of our cells, including brain cells. Little babies may not have the metabolic reserve to pump out sugar from their liver when blood sugar drops, and their kidneys aren't mature enough to regulate these blood chemicals as well as an adult could.

Also, any kind of brain injury or problem can cause seizures. Prenatal factors can lead to problems with brain development, including cysts or excess fluid in the spaces around the brain. Even with no clear history of birth trauma, there can be periods of insufficient oxygen to the baby's brain during or before labor, and that can lead to damage that may not be apparent until seizures begin later in life. There are also infections, including encephalitis and meningitis, that can cause seizures, especially in babies.

Fevers of any cause can sometimes trigger seizures in young children. These are called febrile seizures when there is no other apparent cause, and they affect about 1 in 25 children, typically from six months to three years in age. Febrile seizures are brief and harmless, though they can be quite frightening for the family. Almost all children with febrile seizures outgrow them, often by age three or four, and family education and reassurance are really the only necessary therapy. One other cause, a sad one, but one not to overlook, is trauma. It may be non accidental and can lead to bleeding in the brain and seizures.

There are also a large proportion of seizures that remain unexplained, probably 25 to 30 percent in babies. They're probably caused by a problem with the brain that is too small to see on MRI, but nonetheless interferes with the normal flow of electrical information. Or, perhaps they're caused by an issue with the neurotransmitters between neurons, which we cannot easily measure. Children or adults with recurrent seizures are said to have epilepsy, and the cause of epilepsy is not always apparent.

So let's start our workup. The most important diagnoses to evaluate first are metabolic problems and infection, because with these, we can intervene quickly to help, and if we don't fix them soon, they may get worse. We don't really have much other evidence of infection; Sammi has had no fever, and honestly, she looked great until the seizure started, but nonetheless, let's get a CBC, and we may have to do an LP. That's a lumbar puncture, or spinal tap, to test for meningitis or infected fluid around the brain. We may also have to get an imaging study of the brain, quickly, to make sure that there isn't some kind of bleed or other hidden trauma that's unfolding.

But first, even before these tests, the results of our first blood tests come back; those were the ones drawn when the IV was first started. Sammi's blood glucose is normal, as is her serum sodium. But her blood calcium is very, very low; normal would be from 9 to 11, in that range, and Sammi's is 6.5. Can that cause seizures? You bet.

The question, now, has changed. We know why Sammi is having seizures, but why does she have such a low calcium? We need to start thinking about that here, but first things first. We'll order some IV calcium to bump that up, and we'll keep her on monitors, and we'll plan to repeat the labs in a few hours to make sure we're heading in the right direction.

Just for completeness, the CBC was unremarkable, and since there's no fever and really no other signs of infection, we'll skip the LP and CT scan for now. We already have our explanation for the seizures. But if things don't improve as expected, we could go back and do those other tests later.

Now the parents are asking too, why is Sammi's calcium so low? They say she nurses well, she's been gaining weight fine, shouldn't she get plenty of calcium from mom's milk? Yes, in fact, they're right, milk is loaded with calcium. Sammi is getting plenty, or at least plenty is going into her digestive system. Why isn't enough calcium in her blood? We're not here to spend a lot of time reviewing basic physiology, but a quick calcium physiology lesson will help you understand what's going on with Sammi.

Calcium is essential for life and for growth, and there are elaborate and interconnected mechanisms for ensuring that the right amount of calcium is absorbed and maintained in the body. Ingested calcium is actively taken up by cells in the small intestine and transported within these cells by a specific calcium-binding protein. That protein acts as a little carrier, and the more of these proteins there are in each absorptive cell, the more calcium will make its way from the gut into the body. The amount of these carrier proteins produced in each cell is regulated by Vitamin D. Even if there is plenty of calcium in the diet, if there is not enough activated vitamin D, the gut will not efficiently absorb calcium.

Vitamin D itself comes from two sources. It can be ingested as part of the diet, or the human body can essentially manufacture in it's own skin cells when exposed to sunlight. Now, natural sources of vitamin D are actually very, very scarce. It can be found naturally in fish and fish liver; there's some in beef liver; there's a small amount in eggs; some in mushrooms. That's it. Now, many foods are fortified with added vitamin D, that is, they add it. That includes milk, commercial baby formulas, some juices, some breakfast cereals too. Dairy products other than milk are not typically fortified with vitamin D.

Babies, of course, they don't get much liver in their diets, and Sammi was relying on mother's milk, which, like unfortified cow's milk, has almost zero natural vitamin D. Can Sammi get enough vitamin D from sunlight exposure? In this case, I don't think so. We know children with darker skin need longer sunlight exposures to make the same amount of vitamin D as Caucasian children. So Sammi had all of the pieces in place to put her at risk for low vitamin D. She has dark skin; it's winter, so there's less daylight and less time spent outside; and she's been fed exclusively breast milk which has no vitamin D. She's also four months old, and by then, babies have often used up their stored vitamin D from birth.

To confirm our diagnosis, we draw a vitamin D level. It's actually measured as 25-OH-vitamin D—that's a marker for the most active form. We expect a level of 30 to 35, that would be sufficient. Sammi's is 3. Over the next few days, Sammi is continued on first IV then an oral Calcium supplements, plus a big oral dose of vitamin D. She has no further seizures, and she is sent home to continue nursing, with supplemental vitamin D. She was actually a little low iron in other lab studies, so it was suggested that she start some complementary foods, including iron-rich meats and fortified cereals.

Will Sammi suffer any long-term effects from this? Probably not. Her seizures were brief, and she probably only had them a few days. Short and infrequent seizures do not cause brain damage, though any seizure should be investigated and prevented when possible. Keeping Sammi on a diet with adequate vitamin D and calcium should now ensure that there are no further seizures and her bones develop normally.

Now, just about every pediatrician recommends nursing as the best nutrition for most babies, unless there is a medical or other reason for choosing formula. Human milk is a great source of nutrition, it's easy to digest, it's cheap, and it provides unique immune benefits. However, human milk isn't perfect. We know it is not a sufficient source of vitamin D. That's why it's recommended that exclusively nursing babies begin an oral vitamin D supplement at birth and continue it until they're consuming vitamin D enriched foods, like milk or formula. This recommendation is especially important for babies with the risk factors we've mentioned—dark skin, winter time, not spending time outside, and living in cooler climates. It's also crucial for babies born pre term, because they've had less chance to store absorbed calcium and vitamin D from mom.

Calcium is an interesting little molecule, and it's essential for many life functions. Along with phosphorus, it makes up the mineral matrix of bones, so prolonged vitamin D deficiency can cause rickets in children. The symptoms of rickets can include delayed growth, bone pain, and muscle weakness, along with skeletal deformities, like bowed legs.

Adults don't develop rickets because their bones aren't growing, but if vitamin D or calcium deficient, adults can have decreased mineral density, which can lead to osteoporosis and fracture. Regular exercise, especially weight bearing exercise or resistance training, is also required to keep bones well mineralized. Calcium is also essential for normal muscle functioning, clotting of the blood, normal heart contraction and rhythms, and, as Sammi's case illustrates, normal functioning of nerve cells and the brain.

We talked about the role of vitamin D in calcium absorption, but the control of calcium levels is actually quite a bit more complicated than that. Vitamin D has to be activated by metabolism in the kidney and the liver, and that step of activation itself is regulated by hormones from the parathyroid gland. Parathyroid hormone, along with vitamin D, and another hormone, called calcitonin, regulate the uptake of calcium from cells that both build and repair bone; they also influence the amount of calcium excreted into the urine. So, there are multiple overlapping feedback loops here, all in place to keep calcium levels controlled in a very narrow range.

And vitamin D, itself, its role goes far beyond calcium metabolism and bone health. Vitamin D modulates cell growth, regulates neuromuscular and immune function, and helps control inflammation. The exact functioning of vitamin D, and optimal levels of intake for health, are active areas of current research.

This case illustrated one way that medical cases proceed. We started with one question, the chief complaint from the parents: "She's shaking, is something wrong?" Then we saw the shaking, and the question became, what are these funny movements? Once we determined they were seizures, the question changed, again, to, why is Sammi having seizures? Then we found our answer, the low calcium. Which led to the next question, why is Sammi's calcium low? Sammi's parents didn't bring her to us reporting a low calcium, but a logical chain developed from her chief complaint, step to step, to a diagnosis and treatment plan. One question, correctly answered, leads to another, and eventually, we reach the final answer.

That's not always the way it works. Real medical cases sometimes have blind alleys and distractions and, frankly, misleading clues that lead to a medical journey that's more of a sideways stagger than a sprint to the finish. And sometimes real patients have multiple diagnoses, sometimes related, sometimes unrelated, that contribute to their symptoms. Again, keep an open mind, pay attention to details, and keep your eye on helping the patient, even when the finish line doesn't seem to be getting nearer. We'll hear more about that kind of story at our next grand rounds.

Hickam's Dictum
Lecture 17

The case presented in this lecture has multiple interconnected diagnoses. It is a good example of the importance of the history and physical exam and of watching for times when the story and presentation can change midway through a case. Patients can best help their doctors by being honest, but doctors also have to keep in mind that the information they have been given may not always be accurate. Mysteries become even trickier when the clues are wrong, and that can be part of the challenge.

Episodic Vomiting

- A 39-year-old woman, Sally, comes into the emergency department with a chief complaint of "I can't stop vomiting." Sally says that she has had episodic vomiting and some abdominal pain on and off for a few months, but it's gotten much worse this week, with frequent vomiting every time she tries to eat or drink.

- Vomiting can be caused by a very long list of problems. We often think first of GI conditions, but there are many other conditions, including intestinal obstructions, appendicitis, gallbladder or liver disease, or really disease of any of the other organs in the abdomen or pelvis—the pancreas, the stomach, or the kidneys.

- Many different medications and toxins cause vomiting, as well as **endocrine** disorders and pregnancy. In addition, anything that increases the pressure in or around your brain, or anything that affects the brain, can cause vomiting—migraine, tumor, stroke, or trauma.

- A more extensive review of systems reveals that Sally has also had some headaches for the past few months and that she feels like she's been unsteady on her feet. She says that her feet get numb sometimes and make it hard to stand.

- Sally has high blood pressure and was severely obese but had a gastric bypass operation four years ago. Since then, she's lost about 120 pounds. She takes pills for her cholesterol and high blood pressure, a prescription **vitamin**, and ibuprofen. She smokes cigarettes, she says, and has maybe one or two alcoholic drinks per week.

- The most notable things from her physical exam are high blood pressure and fast heart rate; overall, also, she just doesn't look very well. There are several indications of dehydration: She's been vomiting for a week, her heart rate is fast, and she has dark urine and infrequent urination. We order an IV and some fluids and give her a dose of a safe antinausea medication.

- A head CT comes back normal, and a pulse oximeter shows normal oxygenation. However, her hemoglobin is very low; it's 8 when it should probably be more than 12. In addition, her chemistries show elevated liver enzymes and a positive test for amylase, indicating inflammation in her pancreas. A pregnancy test comes back negative.

- Sally is bleeding in her gut, is vomiting up blood, and is already markedly anemic. It turns out that Sally has bleeding ulcers and anemia requiring transfusions, but both are addressed. At this point, she also has an unsteady gait, complaints of numb feet, odd eye movements, and trouble with memory. In addition, her liver or pancreas problems haven't been explained yet.

- On her neurological exam, Sally has evidence both of **encephalopathy**—brain problems—but also of neuropathy, or myeloneuropathy, which are problems with the nerves or spinal cord. Her memory issues have to involve her brain, and her reduced reflexes and reduced sensation below the knees have to involve nerves or spinal cord.

- This constellation of findings, together, don't seem to be caused by a stroke, which affects only one area of the brain or spinal cord; or a tumor; or a neuropathy that might be caused by something like diabetes. Something more widespread is going on—something that affects both the brain and the nerves.

Wernicke's Encephalopathy

- Sally finally admits that she has a bottle or so of gin, every day, and has since her divorce several years ago. Sally's health problems—liver and pancreas disease, vomiting and bleeding ulcers, and neurological problems—are all manifestations of chronic alcohol abuse.

- Her combination of memory problems, confusion, difficulty walking, and abnormal eye movements is called Wernicke's encephalopathy—a condition most often seen in people with alcoholism. It's caused by a deficiency of vitamin B_1, or thiamine.

- A large dose of intravenous thiamine is administered, and within a day, Sally's memory, gait, and most of her neurological problems have improved.

- Thiamine is essential to cellular metabolism. Although it is necessary for the healthy functioning of almost all body tissues, the nervous system seems to be especially sensitive to thiamine deficiency.

- Thiamine must be ingested; humans and other animals cannot manufacture it. It's widely available in many foods, including whole grains and many vegetables. In the developed world, many grain and cereal products are fortified with extra thiamine, making deficiency rare outside of certain high-risk populations.

- A version of thiamine deficiency, Wernicke's encephalopathy, is the combination of mental confusion, unsteady walking, and unusual eye movements. The most common cause of this kind of thiamine deficiency is alcoholism, which interferes with thiamine absorption and utilization.

- Other risk factors for Wernicke's encephalopathy from thiamine deficiency include starvation, AIDS, frequent vomiting during pregnancy, and incorrect baby formulas.

- A growing risk group is people who have undergone bariatric surgery, like Sally. Because the surgery bypasses some of the absorptive part of the gut, patients who have had weight-reduction surgery are at risk for deficiencies of many nutrients, including thiamine.

- Sally probably wasn't taking her high blood pressure medication or her prescribed vitamin supplements. Therefore, she had multiple risk factors for thiamine deficiency: alcoholism, bariatric surgery, and poor compliance with her medications.

- The prognosis of Wernicke's encephalopathy can be difficult to predict. When treated early, many of the symptoms can improve dramatically and quickly with thiamine administration. However, many patients will continue to have some neurological impairment. Some will go on to develop permanent and pervasive cognitive and memory problems that may require institutional care.

- Sally had evidence of other complications of alcoholism. She had abnormal liver tests, and her CT scan confirmed liver damage. Advanced scarring of the liver, called cirrhosis, is most often caused by prolonged alcohol abuse. Cirrhosis can also be caused by infections like chronic hepatitis or by obesity. Cirrhosis may lead to liver failure, requiring transplantation, or it may lead to cancer of the liver.

- There was also inflammation of the pancreas, called pancreatitis, which can also be caused by alcoholism or obesity. Pancreatitis causes intense abdominal pain and vomiting. Sally may have had multiple causes of her GI symptoms—direct stomach irritation from alcohol, gastric ulcers, pancreatitis, liver disease, and thiamine deficiency itself. All of these can cause stomach upset and vomiting.

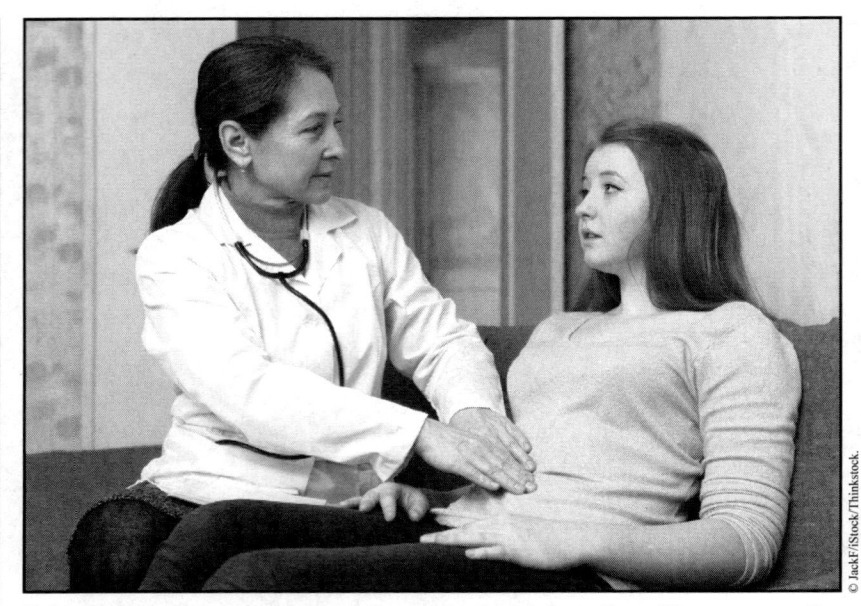

Gastrointestinal symptoms, including abdominal pain and vomiting, can result from excessive alcohol consumption.

- Alcoholism can also contribute to gastric ulcers, which led to Sally's abrupt deterioration. There can be multiple, overlapping factors; alcohol itself can damage the stomach lining and prevent healing. Alcoholics may not consume regular meals, including fat and protein that protect the stomach.

- And if cirrhosis has begun, the liver disease can lead to a decrease in clotting proteins, so the ulcers bleed more. Liver disease can also lead to increased pressure in the blood vessels in the stomach and esophagus, which may further increase bleeding.

- The effect of alcohol consumption on heart disease and stroke is still being researched. It appears that moderate alcohol consumption, about one drink per day, may improve cardiac risk factors, perhaps by its effect on cholesterol metabolism. But excessive drinking directly damages the heart muscle and increases the risk of heart attacks and stroke.

- People with alcoholism also have an increased risk of some cancers, pneumonia, osteoporosis, diabetes, neuropathy, and mental illness. There are also increased risks of death by suicide and motor vehicle accidents, domestic violence, and other addictions.

- Alcoholism is frequently associated with obesity, too; alcohol is a significant source of calories, though it doesn't offer much in the way of actual nutrition, and it will make you fat. And, of course, obesity then contributes to liver disease, heart disease, diabetes, and everything else that's already going wrong.

Managing Weight

- Obesity is a huge problem in the United States, and it's rapidly becoming the most significant health problem in the entire developed world. In fact, overnutrition—eating too much—may have already overtaken malnutrition as a cause of death, worldwide.

- The causes of obesity are complex. It's tempting to just look at obesity as a simple consequence of eating too much while exercising too little, but there is clearly more to the story. Our weights are also influenced by genetic and environmental factors that go beyond just diet and exercise.

- For now, therapeutic options for patients struggling with obesity are limited. Changes in dietary habits can lead to permanent improvements in weight and health, but they're difficult to maintain and don't usually work.

- Improving exercise habits can improve health (even if weight isn't lost), but that may not be practical, and people who are significantly overweight may not be able to exercise as much as they would like. Still, diet and exercise habits should be part of counseling to help patients of any age reach or maintain a healthy weight.

- There are also some kind-of-overlooked, simple eating strategies that may help.
    - People who eat slower tend to consume fewer calories. So, slow down, chew, drink water, and have a relaxed meal—rather than rushing or eating in the car.

    - Eating out in restaurants increases calories tremendously; portions are large, and restaurants cook with plenty of fat and butter. Order only an appetizer, or split an entrée.

    - The simple step of avoiding calories in soda and other sweetened beverages can have a huge impact on weight. For an ordinary adult, just skipping one 12-ounce soda per day, for a year, will lead to about a 10-pound weight loss.

- At this point, there are no good medicines available to help manage weight. Some may curb appetite a little or interfere with nutrient absorption, but they have significant side effects and may actually increase health risks. We need better ways to control appetite and calorie intake, but so far, we don't have those medicines yet.

- After procedures like bariatric surgery—which is the most aggressive therapy to help with weight loss—patients like Sally are at risk of nutritional deficiencies; they may not be able to absorb enough micronutrients from ordinary food. Deficiencies can include not only thiamine, but also copper, zinc, folate, and vitamin D.

- Patients need to be counseled before and after bariatric surgery on the importance of taking appropriate dietary supplements. Because more and more of these procedures are being done, physicians need to remember the special risks of nutritional deficiencies in patients after weight-loss surgery.

Important Terms

encephalopathy: Dysfunction of the brain from any cause.

endocrine: Relating to glands that secrete hormones into the blood.

vitamin: One of a group of compounds that are essential to be ingested in small quantities to maintain health and life.

Suggested Reading

Carpenter, *Beriberi, White Rice, and Vitamin B.*

Gratzer, *Terrors of the Table.*

Questions to Consider

1. In the developed world, who is at risk for nutritional deficiencies?

2. How can a doctor tell if a patient isn't being truthful?

Hickam's Dictum
Lecture 17—Transcript

Sometimes, a diagnosis follows logically. You get your history, do your physical, think it through, and the diagnosis follows. Frequently, though, in the real world, finding a diagnosis requires patience, persistence, and a little bit of luck. Sometimes, you think you've reached the conclusion, only to find that the patient isn't quite done with you. New problems mean rethinking your diagnosis—or diagnoses. Maybe there is more than one problem. The real world can be messy.

This idea is illustrated by comparing two, we'll call them philosophies of medical diagnosis. On the one hand, there's the very appealing principle of Occam's Razor. This basically means that one ought to strive to find the simplest explanation, or the single diagnosis that fits the picture. On the other hand, counterbalancing Occam's Razor, is what's called Hickam's Dictum, attributed to Dr. John Hickam, who is famously quoted as saying, "Patients can have as many diseases as they damn well please."

A 39-year-old woman, Sally, comes into the ED with a chief complaint of, "I can't stop vomiting." Sally, we learn, she has not had a very good week. She says she's had episodic vomiting and some abdominal pain on and off, maybe for a few months, but this week it's gotten much worse—frequent vomiting every time she tries to eat or drink. Our patient looks pale and uncomfortable, so we don't want to spend a lot of time up front with our initial differential diagnosis.

But just to get started, vomiting can be caused by a very long list of problems. We often think first of GI conditions—infections, the so-called tummy bug. But there are many other conditions, including intestinal obstructions, appendicitis, gall bladder or liver disease, or really, disease of any of the other organs in the abdomen or pelvis—the pancreas, the stomach, or the kidneys. Many different medications and toxins cause vomiting, as well as endocrine disorders, and never forget pregnancy. Also, this is another group to keep in mind, anything that increases the pressure in or around your brain, or, honestly, anything that affects the brain, can also cause vomiting; that would include migraine, tumor, stroke, or trauma. That is a huge list. I think it's best to just say, for now, we'll keep an open mind about Sally.

So, more history, Sally says her abdominal pain is crampy, and it's not severe, but it bothers her. The main thing is the nausea and vomiting, which has lately been many times a day. She says her urine has been dark and infrequent. She's had no fevers and no diarrhea, and has had no known ill contacts, though, she works at a caterer, around a lot of food and food prep equipment. She's been unable to work for the past week. A more extensive review of systems reveals that Sally has also had some headaches for the past few months, and also, that she feels she's been unsteady on her feet. Probably, she says, because she's been working too much, and she's always standing. She says her feet get numb sometimes and make it hard to stand.

Some past medical history from Sally might be important. She has high blood pressure, and because of severe obesity, had a gastric bypass operation four years ago. Since then, she's lost about 120 pounds. She says she's supposed to take pills for her cholesterol and high blood pressure, but doesn't remember what they're called. She also takes a prescription vitamin every day since her surgery, and frequently takes ibuprofen to help with her belly aches and headaches. Sally is divorced and denies any sexual activity in the past few years. Her last period was a few weeks ago. She smokes cigarettes, she says, and has maybe one or two alcoholic drinks a week. OK, there's a lot here already. The main thing is the worsening nausea and vomiting, but there have been headaches and this numb feet complaint to remember as well.

Now, let's see what we find on the physical exam. Sally looks uncomfortable. She's pale; she's sweaty. She weighs 230 pounds. She has no fever, her BP is 174/110, pulse 96, respirations 18 per minute. Her pulses are strong. Her belly seems a little tender to palpation, diffusely, kind of everywhere you feel. You try to get her to sit and then to stand up, but she says she's too weak. There's no edema of her legs, and you don't find anything else on her skin exam. A gynecologic exam is normal. You try to do a neurologic exam, including asking her to move her hands in certain ways and doing brief tests of memory, but she waves you away. She says she feels weak, and she's going to vomit again.

It can be frustrating, but sometimes it can be difficult to do a thorough physical exam. Sometimes it's best to step back and not push but plan to repeat the exam later when the patient is feeling better. So, on our exam, the most notable things are the high blood pressure and fast heart rate. Overall, also, she just didn't look very well. Let's get things stabilized, get the ball rolling, then we'll think about diagnoses.

We' have several indications of dehydration; she's been vomiting for a week; her heart rate is fast; we have dark urine and infrequent urination. And, it's doubtful we're really going to be able to help her rehydrate orally, because she's still vomiting. So we'll order an IV and some fluids, and we'll also give her a dose of a safe anti-nausea medication. While that's getting started, we can try to think this through.

We ended our brief differential, the one we mentioned before the full story, with the possibility that brain problems can cause vomiting. Anything from tumors to brain infections to stroke can trigger vomiting, though more typically, brain problems cause vomiting without a feeling of queasiness or nausea.

Sally is at risk for stroke, with her blood pressure and history of high cholesterol. She's had some headaches, and we cannot get a good neurologic exam. There's also that weird numbness symptom in her legs. So do we need to image her brain? I think so. Let's get a quick head CT, it's normal.

What about the gut itself? Intestinal obstruction is an emergency; if she has a blockage for some reason, that has got to be fixed, or resulting damage to her GI system can be catastrophic. Remember, Sally had that gastric bypass operation a few years ago. Anyone who's had surgery inside the abdomen is at risk for adhesions, basically, bands of scar tissue that can later lead to an intestinal obstruction. And the surgery Sally had could have left tissue in her intestine that could scar down, causing a tight spot or stricture that could obstruct the gut. So among the first studies to rule out things that need immediate attention, Sally gets an abdominal CT scan. It doesn't show any strictures, no obstructions, though it does reveal some inflammation in her liver and pancreas, with tissues lighting up brighter than normal on the CT scan.

We'll have to get back to these findings later, because Sally is getting sicker. She's thrown up a few more times, and now, in the ED she's just throwing up repeatedly. The vomit is full of blood. Sally is becoming hard to wake up, alternating between kind of thrashing around and pushing people away and just lying still. Her vital signs remain about the same, and we check a pulse oximeter, too. That's normal, showing normal oxygenation.

Some labs come back. Her hemoglobin is very low, it's 8, probably should be more than 12. And her chemistries show an elevated liver enzyme and a positive test for amylase, indicating inflammation in her pancreas. We also had ordered a pregnancy test; that's negative. Sally had said that she wasn't sexually active, but we know that people aren't always honest in the ED.

There's some unanswered questions, now, I know, but in the ED we often have to act before we get answers. The main things, she's bleeding in her gut, she's vomiting up blood, and she's already markedly anemic. We need to replace lost blood, and we need to stop the bleeding.

Things move fast. Additional blood tests are done to make sure that her clotting factors are normal. That's important, because we don't know why she's bleeding yet, and there have been labs and that CT that showed some kind of liver disease. The liver is where clotting proteins are made, and if she's not able to clot normally, that's going to make bleeding worse. Those blood tests are reassuring. We also checked an ammonia level; that's another way of making sure that the liver is functioning OK, that it's metabolizing the ammonia in the body so it doesn't accumulate. In severe liver disease, ammonia levels increase, and that leads to problems with brain function, including delirium and coma.

The surgical and GI teams are called in, and medicine is given to reduce stomach acid. A blood transfusion and extra fluids are given, and after sedation, an endoscope is put down into her stomach, where three large, bleeding ulcers are found. Those are cauterized, and it looks like the bleeding has stopped. A whole lot of blood is also suctioned out of her stomach. Sally is admitted into the ICU for continued observation.

Now, technically, Sally is off of our service. We're the ED doc tonight. But we peek in into the ICU; we follow her chart, just to see how she's doing. The bleeding ulcers explain a lot of her symptoms, but something isn't quite right, yet. The pancreas is inflamed; the liver tests were abnormal. Is there more to this story? You leave a message for the GI doc to keep you in the loop. He's now taken over care, since the main diagnosis is the gastric ulcers. Sally is also started on medication to lower her blood pressure.

The next day, though, doesn't go so well. Sally's color is better, and her blood tests show that her anemia has improved, but she still can't seem to get out of bed. She seems kind of confused, and she can't remember where she is. You stop by to see her, and she kind of squints at you; she doesn't know who you are. She also starts complaining of double vision.

In the ICU, they remain worried about a possible stroke; she had had high blood pressure, and anemia, that could have worsen a stroke. A head MRI is performed, which can detect even subtle strokes, as well as other brain injuries, but that's normal. Since she's complaining of visual problems, the team tries to get her up and wheel her over to the ophthalmology clinic in the professional building next door, but she can't seem to stand up straight. Her gait is very unsteady, and she's very reluctant to even take a few steps, holding her feet widely apart.

They use a stretcher, and they get Sally next door, and the vision exam is normal. The ophthalmologist, though, notes that her eyes are kind of darting back and forth, back and forth. She has nystagmus, that finding we talked about before during our patient with dizziness. Nystagmus can be caused by brain or inner ear disease that affects the sense of balance.

It's time for a quick recap, Sally had bleeding ulcers and anemia requiring transfusions, though that's been addressed now. At this point, she also has an unsteady gait, complaints of numb feet, odd eye movements, and trouble with memory. Plus, we really haven't explained the liver or pancreas problems. I've said it before, when things get confusing, go back to the history and physical exam. Things were rushed the first time. Let's do it again. We'll go ahead; we'll lave the ED; we'll head down to the ICU. Let's talk to Sally.

She says still doesn't remember last night, but she doesn't mind repeating herself. She says she's had all of this vomiting, but can't really recall much else from the history. Then she says, "Boy, I could use a drink." "How much do you drink, Sally?" you ask. "Not much," she says.

We move on and try to do a more detailed, thorough physical exam, focusing on the nervous system. Tests of memory and concentration, Sally doesn't do so well on those. She can't seem to remember things from even a few minutes ago. Her strength seems OK; she can move her muscles against the pressure from your hand, but when you try to get her to stand up, again, she seems very unsteady on her feet. You also carefully test those reflexes; they're sluggish and reduced, and do tests of sensation by pricking her with a pointy edge of a tongue depressor. Sally seems to have reduced sensation in both of her legs, starting about below her knees.

Now, a detailed neurologic exam done by an experienced neurologist is very valuable; they're really good at focusing from the exam on where anatomically the lesion is. That is, where in the brain or spinal cord or nerves could there be a problem that explains the physical examination. Now, today, we're ED doctors, we're not neurologists, so I'm not going to go into the details of the neuroanatomy here, but one thing, a simple and important thing is clear from the exam, Sally couldn't have just one simple lesion somewhere.

On her exam, Sally has evidence both of encephalopathy, brain problems, but also of neuropathy, or myeloneuropathy, problems with the nerves or the spinal cord. Her memory issues have to be a brain thing, and her reduced reflexes and the reduced sensation below the knees have to be a nerve or spinal cord thing. I don't think this constellation of findings, together, could be caused by a stroke, which affects only one area of the brain or spinal cord, or a tumor, or a neuropathy that might be caused by something like diabetes. No, something more widespread is going on, something that affects both the brain and the nerves—and the liver, and the pancreas, and maybe, could the same something cause gastric ulcers as well?

You're talking with Sally, now, she's scared, now. She's stopped vomiting blood, but she's weak; she can't walk, and she can tell you're worried, too.

"We want to help you feel better," you say. "I think you're going to be OK. But it will really help us if we can work together to figure this out." You ask one more time, "How much are you drinking, Sally?" Sally tells you she has a bottle or so of gin every day, and has had that since her divorce several years ago.

That was the last piece of information we needed. Sally's health problems—the liver and pancreas disease, the vomiting and bleeding ulcers, and now these neurologic problems—they're all manifestations of chronic alcohol abuse. Her combination of memory problems, confusion, trouble walking, and abnormal eye movements is called Wernicke Encephalopathy. This is a condition most often seen in people with alcoholism. It's caused by a deficiency of vitamin B-1, or thiamine.

A large dose of intravenous thiamine is administered, and within a day, Sally's memory, gait, and most of her neurologic problems have improved. Thiamine is essential to cellular metabolism. Though it is necessary for the healthy functioning of almost tissues, the nervous system seems to be especially sensitive to thiamine deficiency. Thiamine must be ingested; humans and other animals cannot manufacture it. It's widely available in many foods, including whole grains and many vegetables. And in the developed world, many grain and cereal products are fortified with extra thiamine, making deficiency rare outside of certain high-risk populations.

In the developing world, where dietary thiamine may be scarce, deficiency can cause the disease Beri Beri. Manifestations of Beri Beri include neurologic problems, lethargy, impairments of memory and cognition, heart disease, and GI problems. It is fatal if untreated. The name Beri Beri is interesting; it may refer to the word for sheep, because it looks like people with Beri Beri walk with an odd gait, lifting their feet high up, and that kind of looks like the walk of sheep somehow. The name may also mean the phrase "weak, weak," which is the name, in Beri Beri it's said twice for emphasis. It's not just weak, it's weak, weak.

OK, in the United States, Beri Beri itself is not common, because of the widespread dietary fortification of many foods. However, we do see a version of thiamine deficiency called "Wernicke encephalopathy," which is the combination of mental confusion, unsteady walking, and unusual eye movements. The most common cause of this kind of thiamine deficiency, Wernicke's encephalopathy, is alcoholism, which interferes with thiamine absorption and utilization.

Other risk factors for Wernicke encephalopathy from thiamine deficiency include starvation, AIDS, frequent vomiting during pregnancy, and incorrect baby formulas. A growing risk group that we need to watch out for is also people who have undergone bariatric surgery, like Sally. Because the surgery bypasses some of the absorptive part of the gut, patients who have had weight-reduction surgery are at risk for deficiencies of many nutrients, including thiamine. Sally probably wasn't taking her blood-pressure medication, and probably wasn't taking her prescribed vitamin supplements, either. So Sally had multiple risk factors for thiamine deficiency—alcoholism, bariatric surgery, and poor compliance with her medications.

The prognosis of Wernicke encephalopathy can be difficult to predict. When treated early, many of the symptoms can improve dramatically and quickly with thiamine administration. However, many patients will continue to have some neurologic impairment. Some will go on to develop permanent and pervasive cognitive and memory problems that may require institutional care.

Sally had other evidence of other complications of alcoholism. She had abnormal liver tests, and her CT scan confirmed liver damage. Advanced scarring of the liver, called cirrhosis, is most often caused by prolonged alcohol abuse. Cirrhosis can also be caused by infections, like chronic hepatitis, or by obesity. Cirrhosis may lead to liver failure, requiring transplantation, or it may lead to cancer of the liver.

There was also inflammation of the pancreas, called pancreatitis, which can also be caused by alcoholism or obesity. Pancreatitis causes intense abdominal pain and vomiting. Sally may have had multiple causes of her GI symptoms—direct stomach irritation from alcohol, gastric ulcers, pancreatitis, liver disease, and thiamine deficiency itself. All of these can cause stomach upset and vomiting.

Alcoholism can also contribute to gastric ulcers, which led to Sally's abrupt deterioration. There can be multiple, overlapping factors here. Alcohol itself can damage the stomach lining and prevent healing. Alcoholics also may not consume regular meals, including fat and protein that protect the stomach. And if cirrhosis has begun, the liver disease can lead to a decrease in clotting proteins, so the ulcers bleed more. Liver disease can also lead to increased pressure in the blood vessels in the stomach and esophagus, which may further increase bleeding.

The effect of alcohol consumption on heart disease and stroke is still being researched. It appears that moderate alcohol consumption, about one drink a day, may improve cardiac risk factors, perhaps by its effect on cholesterol metabolism. But excessive drinking directly damages the heart muscle, and increases the risk of heart attacks and stroke. It certainly can't be good for people who already have the risks of obesity, high blood pressure, and elevated cholesterol to add on the risks of excessive alcohol.

People with alcoholism also have an increased risk of some cancers, pneumonia, osteoporosis, diabetes, neuropathy, and mental illness. There are also increased risks of death by suicide and motor vehicle accidents, domestic violence, and other addiction. Alcoholism is frequently associated with obesity, too; alcohol, itself, is a significant source of calories, though it doesn't offer much in the way of actual nutrition. It can make you fat. And, of course, obesity then contributes to liver disease, and heart disease, and diabetes, and everything else that's already going wrong.

Let's return to Sally. She was admitted for vomiting and abdominal pain and turned out to have alcoholic cirrhosis, pancreatitis, gastric ulcers, and Wernicke's Encephalopathy from thiamine deficiency. Treatment in the hospital included endoscopy for her ulcers, blood transfusions, and medical and nutritional support. She's ready to go home now, with instructions to take ulcer medication, high blood pressure medication, plus several dietary supplements, Close follow-up has been scheduled with several medical specialists and her primary doctor.

And, we've had a heart-to-heart talk with Sally about her drinking. She's agreed to enroll in an alcohol treatment program. We'll want to get her re involved in a weight-control program as well. With the help of bariatric surgery she's lost a lot of weight, but for good health, she still has a ways to go. Continued weight loss will help prevent the complications of high blood pressure, and may also help her liver, pancreas, and stomach disease.

Obesity is a huge problem in the United States, and it's rapidly becoming the most significant health problem in the entire developed world. In fact, over nutrition—too much to eat—may have already overtaken malnutrition as a cause of death, worldwide. The causes of obesity are complex. It's tempting to just look at obesity as a simple consequence of eating too much while exercising too little, but clearly there is more to the story. Our weights are also influenced by genetic and environmental factors that go beyond just diet and exercise.

For now, our therapeutic options for patients struggling with overweight are limited. Changes in dietary habits can lead to permanent improvements in weight and health, but they're difficult to maintain and don't usually work. Improving exercise habits can improve health (even if weight isn't lost), but again, that may not be practical, and people who are significantly overweight may not be able to exercise as much as they would like. Still, diet and exercise habits should be part of counseling to help patients of any age reach or maintain a healthy weight.

There are also some kind of overlooked eating strategies, simple things really, that may help. People who eat slower tend to consume fewer calories—so slow down, and chew, and drink water and talk and have a nice relaxed meal, rather than rushing or eating in the car. Eating out in restaurants increases calories tremendously—portions are large, and restaurants cook with plenty of fat and butter. Order only an appetizer, or split an entrée. Also, the simple step of avoiding calories in soda and other sweetened beverages can have a huge impact on weight. For an ordinary adult, just skipping one 12-ounce soda a day—one can a day, for a year—will lead to about a 10 pound weight loss.

OK, there's diet and exercise, what about medications for obesity? The bottom line, at this point, is that there are no good medicines available to help manage weight. Some may curb appetite a little, or might interfere with nutrient absorption, but they have significant side effects and may actually net increase health risks. We need better ways to control appetite and calorie intake, but so far we don't have those medicines yet.

Now, Sally had had the most aggressive therapy to help with weight loss, bariatric surgery. After this kind of procedure, patients like Sally are at risk of nutritional deficiencies—they may not be able to absorb enough micronutrients from ordinary food. Deficiencies can include not only thiamine, but also copper, zinc, folate, and vitamin D. Patients need to be counseled before and after bariatric surgery on the importance of taking appropriate dietary supplements. Since more and more of these procedures are being done, physicians need to remember the special risks of nutritional deficiencies in patients after weight-loss surgery.

There are a few other loose ends I wanted to come back to in this complex case. Sally had gastric ulcers, which are erosions in the lining of the stomach. In the past, it's been thought that these kinds of ulcers were caused by stress, or that they usually occurred in certain individuals with strong tempers, the "Type A" people. That's really not true. Ulcers in adults are usually caused actually by an infection, a chronic infection in the stomach wall caused by the bacteria *Helicobacter pylori*. So treatment for ulcers should include testing for this bacteria, and treating it with antibiotics if it's present. Treatment should also include medications to reduce stomach acid, and avoiding especially medications like ibuprofen or aspirin that thin the gut wall and contribute to ulcers. Ironically, Sally had been taking ibuprofen for her headaches, which may have made her ulcers worse.

I also wanted to come back to clarify some terms I used about Sally's liver disease. Hepatitis means liver inflammation—similar to how appendicitis means appendix inflammation, or pancreatitis means pancreas inflammation. In common use, hepatitis is often thought to refer only to chronic infections, the ones with letter names like hepatitis A or B or C—but other viral infections can also cause hepatitis, or toxins like alcohol or adverse drug reactions, or autoimmune illnesses, or other things as well. The blood tests we commonly use to test for liver inflammation are commonly called "liver enzymes" or "LFTs," which is short for "liver function tests"—though they don't in fact test for functioning of the liver, they only test for chemicals released into the blood when liver cells die (or, actually, sometimes when other kinds of cells die as well). If hepatitis continues, eventually there will be permanent scarring and fibrosis of the liver, called cirrhosis. Sometimes the line between hepatitis and cirrhosis is blurry, and sometimes patients have elements of both at the same time.

This was quite a case today, with multiple interconnected diagnoses. It was a good example of the importance of the history and physical exam, and of watching for times when the story and presentation can change midway through a case. Sally wasn't entirely truthful, at least at first, about her alcohol habit, and that misdirected the initial workup—a good reminder that patients can best help their doctors by being honest, but also that doctors have to keep in mind that their information they've been given may not always be accurate. Mysteries get even trickier when the clues are wrong, and that can be part of the challenge.

Medical stories can take unexpected turns, but it's still the physician's job to follow the path even when it goes sideways. Or even when the news, and the prognosis, is not very good. More about that, next time.

Forgetting Jerusalem
Lecture 18

You have about a three-hour window after a stroke where clot-busting medicines can help, and the quicker the evaluation, the better. This is not something that can be done at your doctor's office or something you would call for an appointment about. Call 911, or get to a hospital emergency department as quickly as possible. Overall, about 50 percent of strokes could be prevented though better lifestyle choices: not smoking, maintaining a healthy weight, and exercising regularly.

A Stroke?

- In the emergency department, an older man is being pushed in a wheelchair. He's with his daughter, who gives us the chief complaint: "I think my Daddy is having a stroke." Our patient's name is Ramesh, and they're hooking him up to monitors while we get some basic history.

- Ramesh's daughter tells us that he is 61 years old, and he's a barber. She says that he was working, and all of a sudden, he kind of slumped to the floor. His right hand and arm got kind of loose, and since then, he can't talk. This happened only eight minutes ago.

- It's likely that Ramesh had a stroke, but we shouldn't assume that yet. There is a differential diagnosis, a list of so-called stroke mimics—including seizure, fainting, hypoglycemia, brain tumors, and migraines.

- This is a situation where it is better to immediately deal with what's most likely, a stroke, because immediate recognition and treatment can really make a difference. If it ends up not really being a stroke, there is no harm done in waiting to diagnose something different.

- Ramesh's daughter says that her dad is really healthy. He has type 2 diabetes but has been really good about his medications; his blood sugars have been mostly normal. He also has high blood pressure and takes a water pill for that.

- Suddenly, Ramesh looks much better. He's sitting up, smiling, and holding up his right arm. He says that he feels fine. So this wasn't a stroke, after all—it was the beginning of a stroke, but it stopped on its own. What Ramesh had is sometimes incorrectly called a ministroke, but its real medical name is a transient ischemic attack (TIA).

- A stroke, or **cerebrovascular accident**, occurs when there is inadequate blood flow to an area of the brain. Neurons or brain cells in the affected area die, resulting in permanent (or near-permanent) loss of functioning. The exact symptoms will depend on what had been the functioning of that area of the brain.

- A stroke in the stripe of brain that controls motor functioning will cause weakness; a stroke in the back of the brain, the occipital area, will affect vision. Strokes don't have to follow exact functional boundaries; sometimes these symptoms overlap. Strokes can cause problems with emotional control, attention, drawing ability, memory, speech, and more.

- In Ramesh's case, what happened was a brief, temporary blockage of flow—long enough so that the brain cells in that area were affected and stopped functioning, but short enough so that when the blood supply resumed, the cells survived and returned to normal. This is most typically caused by a clot in one of the arteries that supplies the brain. These clots, if you're lucky, can dissolve or get dislodged, allowing blood flow to quickly resume.

- While a general examination of Ramesh is absolutely normal, when we listen over his neck, to his blood vessels, we hear a humming sound called a **bruit**, which is a noise, kind of a rushing or blowy sort of sound, that's heard over an artery when there is some kind of occlusion.

- In this case, we're concerned about a blockage from a clot in the brain, and it could have come from a plaque that's accumulated in the carotid artery, in the neck. A bruit isn't a great, reliable physical finding, but hearing this bruit in Ramesh makes us more suspicious that in the carotids there's a blockage that could have led to his symptoms.

- The physical exam is normal. In addition, Ramesh had a CT scan of his head to make sure that there isn't a hemorrhage, or bleed in the brain. The CT is normal. Ramesh wants to go home.

- The risk of a full-blown stoke after a TIA is probably about 20 percent within the first year; the risk for a stroke within the next few days might be as high as 5 percent overall, but there are some known risk factors we can assess.

- The highest risk for a stroke within days of a first TIA occur in elderly patients. Recurrent stroke risk is also higher in people with poorly controlled high blood pressure and also those whose TIA symptoms lasted longer the first time.

- Overall, Ramesh would seem to fit into the lower-risk category, and with good, reliable follow-up and some initial preventive care steps in the emergency department, it's reasonable to send Ramesh home.

- Three days later, the results of the neck ultrasound show that Ramesh has some blockage, in the 50 to 70 percent range, on the left side of his neck. What to do about this is actually controversial. Whether to intervene is a decision he'll have to make with his own family physician, in consultation with a vascular surgeon.

- Because we know that Ramesh has vascular disease in his neck, it will be a good idea for him to have a cardiac stress test to look for potential blockages in his coronary arteries. And, of course, it will be especially important for him to control his diabetes and high blood pressure and to stay on the aspirin.

TIA versus Stroke

- The risk factors for TIA and stroke are the same, and they overlap with the risks for coronary artery disease and blockages in other blood vessels. All of these are related to age; the risk of stroke doubles every decade of life, starting at 55.

- Men are at higher risk than women, and there are inherited risk factors as well. African Americans, Hispanics, and Asians are all at higher risk than Caucasians (perhaps because they all have higher rates of hypertension).

- Stroke risk is increased not only by high blood pressure, but also by obesity, diabetes, and high cholesterol. Lifestyle choices like smoking, staying sedentary, and excessive alcohol consumption all increase the risk of stroke, as do some medications. Taking oral contraceptives, especially when combined with smoking in women over 35, can further increase stroke risk.

- The symptoms of a TIA or stroke can start out exactly the same, but the risk of a stroke within seven days of a TIA is doubled among those who don't seek treatment.

- Aftercare of a stroke, after clot-busting medicine or treatment of hemorrhage, often includes prolonged rehabilitative care and supportive care. Some functioning can return.

- Immediately after a stroke, there is a window of a few days or weeks where there can be a fairly rapid recovery of function, at least partially. More functioning is more likely to return with a stroke that affected a smaller area of brain and in people who got medical care quickly.

- The location of the stroke is also a predictor; some areas of the brain seem to be more or less fragile than other parts. Improvement will also depend on the overall health of the patient and whether there were complications.

- The recovery period immediately after a stroke occurs when cells near the area of ischemia start to recover. These are cells that were damaged, but not killed, by the stroke.

- After this initial period, there can still be improvement and recovery—though recovery becomes slower after the first few weeks. After that initial period, brain recovery probably isn't related to individual cells recovering their function, but from other mechanisms.

- To some extent, the brain can rewire connections around an area of damage. Past six months after a stroke, though, there is typically not a lot of further recovery possible. The exact extent of recovery within that six-month window is difficult to predict, but it can be substantial. However, 100 percent recovery is rare.

Treatment and Prevention
- There's quite a bit of research going on into brain recovery after stroke, looking for ways to maximize what's called the plasticity of the brain—the ability of the brain to recover function. Children, especially the youngest children, have the best ability to recover after a stroke, probably because their brains are still growing and developing. Even a massive stroke in a young child can end up leading to minimal long-term disability.

- There seem to be important genetic switches on neurons that control their growth and development and, therefore, the ability of brain tissue to recover. A goal of research is in turning these switches back on, effectively making an adult brain, or parts of an adult brain, think it's young again so that it can better grow and recover.

- For the time being, though, the best stroke treatment is stroke prevention. Control high blood pressure, high cholesterol, diabetes, and overweight; eat a healthy diet with plenty of fruits and vegetables; quit tobacco use; and exercise regularly. People at high risk should consider taking anti-stroke medications, typically medicines that prevent clotting, including aspirin or prescription medications. These have both benefits and risks, so their use should be discussed with a doctor.

- Another potential preventive therapy for stroke is an omega-3 supplement—a supplement of so-called healthy fats, often derived from fish oils. Some studies have shown that fish oil taken as a supplement can reduce strokes, but other studies haven't been as persuasive.

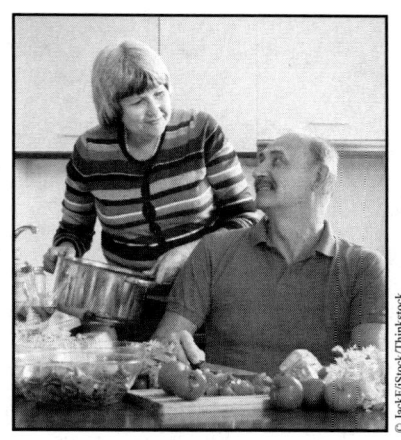

Eating healthy food and exercising regularly could help prevent stroke.

- People who experience early signs of stroke or TIA need to be evaluated as quickly as possible, but there is sometimes a delay. Any sudden symptom of neurological dysfunction—including weakness, speech problems, altered sensations, loss of consciousness, trouble seeing or walking—is a potential stroke symptom that needs to be evaluated very urgently.

- Sometimes an individual experiencing a stroke seems to not notice the symptoms or **deny** symptoms that are really obvious to other people, so it may be up to friends or loved ones to insist that people with stroke symptoms seek care.

Important Terms

bruit: A noise caused by turbulent flow in a blood vessel.

cerebrovascular accident: Stroke—brain damage caused by insufficient blood flow.

deny: In medical lingo, "deny" means that the patient says the symptom in question did not occur. It does not imply that the patient is being untruthful.

Suggested Reading

Lindley, *Stroke*.

Sacks, *The Man Who Mistook His Wife for a Hat*.

Spence and Barnett, eds, *Stroke Prevention, Treatment, and Rehabilitation*.

Questions to Consider

1. What information is needed to decide whether or not to perform a medical procedure or test?

2. What sorts of medical problems mean that a patient should go directly and immediately to the hospital?

Forgetting Jerusalem
Lecture 18—Transcript

Medical students learn medicine from the most recent texts they can get, but there are some diseases that we've known about for a long time. "If I forget you oh Jerusalem, my right hand shall also be forgotten. My tongue shall stick to my palate, if I do not remember you." That's from Psalm 137, probably written about 500 or 600 years before the birth of Jesus. It's an admonishment to keep the Holy Land close at heart, and it's also a good medical description of something that must have been well known in antiquity, and is still a common problem today. And it's what's happening to our first patient. We just came on duty at the ED, and our next patient is being brought back.

He looks to be an older man, being pushed in a wheelchair; he's with a younger woman, maybe his daughter, and she's the one doing the talking. She gives us the chief complaint: "I think my Daddy is having a stroke." Our patient's name is Ramesh, and they're hooking him up to monitors and things while we get some basic history. His daughter's kind of breathless and upset, but what we've learned is that Ramesh is 61 years old, he's a barber, and his daughter works at his barber shop doing hair dyeing and coloring. She says he was working, and all of a sudden he kind of slumped to the floor, and his right hand and arm got kind of loose, and since then, he can't talk. This happened only eight minutes ago—Ramesh's customer was actually an off-duty EMT, who grabbed Ramesh, threw him in his car, and raced to the hospital. EMT, by the way, is Emergency Medical Technician; those are the people who ride the ambulances. If you're going to have a stroke, try to do it right in front of an EMT. They know how to handle emergencies.

What's going on with Ramesh is exactly like that bible passage I started with. My right hand will be forgotten, and my tongue will stick to my palate. The bible here is describing a stroke, specifically a common kind of stroke where there is blockage of the left middle cerebral artery, with resulting damage to the left part of the brain that controls the right arm and the speech center. It's striking how well that 2,500-year-old passage correctly and succinctly sums up the symptoms of this kind of stroke.

Has Ramesh definitely had a stroke, then? It's likely, but we shouldn't assume so, not yet. There is a differential diagnosis, a list of so-called stroke mimics. A seizure can cause sudden neurologic symptoms, and even in the period right after a seizure, there can be lingering effects, including what can seem to be paralysis. Sometimes a faint can kind of seem like a stroke. They're sudden, but of course, pretty soon after someone wakes from a faint, it's clear that they're OK; there's no lasting neurologic or other symptoms.

Hypoglycemia can cause a loss of consciousness and sometimes other neurologic symptoms. One of the first things done on the ambulance or in the ED with a potential stroke is to very quickly check blood sugar. Brain tumors more typically cause slower-onset symptoms, but sometimes they can cause sudden manifestations, including seizures or stroke-like symptoms. And migraines—we've mentioned migraines before—migraines can be very odd, and sometimes they cause sudden neurologic symptoms that really can mimic strokes.

But think about that list of mimics. Really, the only one on the list that needs immediate diagnosis and treatment is hypoglycemia. The rest of those things, migraines, tumors, fainting, seizures, all of that can wait. This is a situation where it is better to immediately deal with what's most likely—a stroke—because immediate recognition and treatment can really make a difference. If, as things turn out, it's not really a stroke, no harm done in waiting to diagnose something else.

One test has already been done; Ramesh's glucose finger stick is normal. It was actually a little high, 180. But you've been lingering at the back of the room while the nurses get their IV started, the monitors on, and a few labs drawn. Ramesh is breathing OK, his initial vitals look OK from across the room, so you get a little more history from his daughter for now. By the way, the ED staff really likes it when the doctor takes the family away for a few minutes; it helps them concentrate on the patient. So we step out in the hall with the daughter; the nurses stay with the patient to do what they need to do. It all works out.

Ramesh's daughter, she's still trembling, she says her dad is really healthy. He has type 2 diabetes, but has been good about his medications; his blood sugars have been mostly normal. The history of diabetes, now that we know about it, that helps explain that highish blood glucose measurement of 180. He also has high blood pressure and takes a water pill for that. He's been married for 39 years, used to smoke, but quit 15 years ago. She says he never drinks or uses drugs, and that he works really hard and keeps his barber shop open seven days. He only takes one vacation a year to fish for a week with his buddies.

A nurse comes out of the room, and she smiles at the two of you, and she says, "I think he's going to be alright." You head in, and sure enough, Ramesh looks much better. He's sitting up, he's smiling, and he's holding up his right arm. And he says, "I feel fine!" So this wasn't a stroke, after all; it was the beginning of a stroke, but it stopped on its own. What Ramesh had is sometimes incorrectly called a mini-stroke. Its real medical name is a TIA, or transient ischemic attack.

A stroke, or cerebrovascular accident, occurs when there is inadequate blood flow to an area of the brain. Neurons, or brain cells, in the affected area die, resulting in permanent, or near-permanent, loss of functioning. The exact symptoms will depend on what had been the functioning of that area of the brain. A stroke in the stripe of brain that controls motor functioning will cause weakness; a stroke in the back of the brain, the occipital area, will affect vision, because the back of the brain is where visual information is decoded and processed. Strokes don't have to follow exact functional boundaries; sometimes these symptoms overlap. Strokes can sometimes cause problems with emotional control, attention, drawing ability, memory, speech. Really, anything the brain does, that functioning can be damaged by a stroke.

In Ramesh's case, what happened was a brief, temporary blockage of flow, long enough so the brain cells in that area were affected and stopped functioning, but short enough so that when the blood supply resumed, the cells survived and returned to normal. This is most typically caused by a clot in one of the arteries that supplies the brain. These clots, if you're lucky, can dissolve or get dislodged, allowing blood flow to quickly resume. So, what's next with Ramesh. His daughter starts bawling. He's smiling, and he says,

"OK, doc, I'm alright, and I need to get back to work!" You know, I kind of like this Ramesh guy.

OK, Vital signs are temperature 98.6, pulse 88, blood pressure 152/82, respirations 12, pulse ox 99 percent on room air. Ramesh looks healthy; he's of Indian descent. A general examination is absolutely normal, but I want to highlight some specific things we're going to look for that are important. His pulses are all normal and strong, including the pulses in his wrists and ankles, showing good blood flow. There's no murmur, and his heart rhythm is normal. A careful neurologic exam is normal, including tests of memory and concentration. His vision, strength, reflexes, and sensation, those are all normal too.

Listening over his neck, to the blood vessels, we hear a humming sound called a bruit. That's something we haven't run across before. A bruit is a noise, kind of a rushing or blowy sort of sound, that's heard over an artery when there is some kind of occlusion or a blockage. You can hear them occasionally over the belly, if there is blockage in the descending aorta, and in children, we sometimes listen for them over the skull. In this case, we're concerned about a blockage from a clot in the brain, and it could have come from a plaque that's accumulated in the carotid artery in the neck.

Now, a bruit isn't a great, reliable physical finding; people can have significant blockages, and there may not be a bruit; or sometimes a turbulent sound can be heard just from the way the artery flows, without there being any true blockage. But hearing this bruit in Ramesh makes us more suspicious that in the carotids, there's a blockage that could have led to his symptoms.

Ramesh feels fine now. So what other workup, if any, do we need? Some basic blood tests were sent off, including a CBC; that was normal, and chemistries, that was normal, and these are important. Strokes can be set off by hematologic conditions that increase clotting risk, including leukemia or multiple myeloma. And those chemistries, those are important too to make sure the kidneys and liver are working OK. We also check some tests for bleeding problems; they're normal, and an EKG; that's to make sure Ramesh doesn't have a problem with the heart rhythm that could allow clots to form in his heart, leading to stroke. The physical exam didn't reveal an abnormal heart rate, but it's best to be sure. All of these tests are normal.

Ramesh also had a CT scan of the head. That's not really to evaluate for the stroke; a CT scan won't reliably show brain damage from ischemia or lack of oxygen for at least until 6 to 24 hours after a stroke. The main reason to do the CT scan is to make sure that there isn't a hemorrhage, or bleed, in the brain. Since Ramesh's symptoms are 100 percent resolved, and he doesn't even have a headache, one could make a case for not doing that CT, but it's also a reasonable screen for brain tumors, and will provide a baseline to compare with future CT scans if Ramesh has more problems. In any case, the CT was done; it was normal, and now Ramesh really wants to go back to his barber shop.

What do you think? Do you think that's safe? Do you think that's a good idea? Overall, the risk of a full-blown stoke after a TIA is probably about 20 percent within the first year, that's without preventive therapy, we'll get to that in a minute. The risk for a stroke within the next few days might be as high as 5 percent overall, but there are some known risk factors we can assess. The highest risk for a stroke within days of a first TIA occur in elderly patients. Now, Ramesh is 61, so he refuses to consider himself in that category. Recurrent stroke risk is also higher in people with poorly controlled high blood pressure. Ramesh's was a little high, but not too bad. The risk is also higher in those whose TIA lasted longer, the first time. Symptoms longer than 60 minutes are especially concerning. Overall, Ramesh would seem to fit into the lower risk category, and with good, reliable follow-up and some initial preventive care steps in the emergency department, it's reasonable to send Ramesh home, or back to work.

Some people probably should be admitted after a TIA; those who are judged to have less reliable follow up, or those unable to manage their own initial therapy, or those without good family support. Inpatient care means that some of the follow-up tests could be done more quickly, too. But in this case, especially because Ramesh himself seems confident, and his daughter is here, she agrees with the plan, we'll send him out after beginning some initial therapy.

First, we'll contact his physician, a family physician who has been seeing Ramesh for years. She confirms that he's always been good about follow up, and suggests an adjustment for his high blood pressure meds; it's especially important after a TIA to keep that blood pressure in a healthy range. She had just checked blood lipids, including cholesterol, a few months ago, and that was fine. Again, we'd want to aggressively treat elevated cholesterol if that were a problem for Ramesh, to help prevent future clotting and vascular disease. She also asks us to send the paperwork to radiology to schedule a Doppler ultrasound of the blood vessels in his neck. We agree on a plan to start Ramesh on an aspirin a day to help prevent future clots. His doctor will see him in her office in two days. Ramesh snips off the hospital wristband. I don't know how, but he snuck in his barber's shears in his back pocket or something, and he leaves with his daughter.

Three days later you happen to see the results of his neck ultrasound. The idea of this study is to look where the source of blood clots might be, these large vessels in the neck that supply the brain. That's where we had heard that bruit. Ramesh does have some blockage, in the 50 to 70 percent range, on the left side here. What to do about this, it's actually controversial. Options for therapy include endarterectomy, which is surgery to remove clotted material blocking up the inside of the carotid arteries, or carotid artery stenting, which is inserting a hollow tube into the carotid artery to keep it open. These are not easy procedures, and they carry a significant risk of triggering a stroke or other problems.

Clearly, higher-grade blockages in a patient who is continuing to have symptoms need to be removed, at least, if it's safe and possible; but for Ramesh, who has had no further symptoms and has what's considered a moderate blockage, it's not clear that aggressive therapy is a good idea. Counterbalancing this, he's only 61, he's in overall good shape, and he can have many healthy years ahead of him. Whether to intervene is a decision we'll have to make with his own family physician, in consultation with a vascular surgeon.

Since we know that Ramesh has vascular disease in his neck, it will be a good idea for him to have a cardiac stress test to look for potential blockages in his coronary arteries. And, of course, it will be especially important for him to control his diabetes and high blood pressure, and to stay on the aspirin.

That brings us back to risk reduction. Why did Ramesh have a TIA, and can he reduce his future risk? The risk factors for stoke and TIA are the same, and they overlap with the risks for coronary artery disease and blockages in other blood vessels. All of these are related to age. The risk of stroke doubles every decade of life, starting at about 55. Men are at higher risk than women, and there are inherited risk factors as well. African-Americans, Hispanics, and Asians are all at higher risk than Caucasians, perhaps because they all have higher rates of hypertension.

Stroke risk is increased not only by high blood pressure, but by obesity, diabetes, and high cholesterol. Lifestyle choices, like smoking, staying sedentary, and excessive alcohol consumption all increase the risk of stroke, as do some medications. Taking oral contraceptives, especially when combined with smoking in women over 35, can further increase stroke risk.

Ramesh had quit smoking 15 years ago. Does that help, to quit? Yes, it does. Within two years of quitting smoking, even long term smokers' risk of stroke starts to decline. By 5 years after quitting, their risk may be comparable to non-smokers' risk. Overall, about 50 percent of strokes could be prevented though better lifestyle choices—not smoking, maintaining a healthy weight, and exercising regularly.

Let's back up to one potentially confusing part of Ramesh's story—that left versus right business; let me clear that up. It turns out that your brain is wired to your body with nerve fibers that cross over from one side to the other. So the right side of your brain controls motor function on the left side of your body, and the left side controls the right. Sensory fibers also cross over. In Ramesh's case, the left-sided blockage led to right-sided weakness. It also affected the speech area of the brain, called Broca's area, which is on the left side, kind of the middle-side area, here.

The symptoms of a TIA, or stroke, can start out exactly the same. In Ramesh's case, the symptoms very quickly resolved, and he did well. With follow up and monitoring, and if he keeps his risk factors of high blood pressure and diabetes under control, he may never have problems like this again. But what if Ramesh didn't seek care at al;? What if he'd just stayed at work and the symptoms of his TIA resolved? That wouldn't have been a good idea. The risk of a stroke within seven days of a TIA is doubled among those who don't seek treatment.

Ramesh was lucky that his symptoms resolved, and this transient ischemic attack provided some warning about his stroke risk in time for him to make lifestyle changes and other steps to prevent a full-blown stroke. What if his symptoms didn't improve? Let's say we're in the ED, here's Ramesh again, but this time two hours have passed since the start of his symptoms of right-arm weakness and difficulty talking. This time, he's not getting better.

We'd then have to think about the different kinds of stroke, which one Ramesh has, because the treatments aren't the same. The most common kind of stroke is caused by a clot, most commonly, a clot directly in the arteries of the brain, a so-called cerebral thrombosis. This is the kind of stroke that's most commonly preceded by one or more TIAs.

A stroke can also be caused by a clot when it acts as an embolus, a clot from somewhere else that breaks off, travels through the circulation, and lodges suddenly in an artery supplying the brain. The most common situation leading to this is atrial fibrillation, where the upper chambers of the heart kind of quiver, instead of pumping. The stagnant blood in A-fib forms little clots. They form in the heart itself, and they can then travel up towards the brain. People with atrial fibrillation need to stay on clot-preventing medicines to prevent strokes.

Whether the clot is directly in the brain or traveled up to the brain, clots cause the majority of strokes. However, a second group of strokes is caused not by clotting, but by bleeding, or hemorrhage. The bleed can be from a burst blood vessel in the brain, or from a blood vessel between the brain and the skull. Any bleeding can lead to damage to the brain by both increasing pressure within the skull, and by disrupting normal blood flow. Some strokes can actually involve areas of both clot, called thrombosis, and bleeding.

Bleeding inside or outside of the brain can very easily be seen on CT. Now, Ramesh's CT scan is normal, so we know there is no bleeding. So, if he had had a stroke, that is, if his symptoms from his TIA didn't improve, he would be a good candidate for what's called thrombolytic, or clot-busting, therapy. Most commonly, an IV medicine called tPA is used. It has to be given within three hours of the beginning of symptoms to be effective. By three hours, even if the clot can be broken down, the brain cells affected will not be recoverable. That three-hour limit can be problematic for people who wake up in the morning with symptoms of stroke. They don't know when it occurred. The clock starts ticking at the last time the patient was known to be normal, even if that was the night before.

There are some other problems with tPA. Though it can improve recovery and reduce long-term disability, because it's an anti-clot medicine, it can actually cause bleeding in six or seven percent of patients, turning a thrombotic stroke, a clot stroke, into a hemorrhagic or bleeding stroke. It also can't be used in people with very high blood pressure because they're at risk for bleeding, nor in people who have bleeding disorders, aneurysms, or prior strokes.

Aftercare of a stroke, after clot busting medicine or treatment of hemorrhages, often includes prolonged rehabilitative care and supportive care. Some functioning can return. The old teaching—that brain cells, once dead, do not recover—that's kind of an oversimplification, and it's not really true.

Immediately after a stroke, there is a few days or weeks window where there can be a fairly rapid recovery of function, at least partially. More functioning is more likely to return with a stroke that affected a small area of brain, and in people who got medical care quickly. The location of the stroke is also important; some areas of the brain seem to be more or less fragile than other areas. Improvement will also depend on the overall health of the patient and whether there were complications, like a prolonged period of increased pressure in the brain, perhaps from bleeding. This period of recovery, the recovery immediately after a stroke, occurs when cells near the area of ischemia start to recover. These are cells that were damaged, but not killed, by the stroke.

After this initial period, there can still be improvement and recovery, though recovery becomes slower after the first few weeks. After that initial period, brain recovery probably isn't related to individual cells recovering their function, but from other mechanisms. To some extent, the brain can rewire connections around an area of damage. If this area of brain was damaged, in time, the neurons nearby can start to transmit signals around that damaged area.

A second mechanism of improvement, again, it's a gradual one, is that completely different areas of brain can slowly start to take over the functioning of the damaged part. For instance, at least some patients who have Broca's Aphasia, that's damage to the speech center on the left side of the brain, can have some improvement in speech and articulation over several months, as other areas of the brain seem to take over some of the speech processing that used to occur in Broca's area. These mechanisms of slow recovery progress over about six months after a stroke, but past that time, there is typically not a lot of further recovery possible. The exact extent of recovery within that six-month window is difficult to predict, but it can be substantial; 100 percent recovery, though, that's rare.

There's quite a bit of research going on into brain recovery after stroke, looking for ways to maximize what's called the plasticity of the brain, this ability of the brain to recover function. We know that children, especially young children, have the best ability to recover after a stroke, probably because their brains are still growing and developing. Even a massive stroke in a young child can end up leading to minimal long-term disability. There seem to be important genetic switches on neurons that control their growth and development, and therefore, the ability of brain tissue to recover. A goal of research is in turning these switches back on, effectively making an adult brain, or parts of an adult brain, think it's young again, so it can better grow and recover.

For the time being, though, the best stroke treatment is actually stroke prevention. Control high blood pressure, high cholesterol. Control diabetes, and prevent overweight; eat a healthy diet with plenty of fruits and vegetables; quit tobacco use, and exercise regularly. People at high risk should consider taking anti-stroke medications, typically medicines that prevent clotting, including aspirin or some prescription medications. These have both benefits and risks, so their use should be discussed with the family's doctor.

One other potential preventive strategy for stroke I wanted to mention is an omega-3 supplement. This is a supplement of so-called healthy fats, often derived from fish oil. We know that populations that consume more fish tend to have fewer strokes, and some studies have shown that fish oil taken as a supplement can reduce strokes. However, other studies haven't been as persuasive, with some even showing some increased risk of at least the hemorrhagic kind of stroke. So, routinely, use of fish oil supplements to prevent strokes really isn't supported. It's a good example, though, of how sometimes promising ideas from initial studies sometimes turn out to not work out as well as hoped. There is still some evidence for other benefits from fish oil, but it's probably not the stroke preventer that some people had been hoping for.

People who do experience early signs of stroke or TIA need to be evaluated as quickly as possible. Yet, there is sometimes a delay. Any sudden symptom of neurologic dysfunction—that could be weakness, or speech problems, or altered sensations, a loss of consciousness, trouble seeing, trouble walking, or sometimes things other people notice, like a droopy face, or eye, or altered speech—any of these things are potential stroke symptoms that need to be evaluated very urgently. Sometimes an individual experiencing a stroke seems to not notice the symptoms or deny symptoms that are really obvious to everyone else. There's even a word for that phenomenon—anosognosia—which may actually be caused by damage to brain areas involved in self-awareness. So it may be up to friends or loved ones to insist that people with stroke symptoms seek care.

Remember, you have about a three-hour window after a stroke where clot-busting medicines can help, and the quicker the evaluation, the better. This is not something that can be done at your doctor's office or something you would call for an appointment about. Call 911, or get to a hospital emergency department as quickly as possible.

Next up, a case that takes some unexpected turns. Sometimes it takes more than one visit to the doctor to get it right; that doesn't mean the doctor did anything wrong. It just means that sometimes you don't see the whole picture at once. Again, an open mind, and a humble willingness to go back and question your own assumptions, that's what it takes to be a good doctor. See you at our next grand rounds.

Sherlock's Investigation
Lecture 19

As either a doctor or a patient, don't decide on a diagnosis and then look for the observations and tests that fit your theory. Instead, you should collect your data, keeping an open mind, and then see if there's a theory that fits the facts you've collected. In other words, every diagnosis is a working diagnosis. As the facts change, your diagnosis might change, too. Don't paint yourself into a diagnostic corner, and don't assume that your diagnosis, even if it made sense when you came up with it, is still correct. When there's new data, it might be time to think again.

Feeling Nauseous, Dizzy, and Weak

- We're working at the student health center of a big university today, seeing college students and faculty. Our patient is a 22-year-old Hispanic woman named Elena whose chief complaint is "I feel terrible."

- Elena says that she has felt nauseous for several days, started throwing up today, and now she feels dizzy and weak. There have been no fevers and no sick contacts. There has been no diarrhea and no abdominal pain—just nausea.

- Elena has a fairly straightforward history, and her vital signs are normal. Her physical exam is normal, and so is a urine test. You give Elena a dose of a medication to decrease nausea and have her stay in your office for a few hours.

- You recheck on her a few times. There's no more vomiting, and she says that she feels better. Still, when she gets up to leave, she seems unsteady on her feet, almost like she might faint. This could be from losing fluid from the vomiting. She is a little dehydrated, but fluids perk her up.

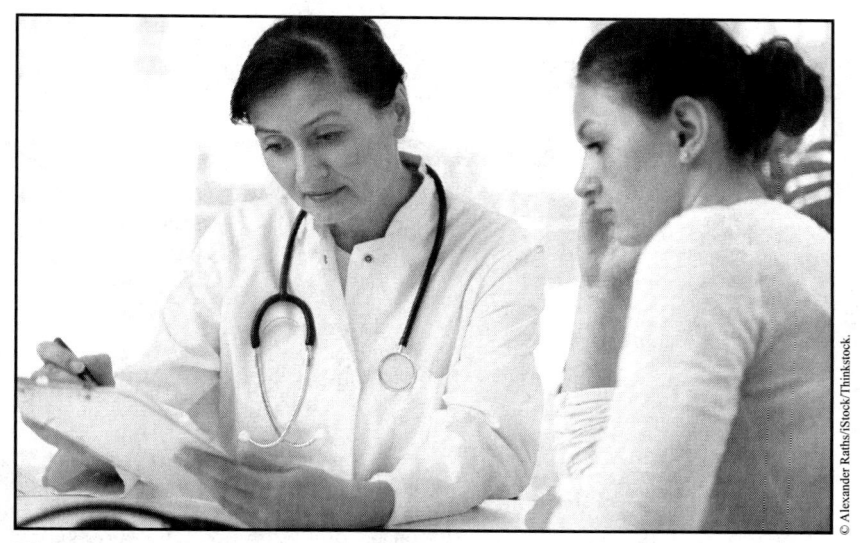

When a patient is diagnosed with multiple sclerosis, it can be shocking, but the disease is common, and support groups are available.

- Four weeks later, Elena returns, saying "I can't see straight." She thinks her vision has become fuzzy over the last few days, especially when reading. It's sort of gradually gotten worse and has maybe been worse toward the end of the day. She says that she just thinks she needs glasses. By the way, her nausea has stopped, and she feels much better in that regard.

- Elena's vital signs are normal, and her eye exam is normal. Her vision is fine when she covers one eye; in other words, one eye at a time, everything was clear. However, she came into the clinic worried that she wasn't seeing right when she was reading. Something isn't right. She thinks it's due to stress and leaves the clinic.

- Three weeks later, Elena returns to the clinic. She says that she's been having urinary accidents, or urinary incontinence, for a few days, and she's assuming that it is a urinary tract infection (UTI). In fact, she's had this same symptom before and was treated for a UTI. But the facts—the history and physical exam and normal urine tests—don't support the diagnosis of UTI. They support the diagnosis of a neurological problem.

- Elena seems to have had one problem that kind of gets better, and then a different one. Her symptoms are occurring at different times. The incontinence has happened a few times before, and it's gotten better and then worse again. This is kind of an unusual kind of pattern.

- Stroke, brain tumor, infection, and migraines can all be ruled out. A young, healthy woman with neurological manifestations that differ and come and go over time leads to only one kind of diagnosis at this point: It is likely that Elena has multiple sclerosis (MS).

Confirming the Diagnosis and Breaking the News

- There are a few tests that Elena needs to confirm the diagnosis. A more thorough neurological exam should be done, including tests of balance, strength, coordination, and memory.

- Before breaking the news to her, we'd like to more about her social support and who she'll be depending on to help her through this. Family and friends are going to be crucial.

- We'll want to schedule an MRI, and Elena will probably need a **lumbar puncture (LP)**, though this will probably be done after referral to a neurologist for specialist-level care. Many centers have multidisciplinary clinics for MS patients to provide the services of neurologists, advanced-training nurses, social workers, psychologists, and other medical professionals. That's where Elena needs to be.

- We have to tell Elena what's going on—she needs to know—but we don't want to be just a fire hose of information. After gently breaking the news to Elena, we'll give her some time and answer her questions. We'll make sure to ask her whether she's heard of MS and what she knows about it.

- Elena may have an idea of what MS is, but we need to tell her that every case is different and that her symptoms may be nothing like those that she may have heard about. We don't want to list every possible symptom that anyone with MS has ever had; instead, we'll stress that there is a tremendous amount we've learned about MS, and a lot of new treatments have become available, and there are more on the horizon.

- MS is common, and we'll try to connect Elena to appropriate support groups that include young women her age. We're going to help Elena get plugged into the MS clinic, and we're going to help make sure she gets the care she needs. And even though a specialist neurologist will be in charge, we're still going to be there to help.

Multiple Sclerosis
- Multiple sclerosis is the most common debilitating neurological disease that affects young adults. Most cases manifest between the ages of 20 and 40, and women are far more likely to be affected than men. There is a strong genetic component to MS: People from certain ethnic groups, especially Caucasians who may have had roots in Scandinavia, seem to be most vulnerable, and MS is 20 times more common in close relatives of people with MS than in the general population.

- But there is more than genetics. Identical twins have only about a 30 percent concordance, meaning that 70 percent of identical twins of people with MS do not themselves develop MS, despite having identical genetic material.

- In addition to a genetic vulnerability, there must be important environmental factors at work. MS is more common in communities farther from the equator, perhaps because of reduced sunlight exposure, leading to lower vitamin D. People who move from an area of high risk to an area of low risk before puberty, but not afterward, seem to have their lifetime risk reduced.

- There have also been multiple outbreaks or clusters of MS, suggesting a possible infectious contributor; there have been many proposed possible infections, though none seems to be the single cause. Smoking, diet, occupation, and socioeconomic status all may also contribute. The cause of MS, as with many other health problems, likely relates to multiple overlapping genetic and environmental factors.

- MS causes damage to the central nervous system (CNS), meaning the brain and spinal cord. There are two major pathological features; one is the destruction of myelin, the insulation around nerve fibers. Myelin makes a sheath around nerve fibers that dramatically increases the speed and efficiency of the transmission of nerve impulses. Without myelin, basically, nerves don't work at all or might be slow and unreliable. This demyelination had been thought of as the main, characteristic pathological feature of MS.

- However, damage can also occur from injury to nerve cells themselves. The affected areas of brain tissue are called the lesions of MS, and at least some of them can be seen on MRI scans; however, the correlation between what's seen on the scan and the clinical effect of the lesion isn't exact. Small lesions can cause significant symptoms, large lesions can cause minimal or zero symptoms, and sometimes symptoms can occur with no visible lesion at all.

- Lesions in MS can come and go, with apparent healing of affected areas while other areas develop new lesions. That's very characteristic of most MS patients: waxing and waning symptoms as different areas of the CNS become more or less affected.

- MS is thought of as an autoimmune disorder, because there is activation of the immune system and inflammation leading to damage in the brain. Also, like other autoimmune diseases, it affects women more than men and starts relatively early in life.

- However, potent anti-inflammatory medicines that suppress flare-ups of MS don't necessarily prevent the long-term progression of MS, leading some to think that there is more to MS than autoimmunity. There's a lot of research going on, and there is certainly more to learn.

- The symptoms of MS depend on where the lesions are. Vision problems are quite common, usually caused by inflammation in the optic nerve. There can be sensory symptoms, including tingling, numbness, or pain; muscle weakness or spasms; or problems with balance and orientation that may contribute to difficulty walking. Fatigue is also a very common and significant symptom of MS, and fatigue can worsen all of the other neurological manifestations.

- Other common symptoms that can progress or wax and wane over time can include bladder and bowel problems, sexual dysfunction, problems with speech and swallowing, cognitive and memory issues, and depression or other psychiatric problems that can be very debilitating.

- MS symptoms can flare up at any time but often seem to have certain triggers. These can include infections. Even relatively ordinary, mild infections, such as a bladder infection or strep throat, can exacerbate underlying MS symptoms. Environmental stresses like heat, cold, or dehydration can be very problematic, and many patients also find that emotional stress can lead to worsening symptoms of MS.

- MS, itself, is not a fatal disease; most people with MS have a normal or nearly normal life span. But the effects of MS on quality of life can be very substantial. Twenty years after diagnosis, most patients remain independent and ambulatory, though some will use a cane for balance or an electric scooter to help prevent fatigue.

- Some patients, maybe 20 percent, will actually have very little progression after their initial presentation; on the other end of the spectrum, about 20 percent may have rapidly progressive disease.

Most patients fall in the middle, with remissions and relapses and a gradual overall progression.

- Although there is no curative therapy, there are a lot of options for medicines that slow or prevent the progression of MS, and there are many ways to treat at least some of the lifestyle complications.

Important Term

lumbar puncture (LP): Sometimes called a "spinal tap"—inserting a needle between the vertebrae to collect cerebrospinal fluid or instill medication.

Suggested Reading

Jelinek, *Overcoming Multiple Sclerosis.*

Wen and Kosowsky, *When Doctors Don't Listen.*

MS Soft Serve, http://mssoftserve.org/.

Questions to Consider

1. What characteristics do you want your doctor to share with Sherlock Holmes?

2. Does a wrong diagnosis always mean that the doctor made a mistake?

Sherlock's Investigation
Lecture 19—Transcript

Welcome back to grand rounds. We have another famous novelist helping us out today. See if you can sleuth out who it is. "It is a capital mistake to theorize before one has data. Insensibly one begins to twist facts to suit theories, instead of theories to suit facts." That's a quote from Sherlock Holmes, from "A Scandal in Bohemia" by Arthur Conan Doyle. It applies very well to detective problems, and it applies equally well to how doctors and patients ought to think about health. Don't decide on the diagnosis, then look for the observations and tests that fit your theory. It's better to collect your data, your history and physical, keeping an open mind, and then see if there's a theory that fits the facts you've collected.

In other words, every diagnosis is a working diagnosis. As the facts change, your diagnosis might change, too. Don't paint yourself into a diagnostic corner, and don't assume that your diagnosis, even if it made sense when you came up with it, is still correct. When there's new data, it might be time to think again.

We're working at the student health center of a big university today, seeing college students and faculty. Our patient is a young Hispanic woman; she's 22. Her chief complaint is "I feel terrible." Elena says she's felt nauseous for several days, started throwing up today, and now she feels dizzy and weak. There have been no fevers and no sick contacts. There's been no diarrhea, no abdominal pain, just nausea. She lives in a house she shares with a few other college students, and no one else has been sick. Elena did travel to Mexico for spring break a few months ago, but had been feeling well until this week.

So, what are we thinking about at first? Common things are common. This could certainly be what's commonly called a tummy bug, or infectious gastroenteritis, a common viral infection that causes vomiting. What we know so far fits pretty well. Sometimes, infections like these include some fever or some diarrhea, which Elena doesn't have; often, multiple people in the same house get this at about the same time, and that's not going on either. Still, common things happen commonly. What else could this be? We've talked through a brief differential of vomiting before. There is a very,

very long list, including diseases in the abdomen, brain tumors, medications, pregnancy, migraine headaches, lots of things.

So, a little more history. Elena has been in good health, though she has had migraine headaches, actually, in the past; they make her throw up. But today this doesn't feel like her migraine, because she has no headache, and it's lasting too long. Elena sounds pretty smart; she's right about migraines. People who have them learn that each episode is stereotyped. That means, for people with migraines, each of their migraines feels about the same. This illness is different, and Elena is right to suspect something else is going on.

She says her last menstrual period was last week, which should rule out morning sickness from pregnancy. She says she is not sexually active, takes no medications, and has no contributory family history. A fairly straightforward history, I think. Vital signs look normal, with a normal BP of 110/66, pulse 88, respirations 12, her temperature is 99.2°F. But Elena, she doesn't look so good. She's kind of pale and seems sort of wobbly when she tries to get up. How many times have you thrown up, you ask? Maybe four times, Elena says.

The remainder of the exam is OK. You try to look for findings that suggest more severe dehydration, like a dry mouth, or a slow capillary refill, that's a quick test; you squeeze the color out of a fingertip and see how long it takes to come back. Ordinarily, cap refill is quick, in a second or less, but in conditions with poor blood circulation, including dehydration, this capillary refill will be slow. Elena's capillary refill is brisk and reassuring.

You give Elena a dose of a medication to decrease nausea and have her stay in your office for a few hours. You recheck on her a few times; there's no more vomiting, and she says she's feeling better. Still, when she gets up to leave, she still seems unsteady on her feet, almost like she might faint. But she says she's feeling better, and she's holding down the drink you gave her. You do one test, a quick urinalysis, and the urine is not concentrated. So you figure, she can't be terribly dehydrated. That's reassuring, so you send her home with instructions to keep drinking fluids and to call back if she feels worse again. Actually, the next day, you're still thinking about her. You have your nurse give her a call, and Elena says she feels much better, thanks a lot.

OK, a pretty ordinary medical encounter, and our patient is feeling better. But think back to that Sherlock Holmes quote. Did we collect the facts, then come up with a theory? Or did we come up with our diagnosis and ignore the facts? The case was pretty straightforward. Elena had some vomiting, and she was a little woozy or unsteady on her feet, presumably from losing fluid from the vomiting. She was a little dehydrated, and fluids perked her right up. But that doesn't really fit, does it? I mean, if she were really dehydrated, wouldn't her urine have been concentrated? And wouldn't her vital signs be at least a little off, maybe at least with a high heart rate? Even backing up, to the history, throwing up four times, would that make a healthy young woman dehydrated, dehydrated enough to be woozy and unsteady?

Anyway, it's four weeks later, and here's Elena again. She's upset. She's crying, because it's finals week, and she's all stressed out, and she says, "I can't see straight." Elena has never worn glasses before, but with all of this reading she's doing, she's having a hard time now focusing on the paper. Elena says, "Finals start tomorrow!"

She's had no further vomiting, no nausea; she says she's felt fine, but she thinks her vision, this is her word, it's gone "fuzzy" over the last few days. It's sort of gradually gotten worse and has maybe been worse towards the end of the day. She says she just thinks she needs glasses. You ask about those migraines. Elena does have a history of those, and some people with migraines have vision issues, like floaters or sparkling lights during migraines, but she says this isn't a migraine she's having, and she isn't seeing any floaters or lights. Things just look kind of blurry.

So what could cause blurry vision? Of course, an optical problem would be the most common thing; this is also called a refractive error, and it means that your eye isn't focusing the image exactly onto the retina. Refractive errors can include myopia, that's also called nearsightedness, or farsightedness; or astigmatism. All of these are common causes of blurry vision, though it is odd for Elena to first notice these at her age. She may also have a more serious eye condition, like glaucoma, or a detached retina, or dry eyes, or perhaps a cataract, or a lot of other things that either affect the eye itself or the optic nerve that brings information from the eye to the brain.

Vital signs are normal, and her eye exam, itself, is normal. With the ophthalmoscope and other instruments we have in the college health clinic, we can look at her eyes, through her corneas and lenses back to the retina, everything looks normal. Her pupils constrict normally when you shine light in them. Her eyes aren't watery; she has no pain. You do a simple vision chart test, that's technically called a Snellen exam, that's when you cover one eye and then the other from across the room and ask her to read the rows of letters to measure someone's visual acuity.

Vision is expressed as two numbers, with a slash between them, like 20/20. That means the patient can see at 20 feet what most people are expected to see at 20 feet. Vision of 20/40 means that what most people can see at 40 feet away, you need to be up at 20 feet to see it. That second number, after the first 20, the higher it is, the blurrier the vision.

Elena has her vision test, and her right eye measured 20/20, and her left eye measures 20/20. Elena says she's embarrassed, but she noticed it too; when one eye was covered for the test, she could see clearly. So she says it must just be her nerves, or eye strain, or a migraine, and she has to go, and thanks, and Elena takes off to study.

What do you think? Elena's vision was fine when she covered one eye. One eye at a time, everything is clear. Yet she came into the clinic worried that she wasn't seeing right when she was reading. Something here is not right. We have some theories. Maybe it's stress or a migraine? But does that really fit the data? Think, would Sherlock Holmes be satisfied, right now?

Three weeks go by. Elena's back,. She says thanks; she made it through finals, and now she'll be working as a teaching assistant through the summer until grad school. She says, "I'm sorry I kind of freaked out last time," and laughs. She says her vision has been fine. This time, today, all she has is a urinary tract infection. The nurse had already had her give a urine sample to test, and you have the results right there on your clipboard.

But Sherlock Holmes, think that maybe he's sitting on your shoulder this time, he wants the data before he's going to let you make a diagnosis. So you ask about the symptoms. Elena says she's been having urinary accidents for a few days; it's kind of embarrassing. She doesn't even realize she's done it. She's started wearing pads to work. She says she knows it's a urinary tract infection because she's had accidents like this before, and it's been an infection. She denies, again, any sexual activity; there's been no fever and no symptoms like burning or pain with urination.

Elena's vitals are normal, and we do a brief physical examination, really, for a simple urinary tract infection, a minimal exam, you figure, is probably sufficient. Everything seems OK. The urine dipstick result is normal, with no signs of infection. There are no white cells, and there's other things that we can test for on that dipstick, usually positive with an infection. No. They're all normal too. Elena says, I know that dipstick comes up normal. I've had that before. But it's always a UTI, and I get antibiotics, and I get better. Sure enough, you flip backwards in the chart, and Elena has been to the clinic twice before in the last year, seeing another doctor and then a nurse-practitioner, with complaints of urinary accidents. She was treated with antibiotics, and she got better. And her prior urinalyses were always normal.

When a urinary tract infection is suspected, the gold standard test is the culture, basically, incubating the urine to see what bacteria, if any, are growing there. That takes a few days, so we often start treating UTIs based only on the dipstick. For her last two UTIs, though she was started on antibiotics, the cultures came back negative. "I don't think you're having urine infections, Elena," you say. "Of course I am," she replies, "what else could it be?" Well, what would Sherlock Holmes think?

Urinary accidents, of course, are normal in little kids, who haven't learned to hold their urine yet. In a 22-year-old college student, something must be going on. Accidents can happen with urinary tract infections, because irritation in the bladder leads to spasms and urine escaping. But in that case, there is usually pain, especially pain with urination, which Elena has never had. And, of course, her tests for UTIs have been negative. Our UTI theory does not fit the facts.

Let's think more generally. How about a condition that makes a lot of urine, like diabetes? People with diabetes, at least adults, don't typically have urinary accidents; they may urinate frequently, but that's different. Besides, the dipsticks Elena has already had, several times, never showed any glucose in the urine. This is not diabetes mellitus. There is actually a different kind of diabetes, much more rare, called diabetes insipidus, that also causes very excessive urine and frequent urination, but again, not typically accidents. Whatever's going on with Elena, it's probably not a disease that causes excessive urine.

Instead, we have to think about control of the urinary bladder. There are two muscles, or they're sets of muscles, that need to work in a coordinated fashion to both hold urine until an appropriate time, and release it. There's a detrusor muscle, that's in the wall of the bladder, and when activated, it squeezes the bladder closed to expel urine. So this muscle has to be kept inhibited, or relaxed, until the right time. There is also a urinary sphincter muscle that keeps the urethra closed. That muscle needs to be kept active, or tightened, until it's time to urinate; then it relaxes. These two muscles relax and contract under control of the autonomic nervous system. We don't consciously control each one separately, but the higher authority, your conscious mind, can inhibit urination until you make it to the bathroom. That's if everything is working correctly.

But what if there is a problem along the pathway, from the brain through the spinal cord, to the nerves, to the bladder? If it affects the system that keeps the urinary sphincter closed, that sphincter might be open all the time, and urine could painlessly dribble out. That's what Elena is reporting; she doesn't have pain or burning like you'd expect from an infection, but just incontinence. Could this be a neurologic condition?

There are some other things that cause incontinence. Damage to the pelvic floor muscles, say after childbirth or surgery, can lead to urinary accidents, as can bladder stones or some kind of tumor. Children will sometimes have accidents from simply holding their urine too long. But there's nothing in the history or physical that suggests these kinds of problems. I think we are looking at something neurologic, here. We have plenty of data. We have plenty of history. Let's revisit what we know and see if there's a theory that fits all of the facts.

Elena's first illness was vomiting, perhaps from an ordinary gastrointestinal infection. The dizziness and trouble walking that occurred with the vomiting, at the time, we thought was maybe from the dehydration, though even then that theory didn't really fit. What else could cause vomiting, plus dizziness, plus trouble walking? Something neurologic. Something, again, in the brain, that affects the balance centers, causing vomiting for the same reason people vomit when they're sea sick. We thought Elena had a gastrointestinal illness, but a neurologic illness explains her symptoms better.

Her second illness, the second time she came to the clinic, was for blurry vision. But her vision, when we tested each eye separately, was fine. What could cause a sense of blurriness that you only notice if both of your eyes are open? Not many things, really. Any problem with the eyeball itself, a refraction error, like nearsightedness, or a problem like a cataract in the lens of the eye, or a retinal detachment in the back of the eye, or a problem with the optic nerve from the eye to the brain, any problem anywhere along this system, you'd notice a vision deficit if you looked through only one eye at a time.

But what if your eyes weren't looking at the exact same image; what if your eyes were crossed, just a little bit. Maybe not enough to really notice two distinct images, but enough so that your brain sees two images, slightly out of phase. What you would notice would be blurriness at the edges of the image. And if you covered one eye, that blurriness would disappear. Blurring, you see, with two eyes together, that disappears when you look through one eye at a time, means that your eyes are not moving together the way they should. Diplopia is the medical word for this condition.

In children, diplopia can be caused by a muscle imbalance, or by immaturity of the control of the eye, or by other problems, but Elena hasn't had problems like this before. New onset diplopia in an adult can be from a problem with the eye muscles, or their nerves, the nerves themselves or the brain areas that control those nerves. Elena came in with blurry vision, so we assumed it was an eye problem. But it was not. It was a neurologic problem.

And let's recap her most recent visit. The reason she came today is urinary incontinence, and she assumed it was a UTI. In fact, she's had this same symptoms before and was treated for a UTI. But the facts, the history, and physical exam, and urine tests, those don't support the diagnosis of UTI at all. They support the diagnosis of, again, a neurologic condition.

There's something else, maybe a little odd about these neurologic problems. They're not all happening all at once. Elena seems to have had one problem that kind of gets better, then a different one. Her symptoms are occurring at different times. The incontinence has happened a few times before, and it's gotten better and then worse again. This is kind of an unusual pattern, don't you think?

Sherlock Holmes is often portrayed as wearing a distinctive hat, you can picture it; it has two brims, one in the front, one in the back, it's called a deerstalker. We're getting closer here, we've almost earned a deerstalker of our own. By the way, just something interesting, the character of Sherlock Holmes was based on a physician, Dr. Joseph Bell, who Conan Doyle met as a young medical student. A keen observer, Dr. Bell was famous for making diagnoses based on the patient's appearance.

OK, back to Elena. Let's think about what causes neurologic symptoms. Could this be a stroke, or a series of TIAs? As we saw in the last case, we'd expect the sudden onset of symptoms, followed by, hopefully, some recovery. All of her individual symptoms actually started kind of gradually, over hours or days, not all at once, and all of them recovered 100 percent. Could Elena be having a series of small strokes? That doesn't fit the facts well.

How about a tumor, maybe a brain tumor? You'd expect that to cause progressive symptoms, as the tumor grows, symptoms should get worse and worse. They shouldn't come and go. So that doesn't fit. Some kind of infection, maybe? Again, she ought to either get worse and worse, or just recover. How could infection cause these different symptoms that come and go? Migraines? Maybe. Migraines can cause almost any neurologic symptom, but they're typically stereotyped, with individual migraines causing the same symptoms, again and again, with each attack. People with migraines may indeed have double vision or dizziness, but it ought to be about the same every time. Migraines wouldn't cause double vision once, vomiting the next time, and urinary incontinence after that.

No, this illness is something unique. A young, healthy woman, with neurologic manifestations that differ and come and go over time. There's really only one likely diagnosis at this point. Elena likely has Multiple Sclerosis, or MS. Multiple sclerosis is the most common debilitating neurologic disease that affects young adults. Most cases manifest between the ages of 20 and 40, and women are far more likely to be affected than men.

There is a strong genetic component to MS; people from certain ethnic groups, especially Caucasians who may have had roots in Scandinavia, seem to be most vulnerable, and MS is 20 times more common in close relatives of people with MS than in the general population. But there is more than genetics; identical twins have only about a 30 percent concordance, meaning that 70 percent of identical twins of people with MS do not themselves develop MS, despite having identical genetic material.

So we know that in addition to a genetic vulnerability, there must be important environmental factors at work. MS is more common in communities farther from the equator, perhaps because of reduced sunlight expose leading to lower vitamin D levels. People who move from an area of high risk to an area of low risk before puberty, but not afterwards, seem to have their lifetime risk reduced. There have also been multiple outbreaks, or clusters, of MS, suggesting a possible infectious contributor. There have been many proposed possible infections, though none seems to be the single cause. Smoking, diet, occupation, and socioeconomic status all may also contribute. The cause of MS, as with many other health problems, likely relates to multiple overlapping genetic and environmental factors.

MS causes damage to the central nervous system, meaning the brain and spinal cord. There are two major pathologic features. One is the destruction of myelin, the insulation around nerve fibers. Myelin makes a sheath around nerve fibers that dramatically increases the speed and efficiency of the transmission of the nerve impulses. Without myelin, basically, nerves won't work at all, or they might be slow and unreliable. This demyelination had been thought of as the main, characteristic pathologic feature of MS. However, damage can also occur from injury to nerve cells themselves.

The affected areas of brain tissue are called the lesions of MS, and at least some of them can be seen on MRI scans. However, the correlation between what's seen on the scan and the clinical effect of the lesions isn't exact. Small lesions can cause significant symptoms; large lesions can cause minimal or zero symptoms, and sometimes symptoms can occur with no visible lesions at all. Lesions in MS can come and go, with apparent healing of some affected areas, while other areas develop new lesions. That's very characteristic of most MS patients—waxing and waning symptoms as different areas of the central nervous system become more or less affected.

MS is thought of as an autoimmune disorder, because there is activation of the immune system and inflammation leading to damage in the brain. Also, like other autoimmune diseases, it affects women more than men and starts relatively early in life. However, potent anti-inflammatory medicines that suppress flare ups of MS don't necessarily prevent the long-term progression of MS, leading some to think that there is more to MS than auto immunity. There's a lot of research going on, and there is certainly more to learn.

In any case, the symptoms of MS depend on where the lesions are. Vision problems are quite common, usually caused by inflammation in the optic nerve. There can be sensory symptoms, including tingling, numbness, or pain, or muscle weakness or spasms, or problems with balance and orientation that may contribute to difficulty walking. Fatigue is also a very common and significant problem with MS, and fatigue can worsen all of the other neurologic manifestations.

Other common symptoms that can progress or wax and wane over time can include bladder or bowel problems, sexual dysfunction, problems with speech and swallowing, cognitive and memory issues, and depression, or other psychiatric problems that can be very debilitating. MS symptoms can flare up at any time, but often seem to have certain triggers. These can include infections, even relatively ordinary, mild infections, like a bladder infection or strep infection, can exacerbate underlying MS symptoms. Environmental stresses like heat or cold or dehydration can be very problematic, and many patients also find that emotional stress can lead to worsening symptoms of MS.

There are a few tests that Elena needs to confirm the diagnosis. A more thorough neurologic exam should be done. Remember, this visit today was for a suspected UTI, and we skimmed past the neuro exam, but we need to head back in and talk to Elena, and we need to check her exam in more detail, including tests of balance and strength and coordination, tests of memory, a good detailed exam to get more information.

Before breaking the news to her, I'd like to know more about Elena's social support and who she'll be depending on to help her through this. She's a college student, so technically an adult, but family and friends are going to be crucial. We'll want to schedule an MRI, and Elena will probably need an LP, or lumbar puncture, though this will probably be done after referral to a neurologist for specialist-level care. Many centers have multidisciplinary clinics for MS patients to provide the services of neurologists, advanced-training nurses, social workers, psychologists, and other medical professionals. That's where Elena needs to be.

But that's not where she is right now. She's 22 years old, and she's sitting in the college health clinic, and she thinks she has a UTI. Although, by now, she knows something else is on your mind. Patients can tell. This first conversation, it's important. We have to tell Elena what's going on; she needs to know, but we don't want to be just a fire hose of information. Elena does not need to know, for instance, that there's a correlation between MS and vitamin D status. What she does need to know, is this, "Elena, we've met a few times, and we've had a few, different sorts of problems over the last few months. I think they're connected, even though we didn't know it until today. These symptoms you've been having, I think they're from your neurologic system. I think it's likely that you have Multiple Sclerosis."

From there, give Elena some time, and answer her questions. We'll make sure though, to ask her what she knows about MS, and whether she's heard of it. Elena may have an idea of what MS is, and we need to tell her that every case is different, and that her symptoms may be nothing like those she may have heard about. We don't want to list every possible symptom that anyone with MS has ever had.

Instead, we'll stress that there is a tremendous amount we've learned about MS, and a lot of new treatments have become available. There are more on the horizon. MS is common, and we'll try to connect Elena to appropriate support groups that include young women her age. We're going to help Elena get plugged into the MS clinic; we'll make some calls; we'll make sure she gets there, and we're going to help make sure she gets the care she needs. And even though a specialist neurologist will be in charge, we're still going to be there to help.

MS, itself, is not a fatal disease; most people with MS have a normal, or nearly, normal lifespan. But the effects of MS on quality of life can be very substantial. Twenty years after diagnosis, most patients remain independent and ambulatory, though some will use a cane for balance, or an electric scooter to help prevent fatigue. Some patients, maybe 20 percent, will actually have very little progression after their initial presentation; on the other end of the spectrum, about 20 percent may have rapidly progressive disease. Most patients fall in the middle, with remissions and relapses and a gradual overall deterioration. Though there is no curative therapy, there are a lot of options for medications that slow or prevent the progression of MS, and many ways to treat at least some of the lifestyle complications.

Next up, a diagnosis that may have become much, much more common over the last 20 years, or maybe not. There's a lot of controversy about this diagnosis, what causes it, how to treat it, and even how common it is. See you next time.

The Boy Who Doesn't Speak
Lecture 20

Studying how the mind works and how children think is challenging. We know that children can have potentially devastating problems with the way their emotional and cognitive minds develop, but how best to identify and help these children is not always so clear. The challenge with autism is understanding how the human mind develops and functions. There is a lot of controversy about this diagnosis, what causes it, how to treat it, and even how common it is.

Speech Delays
- Our first patient in the pediatric clinic is James, who is coming in for his routine two-year-old checkup. His parents express the chief complaint: "We don't think he talks right."

- Because this is James's well check, or checkup, we go through some basic information first, before addressing the questions the parents have. James's growth is fine, and he hasn't had much in the way of medical problems.

- The parents have concerns in two areas: feeding and communication. They say that James started speaking late, when he was around 18 months old, and that he just doesn't talk as much as other two-year-old children.

- He uses only two words consistently: "ball" and "no." Sometimes, he'll be able to say words back, to repeat back what he heard, but he doesn't really use those words to communicate. They're especially worried because James really hasn't seemed to make much progress since he started talking at 18 months.

- Most two-year-old children can put two or three words together, making a simple sentence. James does seem far behind in at least the expressive part of speech. In pediatrics, we call this a developmental delay—a skill that most children have acquired by now but that our patient seems to lagging behind with.

- Many medical problems can contribute to language or other developmental delays, so we have to keep an open mind, and we have to keep an eye out for other clues, to find the best way to help our patient.

- Aside from preterm birth, James has had no specific risk factors for developmental problems that we've identified. And on the developmental history, we've learned that he's about 12 months behind in expressive language, using only a few rudimentary words. He may be a little behind on receptive language skills; his fine and gross motor skills seem okay. He has many atypical sorts of behaviors in the realms of social interactions and play styles. And, as far as we can tell, he seems to be bright and intelligent.

- Children with an isolated expressive speech delay—that is, there is nothing atypical in the development or history aside from the fact that they're just kind of "late talkers"—have an excellent prognosis. Most of those children do very well and catch up after a bit of a late start.

- But James seems to have more going on here, especially with some of these behavioral and social and interactive skills. In addition to his speech-language delay, he's not really acting like a typical toddler.

- The physical exam is a crucial part of the evaluation of developmental problems. We'll use that time not only to observe James's skills and interactions, but also to look for any sorts of findings that might indicate a specific diagnosis or might hint at a certain kind of diagnosis.

- It was a fairly difficult exam—James did not like to be touched and seemed difficult to distract—but as far as we could tell, the exam seemed normal. A good hearing test is absolutely essential for any child with language delay. This could be a problem with hearing. If he doesn't hear well, it will prevent James from learning words and could also explain some of his behavior, especially the limited way he interacts with others.

- We've become suspicious of a specific diagnosis: autism. James's hearing test comes back normal. It's time to ask James's parents a few more questions and gently discuss with them our concerns.

- We should try to give the parents a brief outline of what autism is and stress that early identification and treatment can really help these children learn these skills. Autism is very much a learning disorder. Some things that most children learn automatically children with autism need to work at and need extra help to learn.

- However, exactly what information to share, and how quickly to share it, really depends on how the family is doing. This kind of diagnosis can be truly life changing or maybe even life shattering.

- The doctor needs to stress that there is good treatment for autism and that most children diagnosed in the first several years of life are able to make big improvements in communication and social skills.

- There are children with more severe autism, and the prognosis for those children is not as good. This includes children who have a low IQ, especially children with Down syndrome or complicating medical conditions. Sometimes there isn't really any reason why one child is so severely affected, at least not a reason we understand yet. But most children with autism are mildly to moderately affected, and therapy and special education can really help.

Autism Spectrum Disorder

- Autism—or, as it's now more formally called, autism spectrum disorder (ASD)—is a complex neurodevelopmental disorder that's characterized by three distinct though overlapping problems: impairments in social interactions; impairments in communication; and a pattern of repetitive, stereotyped behaviors.

- One of the earliest and most characteristic indicators of autism is a failure of the development of what's called joint attention, which is a child's ability to share interests and experiences or to request things from others using gestures, eye contact, and verbal communication.

- For example, children without autism (called "neurotypical") will point at things, usually by 12 to 15 months. They'll point when they want you to look at something, or they'll point when they want something. They'll also understand when other people point to look at the thing that someone else is interested in, to share that experience.

- There are other ways to share like this, too. Neurotypical children will bring toys to caretakers to show them what they're interested in, and during play, neurotypical toddlers will frequently look at their parents to make sure that they're paying attention, and they'll deliberately sort of "show off" to get attention.

- There is some research that shows that failure of joint attention in autism isn't just characteristic, but that it may be the essential early step that leads to other eventual symptoms. Joint attention—paying attention to what parents are paying attention to and enjoying positive feedback for doing this—is exactly how babies learn to communicate and interact. If that shared attention isn't working correctly early on, it may lead to missing out on the learning of all sorts of social and behavioral skills.

- Later on, other typical symptoms of autism develop. These frequently include repetitive, stereotyped behaviors, such as head banging, rubbing, or spinning. Routines can become very rigid, and children with ASDs (and, thus, their parents) may find breaks in routine very difficult.

- Children with autism like to play, and they find their play soothing, but their play tends to be different from that of neurotypical children. They'll perhaps be fascinated by the details of an object

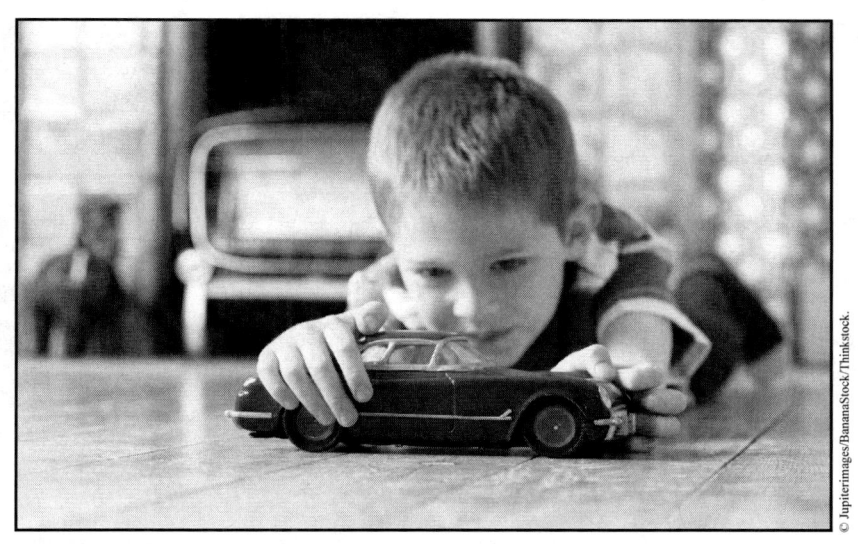

Autism, a disorder that affects physical, social, and language skills, is first detected in infancy.

or find ways to use an object that's not based on pretending or on what the object was meant to be used for. Rather than throw a ball, they'll stare at it as it reflects colors, or rather than push a toy car, they'll spin the wheels.

- There's a tremendous range of autism, which is why we now refer to an "autism spectrum," and not all children with autism will show all of the symptoms. Complicating the picture is that many children with autism will also have genetic disorders (such as Down syndrome) or a history of other medical problems (including fetal alcohol exposure or cerebral palsy), and many also develop psychiatric disorders, including anxiety disorders or obsessive compulsive disorder.

- There's a lot of overlap, and the picture changes as a child develops. One thing is for sure, and it's crucial to communicate this to parents: No two children with autism are the same, and the most important challenges to tackle will depend on the individual child.

Controversies and Early Detection

- There are many controversies surrounding autism. One of them concerns the tremendously increased rates of autism being seen in many areas of the developed world. In the United States, autism affects up to 1 in 88 children.

- Good longitudinal studies, over time, have shown that the incidence of autism hasn't changed much when you use the same diagnostic criteria across age groups. Over the last 20 years, we've really changed the definition of autism to become much broader, so many more children are being caught under an ever-widening umbrella.

- In addition, there is an effect of diagnostic substitution: While the diagnoses of autism have seemed to go up, the diagnoses of mental retardation have gone way down.

- The rates of severe autism haven't changed very much either. Almost the entire increased incidence is seen in more mildly affected children. However, even mild manifestations can be very difficult for children and families, and the treatment can be very costly.

- There is another huge controversy over what is causing autism. Briefly, there seem to be both genetic factors and environmental influences. The environmental clues that seem to be most influential are those that occur very early in life, or even during pregnancy.

- Although children aren't typically diagnosed with autism until maybe even three or four years of age, in retrospect, studies of even very young babies, a few months old, show subtle differences that, though unappreciated at the time, were evidence that something had already happened to cause autism.

- Early identification seems to be the key to treatment. Young babies are especially capable of learning a tremendous amount. Their minds are little sponges. Early therapy to help reinforce the skills of shared attention and early language development can be very effective.

- We need to do a better job of finding children like James early on—to get them into therapy as soon as possible. While there is no medicine that treats the core symptoms of autism, medication can be useful to treat some of the problematic behaviors. What's far better than medicine, though, is early hands-on therapy, engaging the parents, to practice and teach the skills that these children need to learn.

Suggested Reading

Brazelton, *Touchpoints*.

Offit, *Autism's False Prophets*.

Questions to Consider

1. How are children developing differently now than 100 years ago? 1,000 years ago?

2. How can you tell if a disease is caused by environmental exposures, genetics, or both?

The Boy Who Doesn't Speak
Lecture 20—Transcript

I'm a pediatrician, and one thing pediatricians know is that kids can't always tell you what's wrong. With kids, you have to pay careful attention, watch for those clues, and try to take in the whole picture. Of course, that's true for adults too, but it's especially true with kids.

Let me quote from a book published in 1942 by Rose Zeligs, called *Glimpses into Child Life*, about her observations teaching children in Cincinnati, Ohio. "To understand and measure emotional qualities is very difficult. Psychologists and educators have been struggling with that problem for years, but we are still unable to measure emotional and personality traits with the exactness with which we can measure intelligence."

It's now seventy years later, and her observation remains true; studying how the mind works and how children think is challenging. We know that children can have potentially devastating problems with the way their emotional and cognitive minds develop, but how best to identify and help these kids, that's not always clear.

We're in pediatric clinic today, and it should be an easy day. It's summer, and we have mostly checkups scheduled, sports and camp clearance forms, that kind of thing. The practice of office pediatrics is very different, summer versus winter. Wintertime, it's coughing and fevers and congestion and misery; in the summer, our business is typically sunburns and twisted ankles and camp physicals.

Our first patient is James, who is coming in for his routine two-year-old checkup. On the intake form, there's a box for his parents to write any concerns. We'll use their comment as James' chief complaint today. "We don't think he talks right." Let's head into the exam room. James is sitting on the floor, naked except for his diaper, and he's playing with a few of those small rubber bouncing balls, what I called the superball as a child. He's rolling them around under his palm against the floor. James seems completely engrossed with this, so you first introduce yourself to his parents. Ordinarily, we'll try to focus on the children in these encounters, and I personally usually say hi to the kids first, but James doesn't look like he's ready to greet the doctor.

Now, well checks, or checkups, they're kind of different from the other medical encounters we've become experienced with. In an ordinary encounter, the chief complaint drives what we ask about and what we do. Everything, really, starts with the patient's concern, or the parents' concerns, if the child's too young to tell us. We focus on the problem that triggered the visit. A checkup has another focus—surveillance for problems that could be lurking and their prevention and management. Pediatric well visits always include an element of what we call anticipatory guidance, that's a discussion of issues parents can expect to come up, and how to handle them, before they've even become a worry. We also discuss typical growth and what developmental changes to expect and encourage.

Of course, parents and patients at well checks often have a list of their own concerns to discuss. So we have to balance getting through the things the doctor wants to get through, plus the things the family wants to discuss. Well checks, needless to say, take longer than ordinary sick visits.

Since this is James' well check, we go through some basic information first before addressing the questions the parents have. James's growth is fine, he's a little small and slender, but he's growing well. He hasn't had much in the way of medical problems, just a few ear infections, though he was born about six weeks premature and spent a week in the hospital after he was born. We have a developmental questionnaire that parents complete at well checks for young children, to be sure they're progressing as expected, and his parents have checked off concerns in two areas—feeding and communication.

His parents say James started speaking late, when he was around 18 months old, and that he just doesn't talk as much as other two-year-old children. He uses only two words consistently, "ball" and "no". Sometimes, he'll be able to say words back, to repeat back what he's heard, but he doesn't really use those words to communicate. They're especially worried because James really hasn't seemed to make much progress since he started talking at 18 months.

So, our first question, does James have a problem we need to evaluate further? I think so. By 18 months of life, most kids will have about 18 words; by age 2, most kids will have a word for almost everything they see, even if it's not the correct word, it's a word. Most two year olds can also put two or three words together, making a simple sentence. James, he does seem far behind in at least the expressive part of speech. In pediatrics, we call this a developmental delay, a skill which most children have acquired by now, but in our patient, it seems to be lagging behind.

Our second question, what's the diagnosis, or why is James behind in this skill? We need at least a brief differential diagnosis to think about, to help direct our next questions and the physical exam. Many medical problems can contribute to language or other developmental delays. Certainly serious, chronic illness, especially those requiring prolonged or repeated hospitalizations, will set a child behind. There are also specific biologic diagnoses that could affect James' development and developmental potential, including genetic disorders like Down syndrome, or conditions caused by problems in the brain, like cerebral palsy; also problems like hypothyroidism, or deafness, or, honestly, a huge list of other medical diagnoses. External factors may also be very influential, things like psychosocial neglect or maternal depression or lead exposure.

There is also a large category of primary neurodevelopmental disorders, this includes language delay and autism and cognitive disabilities that themselves may or may not have a specific biologic marker. They're all considered primary because they're not caused by a specific, identifiable medical conditions. Sometimes, multiple environmental, genetic, and familial factors contribute to developmental delay. And sometimes there really isn't any more specific diagnosis that can be reached at all. I'm sorry, that wasn't really a brief differential diagnosis, was it? But it illustrates that we have to keep an open mind, and we have to keep an eye out for other clues to find the best way to help our patient.

As always, the history is the key. In this case, we have to take both a general health history, looking for risk factors for delay, but we also have to get a detailed developmental history to see what skills are behind and what the pattern of delay suggests. We'll get to that part next, but first let's see what we can uncover with our general medical history. We start with prenatal factors, maternal illness during pregnancy, use of drugs or alcohol, perhaps a history of prior stillbirths or miscarriages; then we'll focus on the birth itself. Were there obstetric complications? We know that James was born prematurely, which itself is a risk factor for developmental delay, especially if there were complications or a prolonged stay in the neonatal ICU.

We then ask about any prior serious illnesses during James' life, especially focusing on any neurologic illnesses, such as seizures or meningitis or serious head trauma. Has he been exposed to lead or other toxins, possibly from mom or dad's work? Was there any history of very poor feeding, or other reasons for James to have prolonged malnutrition? Is there any contributory family history, perhaps uncles or siblings or anyone else with developmental problems, deafness, blindness, any sort of brain disorder? And the social history, it's crucial here.

We'll ask, gently, but is there any reason to suspect abuse or neglect or family violence? Could one or both parents have mental illness or intellectual disabilities, or has there been very limited social or financial support? I also like to ask about how the parents have encouraged James' development. We know, for instance, that lots of time in front of the TV slows language development, and that children who practice in a walker take longer to learn to walk on their own. That's a whole lot of questions, but none of them, today, uncovered a single concerning answer. They were still worth asking, if for no other reason, than at least to get to know this family. They want to know that you're looking for answers.

Let's move on to our developmental history now. There's a tremendous amount of information we could look for, and sometimes we will refer to a developmental specialist to really nail down these details, but for now, we want to focus on answering a few key questions. Is James delayed only in speech, or is this a broader problem? Children with broad developmental problems, that is, delays in many areas, are of much more concern. We also need to know, what's the pattern here? Is James just slow to acquire skills, moving upwards but not at the expected rate, or had he been zipping along just fine until a certain point, then suddenly slowing down? Or, is he actually regressing; is he losing skills? Children who are regressing or losing skills are more likely to have a specific diagnosis that needs more urgent attention than kids who are lagging behind but gaining skills at their own rate.

We break up developmental skills into several realms. For each one, we'll want to figure out where James stands, where he is in comparison to other children, and his rate of acquiring new skills. Often we'll express developmental skills by comparing him to the average of a certain age, so we might say that James, who is 2 years old, has the speaking ability of a typical 12 month old.

Two major areas of development include fine and gross motor development, so we ask about James' ability to use utensils, to scribble with a crayon, and walk and hop. We can also observe these skills ourselves during the exam. For instance, asking James to stack blocks to test his fine motor skills. James does seem to like to scribble, and he walks easily, but he refused to stack any blocks for us. Instead, he just stared at them and then, swatted them away.

We also ask about language use, both expressive and receptive, that is, both how James has tried to talk to us, but also how well he understands our communication with him. Two year olds might be quite shy in the office, so sometimes it can be helpful to review videos of speech and interactions. James, today, seemed unwilling to speak at all, and pretty much ignored what we said to him. His parents say that he does at least sometimes seem to understand what they say to him at home.

A crucial area of development to assess, though perhaps this is more subtle, are social skills and interactions. All children have behavioral struggles to some degree, especially two year olds. Children certainly have different temperaments and different ways of interacting with each other and with their families. So, what we're looking for here are especially atypical behaviors that are pervasive and repetitive and consistent. We ask about feeding and eating habits, and sleep routines as well.

Has there been excessive anxiety or fearfulness, or on the other hand, a complete lack of fear? How does James respond to noises and sounds and strangers? Does he like typical toddler activities, like being bounced or swung, or playing hide and seek? Is he interested in other children? A favorite question of mine, what are some of his favorite toys, and what does he do with them? For instance, most two year olds like to pretend; they like to play acting games; think about tea parties or pushing toy cars along a track.

When we ask these things, we learn that James is very fussy at mealtimes and will only eat from one favorite plate. He likes a very limited number of foods. His overall behavior is much better if the family follows a set routine, and even on weekends, they kind of set up a fake day care in the basement so he can follow his weekday routine. His parents say he doesn't really take much interest in strangers either way. As long as they don't try to talk with him, he pretty much ignores them. At play dates and at school, he spends very little time playing with others. His favorite toys are three small rubber balls that he brings with him everywhere—he's got them with him right now. And he likes to roll them on the floor under his hand. He has never liked swings; he's never liked being bounced and doesn't seem very interested in hide-and-seek games.

We also need to try to assess James' overall cognitive development. This isn't always easy, at age two. Later, formal intelligence testing can be undertaken, but for now, we'll have to rely on a few observations. For instance, by 12 to 18 months most babies are fascinated by games that include cause and effect, simple things, like dropping a ball so mom has to pick it up. There's also the development of the pretend use of tools or toys by this age, like making soup in a big pot or pushing a toy to pretend to mow the lawn. James's parents recall that he used to laugh at games where he threw a ball and the dog went to get it, and that he definitely remembers where he left things. He remembers, for instance, where his favorite balls are better than his parents do. He also seems to have great problem-solving skills; once he moved a chair to get on top of a table so he could reach a toy, and that he's managed to outsmart every baby-proof lock in the house.

It's important to keep in mind that there are no single, crucial milestones at any age; it's not the single thing that James does or doesn't do, but the pattern of skills. He might not yet know the hand gesture for touchdown, for instance, especially if his family doesn't watch much football, but he ought to know at least some hand gestures, like waving bye-bye or pointing at objects when you name them.

OK, let's catch up and summarize what we've learned. Aside from preterm birth, James has had no specific risk factors for developmental problems that we've identified. And on the developmental history, we've learned that he's about 12 months behind in expressive language, using only a few rudimentary words. He may also be a little behind on receptive language skills. His fine and gross motor skills, those seem OK. He has many atypical sorts of behaviors in the realms of social interactions and play styles. And, as far as we can tell, he seems to be bright and intelligent.

So, how concerned should we be at this point? I think we need to continue to worry. Children with an isolated expressive speech delay, that is, there is nothing else atypical in the development or history, they're just kind of late talkers, they have an excellent prognosis. Most of those kids do very well and catch up after a bit of a late start. But James seems to have more going on here, especially with some of those behavioral and social and interactive skills. In addition to his speech-language delay, he's not really acting like a typical toddler.

The physical exam is a crucial part of the evaluation of developmental problems. We'll use that time not only to observe James' skills and interactions, but also to look for any sorts of findings that might indicate a specific diagnosis, or might hint at a certain kind of diagnosis. For instance, abnormal head growth; a very small head or a very large head could indicate a problem with brain development. Skin findings, including certain kinds of birthmarks can hint at an underlying neurologic disorder, and an enlarged spleen or liver can be a hint that there is a metabolic disease that could affect the brain. Particular attention needs to be paid to the neurologic exam, including muscle bulk and tone and reflexes, or any asymmetric findings. It was a very difficult exam. James did not like to be touched and seemed hard to distract, but as far as we could tell, the exam seemed normal. We let James sit on the floor, rolling those plastic balls under his hand and think about our next steps.

There's one test we know we're going to want, a good hearing test; that's absolutely essential for any child with language delay. Could this be a problem with hearing? Of course it could. If James doesn't hear well, it will prevent him from learning words, and could also explain some of his behavior, especially the limited way he interacts with others. Fortunately, upstairs from our clinic is an ENT specialist, and today, they have their audiologist in the office. So we send the family upstairs for a hearing test while we think about what to do next. We've become suspicious of a specific diagnosis, but we need a little time to think it though and think about how to confirm it.

So James and his family head upstairs; we think about autism. Or, as it's now more formally called, an autism spectrum disorder, or ASD. This is a complex neurodevelopmental disorder that's characterized by three distinct though overlapping problems—impairments in social interactions, impairments in communication, and a pattern of repetitive, stereotyped behaviors. A broad umbrella term, pervasive developmental disorder, had been used to encompass autism and several related disorders, but that's being replaced now with the term ASD, or autism spectrum disorder.

One of the earliest and most characteristic indicators of autism is a failure of the development of what's called joint attention; this is a child's ability to share interests and experiences or to request things from others using gestures, eye contact, and verbal communication. For instance, children without autism—these kids are called neurotypical—they'll point at things, usually by 12 to 15 months. They'll point when they want you to look at something; or they'll point when they want something. They'll also understand when other people point, to look at the thing that someone else is interested in, to share that experience. There are other ways to share like this, too. Neurotypical kids will bring toys and things to caretakers to show them what they're interested in, and during play, neurotypical toddlers will frequently look at their parents to make sure that they're paying attention, and they'll deliberately sort of show off to get attention.

There's some research that shows that this failure of joint attention in autism isn't just characteristic, but that it may be the essential early step that leads to other eventual symptoms. This joint attention—paying attention to what parents are paying attention to, and enjoying positive feedback for doing this—this is exactly how little babies learn to communicate and interact. Think of a four month old who smiles back at mom when she smiles. Then Mommy says the baby's name, and they coo at each other and enjoy each other's attention. This isn't just for fun; it's how babies learn how important their name is, who they are, and how they practice the critical skill of sharing moments together to learn to interact. If that system, that shared attention, isn't working correctly early on, it may lead to missing out on all of the learning and all sorts of social and behavioral skills.

Later on, other typical symptoms of autism develop. These frequently include repetitive, stereotyped behaviors, like head banging, or rubbing, or spinning, or rolling a plastic ball along the floor, over and over again. Routines can become very rigid, and children with ASDs, and thus, their parents, too, may find breaks in routine very difficult. Now, children with autism like to play, and they find their play soothing, but their play tends to be different from that of neurotypical children. They'll perhaps be fascinated by the details of an object, or find ways to use an object that's not based on pretending or on what the object was meant to be used for. Rather than throw a ball, they'll stare at it as it reflects colors, or rather than push a toy car, they'll flip it upside down and spin the wheels.

There's a tremendous range of autism, which is why we now refer to an autism spectrum, and not all children with autism will show all of the symptoms. Complicating the picture is that many children with autism will also have genetic disorders, like Down syndrome, or a history of other medical problems, including fetal alcohol exposure or cerebral palsy, and many also develop psychiatric disorders, including anxiety disorders or OCD. So there's a lot of overlap, and the picture changes as a child develops. One thing is for sure, and it's crucial to communicate this to parents: no two children with autism are the same, and the most important challenges to tackle will depend on the individual child.

By now, James has come back downstairs; he's had a normal hearing test. Pediatric audiologists are very gifted at being able to test kids, even when you'd think they couldn't cooperate. Ophthalmologists, too. It's quite amazing, really. Now that we've thought some more about autism, we have just a few more questions for James' parents.

Does James point to things to show he wants them, or does he look at where his parents point? No, they say. Does he look at where you're looking? His parents kind of shrug at each other. "I don't think so," says Dad. They say that they've learned that if they need James to look at something, they just bring it right to him. Does he ever bring toys to show you, or does he sometimes deliberately smile at you or do cute things just to get your attention, to make you watch what he's doing? No, says mom. She's starting to cry a little.

James is playing on the floor again, kind of in his own world. You give mom a tissue, and this is what you say, "I can tell James is really smart. He solves problems by himself, and he can take care of a lot of things all on his own. I can tell that he's been well taken care of, that you love him, and he loves you. I can tell, though, that there are some things he really hasn't learned on his own, some things that many children learn automatically; he's kind of missed out on some of those skills, like paying attention when you point and using talking to communicate. I think he can learn these things, but it might take him some extra time."

"But what's wrong with him, doctor?" asks his mom. "Everyone says he's just not right. He's going to be OK, isn't he?" I'll tell you that the last time I had this conversation with parents, I cried a little too. It's not against the rules to be yourself, even for a doctor. "He is OK now," is actually what I would say. "He's James, he's himself, he's smart and he can learn things. He does have some challenges, and I'm going to help you through them. What I think he has is something we call an "autistic spectrum disorder," or autism. Are there things you already know about autism?" Asking that question is a very good starting point.

Well, the conversation goes on from there. I would try to give the parents a brief outline of what autism is, and I'd stress that early identification and treatment can really help these children learn these skills. To me, autism is very much a learning disorder. Some things that most children learn automatically, kids with autism need to work at and need extra help to learn.

However, exactly what information to share, and how quickly to share it, really depends on how the family is doing. This kind of diagnosis can be truly life changing, or maybe even life shattering. Parents dream of their child's future, and a diagnosis like this can put everything in doubt. Parents may blame themselves, or each other. Parents may end up divorced, and siblings may end up with their own guilt as families fall apart. This is a time when the family's doctor can be a source of strength and a resource for support, which is probably more important than spending a whole lot of time right now teaching about autism. As the doctor, though, right up front, you want to stress that we have good treatment for autism, and that most children diagnosed in the first several years of life are able to make big improvements in communication and social skills.

Now, there are children with more severe autism, and the prognosis for those children is not as good. This includes children who have a low IQ, especially children with Down syndrome or complicating medical conditions. Sometimes there isn't really any reason why one child is so severely affected, at least, not a reason we understand yet. But that's really the minority of cases. Most children with ASD are mildly to moderately affected, and therapy and special education can really help.

I started this lecture with a quote from Rose Zeligs about the difficulty measuring emotion and personality; it's actually the same quote that Dr. Leo Kanner used in his 1943 paper that first accurately described and named autism. The challenge then, and now, is understanding how the human mind develops and functions.

There are a lot of controversies surrounding autism, and I'm not going to cover them in great detail now. One of them concerns the tremendously increased rates of autism being seen in many areas of the developed world. In the United States, autism affects up to 1 in 88 children. That's a number that pops. Is there an autism epidemic, right now? Actually, maybe not. Good longitudinal studies, over time, have shown that the incidence of autism hasn't changed much when you use the same diagnostic criteria across age groups. Over the last 20 years, we've changed the definition of autism to become much more broad, so many more children are being caught under an ever-widening umbrella. Also, there is an effect of diagnostic substitution.

While the diagnoses of autism have seemed to go up, the diagnoses of mental retardation and other disorders have gone way down.

We also know that the rates of severe autism haven't changed very much. Almost all of the increased incidence is seen in more mildly affected children. I don't mean to downplay that though. Even mild manifestations can be very difficult for children and families, and the treatment can be very costly.

Another huge controversy—what's causing autism? Briefly, there seem to be both genetic factors and environmental influences as well. The environmental clues that seem to be most influential are those that occur very early in life, or even during pregnancy. Though children aren't typically diagnosed with autism until maybe three or four years of age, in retrospect, studies of even very young babies, a few months old, show subtle differences that, though unappreciated at the time, were evidence that something had already happened to cause autism.

Early identification, that seems to be the key to treatment. We know that young babies are especially capable of learning a tremendous amount. Their minds are little sponges. Early therapy to help reinforce the skills of shared attention and early language development can be very effective. We need to do a better job finding children like James early on, to get them into therapy as soon as possible. While there is no medicine that treats the core symptoms of autism, medication can be used to treat some of the more problematic behaviors. What's far better than medicine, though, is early hands-on therapy, engaging the parents to practice and teach the skills that these children need to learn.

Next up, our grand rounds will take place in the frozen Antarctic. You'd better dress warmly. See you then.

Antarctic Adventure
Lecture 21

Appendicitis refers to acute inflammation of the appendix, and it's the most common abdominal surgical emergency. About 250,000 appendectomies are done in the United States each year—though the incidence is much lower in the developing world. About 1 in 14 people will experience appendicitis during their lifetimes and will get their appendix removed. Almost all patients with appendicitis have pain. One recent report showed that a history of increased pain while driving to the hospital over bumpy roads correlates well with an appendicitis diagnosis.

Appendicitis

- The appendix is a small, hollow tube—really more like a small pouch, about four inches long—that comes off the beginning of the large intestine, in the lower right of the abdomen. Sometimes it's referred to as the "vermiform" appendix, meaning that it is shaped like a worm.

- It's thought that the appendix in humans is a vestigial organ—a vestige of a structure that's perhaps important for the digestive processes of other animals, but not for us. There are immune cells in the appendix, so some have speculated that the organ serves to help the immune system develop in the fetus before birth. Removal of the appendix at any age doesn't lead to any loss of function.

- Inflammation of the appendix occurs if anything obstructs its opening. About 30 percent of the time, there is what's called a fecalith, a stonelike piece of stool that you could see on a plain X-ray, but more commonly, it's not specifically known why the opening to the appendix became blocked.

- Whatever blocks that opening, once it's blocked, normal mucus secretions cannot drain, and the appendix swells and becomes distended. Swelling of any of the hollow organ causes pain, which is first sensed by the nerves within the gut itself. This pain is kind of crampy and usually not severe at first. It's usually first felt in the middle or upper belly, near the belly button.

- Continued swelling leads to a decreased blood supply within the wall of the appendix and invasion of normal gut bacteria, which can now multiply unchecked. The inflammation then spreads through the wall of the appendix and presses on the side of the inside of the abdominal cavity—which is when the pain becomes more sharp and focused and intense, localized over the right lower quadrant of the belly.

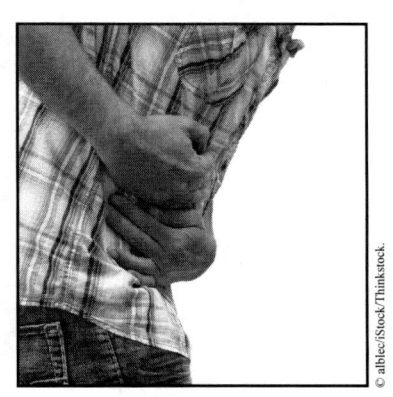

In almost all patients, appendicitis is characterized by pain the abdominal region.

- There are usually signs of **peritonitis**, including marked tenderness. Without treatment, perforation of the wall of the appendix will occur, spilling infected contents into the abdomen. In the past, this was often fatal, but modern surgical techniques and antibiotics mean that the overall mortality even after a perforated appendix is low. Still, it is best to diagnose and treat appendicitis before the appendix ruptures.

- Almost all patients with appendicitis have pain. The classic story (which does not always occur) is pain that begins suddenly in the middle of the abdomen and then, 6 to 24 hours later, moves to the lower right, becoming sharper and more focused.

- The pain, especially once it has moved, is made worse by movement of the patient or tapping on the abdominal wall, so patients with appendicitis, classically, want to lie very still, or if they do walk, they walk slowly, hunching over to their right.

- There is also often nausea, and less often, there is vomiting. **Anorexia**—that is, a lack of desire to eat—is nearly universal and can even be the very first symptom, especially in children. Fever is seen sometimes, most typically low grade. Fever is more common and sometimes higher if the appendix has ruptured.

- Appendicitis doesn't follow the typical pattern of presentation in young children or babies or in elderly people, so those ages have a much higher rate of delayed diagnosis and perforation.

- The diagnosis can also be especially challenging in women, who can have similar symptoms with pelvic conditions including tubal pregnancy, ovarian rupture or torsion, or complications from pelvic infections. Also, some people have somewhat unusual anatomy. Although appendiceal pain is usually in the lower right, the appendix can sometimes refer pain more to the back or on the side—or even be located on the left side in rare cases.

Diagnosis
- There are many tests that a doctor can do to determine whether a patient has appendicitis. When blood tests are done, they almost always show an elevated white cell count for a patient with appendicitis. However, this is considered a nonspecific finding, because many other conditions can also elevate the white count.

- Blood tests can also rule out liver and pancreas disease; in a woman of childbearing age, a pregnancy test is essential. A urinalysis can also be a useful test, though sometimes the inflammation from the appendix, which can lie near the ureter in the back, can cause some white cells to appear in the urine.

- A plain X-ray can be done to help the evaluation. If a fecalith is seen, that can be diagnostic of appendicitis, though it's not usually present. However, an X-ray can help provide clues for other sources of pain, such as a kidney stone—this could show findings that suggest an abdominal obstruction or perforation.

- Advanced imaging is now often used to confirm the diagnosis of appendicitis, or to rule out other conditions. Ultrasound can be used to visualize an enlarged appendix with a thickened wall, though this requires good technique, and the accuracy of ultrasound depends on the operator as well as patient characteristics.

- For example, it is difficult to get a good abdominal ultrasound on an obese patient. Even under ideal situations, often a normal appendix can't be seen on ultrasound, which limits its ability to rule out appendicitis. However, ultrasound may be especially useful in women to look for other pelvic conditions.

- A CT scan is considered the preferred test, if necessary. It is not as dependent on the operator, and it has an overall accuracy of at least 95 percent and can also diagnose abscesses and perforations.

- However, CT scans do expose the patients to some ionizing radiation, and there's growing concern that the overuse of CT scanning, especially in children, could be contributing to the later development of cancer.

- If the diagnosis is unclear, a CT scan may be very useful prior to surgery; when the diagnosis of appendicitis based on the history and physical exam is very likely, it is preferable to go to surgery without any imaging at all.

Appendectomies
- Historically, overall, about 20 percent of patients taken to surgery for suspected appendicitis turn out to have a normal appendix. Extremes of age—children and the elderly—have a higher rate of missed diagnoses, as do women of childbearing age. That 20 percent figure is probably higher than what's seen now, perhaps in part because of the availability of imaging, but there will continue to be a certain rate of false diagnoses, because of the nature of appendicitis.

- Earlier intervention results in simpler, more successful surgery with fewer complications, but the diagnosis is less certain early in the presentation. A reasonable period of observation, while repeating the abdominal exam—about four to six hours—can be a very useful diagnostic tool.

- However, waiting and waiting, until the diagnosis is 100 percent certain, isn't a good idea. Sometimes it's best to go to the operating room, even knowing that there is a chance that the appendix is actually not the cause of the symptoms.

- In the past, every case of appendicitis needed to go to the operating room; a perforated appendix was usually fatal. But we do have other options for selected cases. If surgery is unsafe—either because the patient is too unstable, has another condition that precludes surgery, or because there isn't an available facility—giving intravenous antibiotics is an alternative to prevent complications until surgery can be scheduled.

- With antibiotics, some patients can have complete resolution of their appendiceal inflammation, but many will have recurrences and will eventually need appendectomy.

- In the case of a perforated appendix, treatment can be either an immediate appendectomy or a prolonged course of IV antibiotics, usually after CT- or ultrasound-guided drainage of the infected fluid. An appendectomy can be done a few months later, after the inflammation has settled down.

- The traditional way to perform an appendectomy is open surgery. These days, appendectomies are often performed using minimally invasive surgical techniques, using a laproscope.

- There are a variety of techniques, but the basic idea is to make one or more small incisions through which a scope, basically a camera and light source on a stick, can be inserted. Then, the abdomen is inflated with carbon dioxide gas—which is used because the gas can be reabsorbed by tissues, and it's not flammable. Through the laproscope, the surgeon can see everything.

- Laparoscopy can be especially useful when the diagnosis is less clear, because the surgeon can see throughout the abdomen. If appendicitis is confirmed, the appendix can be removed with the help of additional instruments that can enter the abdomen though one or more other small incisions or alongside the scope. Recovery after an uncomplicated, routine laproscopic appendectomy is very fast, and many patients will go home from the hospital in less than 24 hours.

- Laparoscopic appendectomy has many advantages. There's better visualization of the entire abdomen, smaller scars, and quicker recovery. However, the procedure takes longer, and it's more expensive, requiring more high-tech equipment.

Important Terms

anorexia: Lack of appetite or disinterest in eating.

peritonitis: Inflammation in the lining of the abdomen.

Suggested Reading

Rogozov and Bermel, "Auto-Appendectomy in the Antarctic."

Stern, Cifu, and Altkorn, *Symptom to Diagnosis.*

Questions to Consider

1. Should doctors treat themselves for their own medical problems?

2. What are the red flags of serious abdominal pain that needs immediate evaluation?

Antarctic Adventure
Lecture 21—Transcript

In our grand rounds series, we've met patients in the emergency department and in medical and pediatric clinics. Today, we're going to step out just a little further. We're part of the Soviet Union's Sixth Antarctic Expedition, one of 12 men dropped off in February 1961. Our task is to build a new permanent base station on the Schirmacher Oasis, a plateau about 50 miles inland. The base, named Novolazarevskaya, took nine weeks to build in the balmy Antarctic summer, when temperatures usually hover around freezing. We finished it just in time, and our ship left just before winter descended and the seas froze over. We will have no further support and no contact with the outside world for eight months. In the upcoming long winter, the daily average temperature is about negative 10 degrees Fahrenheit, and there is darkness for about 20 hours a day.

There's only one person in the group with medical training, and that's you, a 27-year-old surgeon who is the team's doctor, driver, and meteorologist. We've got a small medical station with basic tools, some intravenous equipment, some pain medicines, antibiotics, and an autoclave for sterilizing instruments. That's about it. Fortunately, all of the researchers are young, healthy men, and other than frostbite and boredom, we're not expecting much in the way of medical problems during our 12-month stay.

Unfortunately, you wake up this morning, it's April 29, 1961, and you don't feel so good. The first thing you notice is nausea, so we'll use that as our chief complaint. Nausea is not a very pleasant sensation; it's the feeling you have when you think you have to vomit, or you think you're going to vomit. The differential diagnosis overlaps with vomiting, and it's one of those large lists that includes all sorts of problems, from common and minor things to rare but very significant, emergency health concerns. As always, keep an open mind.

Remember, the point of thinking through a differential diagnosis is so you remember to at least consider every possibility. You will not see something that you aren't looking for. When the lists get large, as they so often do, we need some kind of organizational scheme, some way to hold the list together so nothing falls between the cracks. One way you could make a list is to think of the most common things first and sort of work your way down from there. That would work, of course, most of the time, because common things occur commonly. But I'm not so sure that's the best way. The point of the list is a mental reminder, and it's the uncommon things that we're most likely to forget. So I don't think we should leave those for last.

So today, let's start with the most serious conditions, the stuff we really don't want to miss, and then work our way down to less serious things that could be safely diagnosed later. If we first think about the serious things first, we're less likely to miss anything important. As a further memory jog for nausea, let's see if we can come up with two separate lists, one of things within the abdominal cavity, then things outside of the abdomen.

OK, we're ready to think. We'll start with nausea caused by something within the abdomen, remembering first the most serious and immediate disorders. The top one to remember is anything that obstructs the gut and prevents food from traveling through. Those conditions need to be fixed quickly. One example of an anatomic obstruction would be a volvulus, where a section of gut twists around itself and gets blocked. That is a surgical emergency. Intestinal obstruction can be physical, as with a volvulus, or it could be related to damage, infection, or inflammation in the gut wall that prevents normal muscular contractions; this condition is called an ileus. The vomiting that is caused by intestinal obstruction is often described as bilious, that is, showing a green or yellow color from bile. That's not always present, but when vomit does contain bile, it's important to think about the possibility of an obstruction.

We also want to consider any illness of any organ within the abdomen, including all of those kind of itis conditions—hepatitis, that's liver inflammation; pancreatitis; appendicitis; cholecystitis, that's inflammation of the gall bladder. Of course, ordinary mild infections of the gut, viral or bacterial infections, can cause nausea as well, but those aren't going to cause serious harm quickly, so we'll leave them for last on this version of our differential list.

Don't forget, many diseases outside of the abdomen can also cause nausea. These can include very serious things, like a myocardial infarction or a heart attack. Any condition that increases pressure in the brain, including tumors or bleeding, can cause vomiting, though typically without nausea. There are also less serious but still miserable conditions, including inner ear disorders. Many medications cause nausea, almost any medication, really, and nausea can also accompany kidney disease, thyroid illness, diabetes, liver failure, and alcohol or other intoxications.

Do you think all of this was going though your head when you woke up in Antarctica? Probably not, at least at first. But now, a few hours have gone by, and you're not feeling any better. You don't feel hungry, and you skipped breakfast. By noon you're starting to run a fever, and starting to develop more abdominal pain, right around the navel, in the middle. You still feel nauseous, though there hasn't been any vomiting.

You're now running a fever of 100.9 degrees, not too high, but enough to add to your discomfort. Even though you've been stoic and haven't complained, your fellow researchers at the station have commented that you don't look so good. They've also been kind enough to point out that the closest doctor, other than you, is over a thousand miles away. And there's a huge snowstorm, and you don't have any aircraft anyway. You are on your own. Sometimes, time can be one of the best diagnostic tools. It's been about six hours, and the story has evolved. Let's see what's happened to that list of causes of nausea.

Could this still be an abdominal obstruction? I don't think so; there hasn't actually been any vomiting. An infection? That sounds fairly likely, in a way; a fever has started, and that's always suggestive of a possible infection. But, we've been in an isolated Antarctic station for months, and no one else has been sick. Where could an infection have come from? Could this be a heart attack? I doubt it; we're six hours into this, and there really ought to be chest pain or arrhythmias or other symptoms in the chest by now. Instead, we have this worsening belly pain and a new fever. We're taking no medications, and we had a thorough medical exam and a series of blood tests when we volunteered for this mission. None of those tests a few months ago had showed any problems at all. So chronic illnesses, like diabetes, thyroid disease, or kidney problems, all of those seem unlikely.

At this point, it's time for a physical examination. Can we even do an exam on ourselves? We might as well try. Temperature now is 101.1, pulse 100, respirations, well, we can't really count our own respirations; If you concentrate on your own breathing, that always changes the rate, but we're not feeling short of breath, and we're not coughing, so we're not really worried about our chest or lungs. Still, we try to listen to our own heart and lungs, the way medical students do when they practice, and as far as we can tell, everything sounds OK.

Speaking of sounds, we usually use our stethoscope to listen to hearts and lungs, but it's a clever tool for other things too. We're going to listen over the abdomen. Ordinarily, you hear through the stethoscope all sorts of abdominal noises, what are called bowel sounds; they're kind of gurgly sorts of noises. They're normally present all of the time, because even when you're not thinking about it, your gut moves constantly, pushing food around. We listen, now, to ourselves, and we hear nothing, nothing at all.

The gut is not moving. Do you remember what that condition is called? It's an ileus, sometimes referred to as a paralytic ileus. It means that the intestinal tract is in some kind of serious trouble. Now, ileus is not a specific diagnosis; it's more of a marker or a finding that means something serious has gone wrong to shut down the normal movement of the gut. Ileus can be seen after abdominal or pelvic surgery, or during any kind of serious illness. It can be caused by certain medications too, or by muscle or nerve disorders, like Parkinson's disease. But in this case, what fits best with the presentation and worsening abdominal pain is some kind of serious infection or inflammation of the gut itself.

Let's palpate now, gently feeling the abdomen. It seems OK, there's no mass that we can feel, though it kind of hurts everywhere. In fact, it seems to kind of hurt worse when we press down. The belly has become tender. That word, tender, it's a very important thing to look for on a physical exam. Tenderness is different from just pain. Pain means it hurts wherever the patient points. Tender means it hurts even more when you touch and examine that part. For instance, a toe that's stubbed and bruised will hurt, but a toe that's stubbed badly enough to break the bone, that's going to be tender to touch. Or an insect bite or bee sting, that's going to be painful, and maybe with some redness and swelling too, but if the swollen area is actually tender to touch, there might be a secondary infection or a retained bit of the stinger under the skin at the site of the wound.

Tenderness has to be tested carefully; you don't want to just mash around. That's cruel, and it makes people apprehensive. Start gently, deliberately starting with an area of the belly that isn't in pain, and try a little distraction. Watch how patients react when you touch, first lightly, then a little harder. You usually don't have to ask if it hurts; just see what the patient does. You'll know if you've found tenderness. A lot of people have belly pain for a variety of reasons, but belly tenderness—pain when you gently palpate or touch the belly—that means there is inflammation in the abdomen, a finding that suggests peritonitis.

There's a general term, peritonitis, which means inflammation of the lining of the abdomen. The lining of the abdomen is the peritoneum, so inflammation is called peritonitis. This can be caused by infections or serious inflammation within the gut, or can arise spontaneously, especially when there is an immune compromising condition. Peritonitis is serious, and is associated with specific physical findings on the exam, the main one being tenderness. There's other physical findings with peritonitis that we can look for, too, and one of them is a silent belly, or ileus. We have worsening abdominal pain and a silent belly when we listen, that's the sign of ileus, and now tenderness, that's peritonitis, and that's not good. And, again, we're thinking to ourselves: The closest other doctor is over 1,000 miles away.

The pain, now, it's getting worse. It's been a few more hours; it's actually been 10 hours since we woke up with the nausea. Now the abdominal pain is severe and has moved from the middle down to the lower right side of the belly. It hurts especially when you move or when you try to walk, so you just want to lie still. If you could repeat your abdominal exam, you'd find that bowel sounds are still absent, and touching the belly increases the pain; touching on the left side of the belly, increases the pain in the lower right. If you even jiggle the bed a little bit, it hurts in the lower right, even worse.

We've just diagnosed ourselves with appendicitis. By the way, this is a true case. It happened to a 27-year-old Russian physician, Leonid Rogozov, during the sixth soviet Antarctic expedition in 1961. His son, Vladislav Rogozov, himself an anesthesiologist, he collected the details of this case and published it with photographs in the British Medical Journal in 2009. I've embellished and added in some of the details, but what happened next is directly from Dr. Rogozov's account.

This is a quote from his own journal:

> "18:30. I've never felt so awful in my entire life. The building is shaking like a small toy in the storm. The guys have found out. They keep coming by to calm me down…now everyone's running around, preparing the autoclave. We have to sterilize the bedding, because we're going to operate." By which Dr. Rogozov meant, I'm going to operate. On myself."

At this point, he knew his diagnosis, and he had decided, quote, "I just can't fold my arms and give up."

With the help of three other men, he positioned himself on the left side, semi reclining. He injected himself in the skin with a local anesthetic, procaine, similar to the Novocaine commonly used by dentists. Then the patient made about a four inch incision through his own abdominal wall. His assistants held mirrors and handed him sterile instruments as they were needed, though afterwards, Rogozov wrote that he was really doing the surgery by feel. The reversed images in the mirror actually made it more difficult to work. Because of weakness and nausea, he took frequent rests during the procedure.

Rogozov found a grossly inflamed appendix with a small perforation. After pouring an antibiotic solution directly into his abdomen, Dr. Rogozov removed his own appendix. The surgery took just under two hours. His pain and fever resolved within just a few days, and in two weeks he was able to resume his responsibilities. He completed his entire assignment at the Antarctic station after what has become the most famous case of self-surgery ever reported.

Appendicitis refers to acute inflammation of the appendix, and it's the most common abdominal surgical emergency. About 250,000 appendectomies are done in the U.S.A. each year, though the incidence is much lower in the developing world. About 1 in 14 of us will experience appendicitis during our lifetimes and will get our appendix removed. The appendix itself is a small, hollow tube, really more like a small pouch, about four inches long, that comes off the beginning of the large intestine in the lower, right of the abdomen. Sometimes it's referred to as the vermiform appendix, that word meaning shaped like a worm.

It's thought that the appendix in humans is a vestigial organ, a vestige of a structure that's perhaps important for the digestive processes of other animals, though not for us. There are immune cells in there, so some have speculated that the organ serves to help the immune system develop in the fetus actually before birth. We know that removal of the appendix at any age doesn't lead to any loss of function.

Inflammation of the appendix occurs if anything obstructs its opening. About 30 percent of the time, there's what's called a fecalith, a stone-like piece of stool that you could see on a plain X-ray, though more commonly, it's not specifically known why the opening to the appendix became blocked. Whatever blocks that opening, once it's blocked, normal mucus secretions cannot drain, and the appendix swells and becomes distended. Swelling of any of the hollow organ causes pain, which is first sensed by the nerves within the gut itself. This pain is kind of crampy, and usually not severe at first. It's usually first felt in the middle or upper belly, near the belly button.

Continued swelling leads to a decreased blood supply within the wall of the appendix and invasion of normal gut bacteria, which can now multiply unchecked. The inflammation then spreads through the wall of the appendix and presses on the side of the inside of the abdominal cavity, that's when the pain becomes more sharp and focused and intense, localized over the right, lower quadrant of the belly. At this point, there are usually signs of peritonitis, including marked tenderness. Without treatment, perforation of the wall of the appendix will occur, spilling infected contents into the abdomen. In the past, this was often fatal, though modern surgical techniques and antibiotics mean that the overall mortality, even after a perforated appendix now, is low. Still, it's best to diagnose and treat appendicitis before the appendix ruptures.

Almost all patients with appendicitis have pain. The classic story, which, by the way, doesn't always occur, is pain that begins suddenly in the middle of the abdomen and then, 6 to 24 hours later, moves to the lower right, becoming sharper and more focused. The pain, especially once it has moved, is made worse by movement of the patient or tapping on the abdominal wall, so patients with appendicitis, classically, want to lie very still, or if they do walk, they walk slowly, hunching over to their right. One recent report showed that a history of increased pain while driving to the hospital over bumpy roads correlates well with an appendicitis diagnosis.

There is also often nausea, and less-often vomiting. Anorexia, that is, a lack of desire to eat, is nearly universal, and can even be the very first symptom, especially in children. Fever is seen, sometimes, most typically low-grade. Fever is more common and sometimes higher if the appendix has ruptured. Appendicitis doesn't follow the typical pattern of presentation in young children or babies or in elderly people, so those ages have a much higher rate of delayed diagnosis and perforation.

The diagnosis appendicitis can also be especially challenging in women, who can have similar symptoms with pelvic conditions, including tubal pregnancy, ovarian rupture or torsion, or complications from pelvic infections. Also, some people have a somewhat unusual anatomy, though appendiceal pain is usually felt in the lower right, the appendix can sometimes refer pain more to the back or on the side, and even be located on the left side in rare cases.

Our case today relied, of course, on the history and physical examination, and these remain essential to making the correct diagnosis in a timely manner. Though there is no single feature on the history and physical that's 100 percent diagnostic, a combination of findings can be reliable indicators of appendicitis. The most useful findings are, number one, pain in the lower right side; number two, pain that begins in the middle of the abdomen and moves to the lower right side; and number three, findings that suggest peritonitis. Those include some we've mentioned before, like tenderness or pain that's triggered by motion, but also a finding called rigidity that refers to an involuntary tightening of the abdominal muscles. The belly of a patient with peritonitis will feel stiff and firm.

Also, the time course of the pain, that's very suggestive. Dr. Rogozov first noticed symptoms in the morning, when he woke up, and within a few hours he developed the findings of peritonitis. Patients with appendicitis develop severe and worsening pain in a short few hours; someone who has pain lasting for several days or more is less likely to have appendicitis. Keep in mind, though, that these findings, combined, are very suggestive of appendicitis; many patients with appendicitis don't have the entire, classic story. The classic sequence of symptoms is only present two thirds of the time.

If Dr. Rogozov had had access to a modern hospital, other tests would probably have been done. Blood tests would have confirmed an elevated white cell count, that's almost always seen in appendicitis, but it's what's called a non-specific finding, because many other conditions can also elevate the white count. Blood tests could also have ruled out liver and pancreas disease; and in a woman of child-bearing age, a pregnancy test would have been essential.

A plain X-ray can be done to help the evaluation. If a fecalith is seen, that can be diagnostic of appendicitis, though it's not usually present. However, an X-ray can help provide clues for other sources of pain, like a kidney stone, and it could show findings that suggest an abdominal obstruction or perforation.

Advanced imaging is now often used to confirm the diagnosis of appendicitis or to rule out other conditions. Ultrasound can be used to visualize an enlarged appendix with a thickened wall. though this requires good technique, and the accuracy of ultrasound depends on the operator as well as patient characteristics. For instance, it's difficult to get a good abdominal ultrasound on an obese patient. Even under ideal situations, often a normal appendix can't be seen on ultrasound, which limits its ability to rule out appendicitis. However, ultrasound may be especially useful in women to look for other pelvic conditions.

CT scan is considered the preferred test, if necessary. It is not as operator dependent and has an overall accuracy of at least 95 percent, and can also diagnose abscesses and perforations. However, CT scans do expose the patients to some ionizing radiation, and there's growing concern that the overuse of CT scanning, especially in children, could be contributing to the later development of cancers. However, if the diagnosis is unclear, a CT scan may be very useful prior to surgery. When the diagnosis of appendicitis, based on the history and the physical exam is very likely, it is preferable to go to surgery without any imaging at all.

Historically, about 20 percent of the time, overall, patients taken to surgery for suspected appendicitis turn out to have a normal appendix. Extremes of age—children, the elderly, the young and the old—have a higher rate of missed diagnoses, as do women of child bearing age. That 20 percent figure is probably higher than what's seen now, perhaps in part because of the availability of imaging; but there will continue to be a certain rate of false diagnoses, because of the nature of appendicitis. We know that earlier intervention results in simpler, more-successful surgery with fewer complications; but we also know that the diagnosis is less certain early on. A reasonable period of observation, while repeating the abdominal exam, say 4–6 hours, can be a very useful diagnostic tool. However, waiting and waiting, until the diagnosis is 100 percent sure, isn't a good idea. Sometimes it's best to just go to the OR, even knowing that there is a chance that the appendix is actually not the cause of the symptoms.

Does every case of appendicitis need to go to the OR? In the past, yes. A perforated appendix was usually fatal. But we do have other options for selected cases. If surgery is unsafe, either because the patient is too unstable, or has another condition that precludes surgery, or because there isn't an available facility, giving intravenous antibiotics is an alternative to prevent complications until surgery can be scheduled. With antibiotics, some patients can have their complete resolution of their appendiceal inflammation, but many will have recurrences and will need an appendectomy later.

In the case of a perforated appendix, treatment can be either an immediate appendectomy or a prolonged course of IV antibiotics, usually after CT- or ultrasound-guided drainage of the infected fluid. An appendectomy can be done a few months later, after the inflammation has settled down.

Now, Dr. Rogozov performed his surgery the traditional way, called open surgery, through an incision over a classic spot on the abdomen called "McBurney's Point." You draw a line from the anterior superior iliac spine, this hard part in front of your pelvis, up towards the belly button. Go one third of the way up that line, and you're right over the base of the appendix. That's where Dr. Rogozov made his incision. These days, appendectomies are often performed using minimally invasive surgical techniques, using a laparoscope.

There are a variety of techniques, but the basic idea is to make one or more small incisions though which a scope, basically a camera and light source on a stick, can be inserted. Then the abdomen is inflated with carbon dioxide gas; that's used because the gas can be reabsorbed by tissues, and it's not flammable. Through the laparoscope, the surgeon can see everything. Laparoscopy can be especially useful when the diagnosis is less clear, because the surgeon literally can see throughout the abdomen. If appendicitis is confirmed, the appendix can be removed with the help of additional instruments that can enter the abdomen though one or more other small incisions or alongside the scope. Recovery after an uncomplicated, routine laparoscopic appendectomy is very fast, and many patients will go home from the hospital in less than 24 hours.

Laparoscopic appendectomy has many advantages. There's better visualization of the entire abdomen, smaller scars, and quicker recovery. However, the procedure takes longer, and it's more expensive, requiring more high-tech equipment. When you're stuck in the Antarctic, you have to use the traditional, open approach.

By the way, if you're curious about what happened to Dr. Rogozov, his story was a sensation in the Soviet Union, and he was awarded the Order of the Red Banner of Labour. He resumed working as a surgeon and medical instructor, later serving as the head of surgery at a hospital in St. Petersburg. Rogozov himself insisted that there be no glorification of his deed, only a small bulletin about his surgery appeared after his return in 1962. He died in

2,000 at age 66. In 2009, his son published the first comprehensive account of his self-appendectomy in the Antarctic. I don't think many physicians will ever duplicate this story.

Though, actually, one other doctor did do something similar. In 1999 Dr. Jerri Nielsen, working as the only doctor at an isolated station near the South Pole, discovered a lump in her own breast. She performed her own biopsy, and using airdropped supplies, began therapy for cancer.

Next up, not every case starts in the ED or a doctor's office. When you're an emergency physician, you're always on the job. See you next time.

A Sunday Drive
Lecture 22

What happens to a human body when it's pushed to the edge of survival? Imagine that you are in your car on your way to the emergency department for your next shift. A man on a motorcycle passes you, darting into and out of oncoming traffic. He's probably going 60 miles an hour on a two-lane street. Up ahead of you now, you see his back wheel clip the edge of a car. The motorcycle spins out of control and slams into a concrete utility pole. What do you do?

Motorcycle Accident

- After an accident occurs, the first step is to clear the area. You need to ensure your own safety, making sure that no one is going to drive into you or the victim when you stop to help. You pull over, leaving your blinkers on and leaving enough of your car in the lane to slow traffic.

- Then, you call for help. You're going to do what you can, but you already know that you're going to need an ambulance, and the faster they get here and get the cyclist to the hospital, the better his chance of survival. If other people have stopped to help, you can split up the jobs. Say to someone else, "You, call 911"—don't assume that somebody else has already called.

- Once the ambulance is on its way and the area seems safe, you approach your patient. He's lying on the ground, on his back; his motorcycle helmet has been crushed and knocked off his head. You can see the name "Tommy" airbrushed across the back of the helmet. Tommy is lying awkwardly; his legs look broken, and one shoulder is pushed backward unnaturally.

- The initial care of a trauma or a critically ill patient—including any trauma patient, from any kind of trauma—starts with what's called the primary survey. Medical personnel go through five items, in order; they always address the step they are on before they go on to the next step. There's a handy mnemonic to remember the five steps of the primary survey: ABCDE.

- The point of this primary survey is to identify and immediately deal with life-threatening problems. In the field, if there is something that is an immediate threat to life, do what you can to fix it; if you can't fix it, continue support and get the patient transported as quickly as possible.

- This primary survey is for medical people—emergency medical techs and nurses, respiratory therapists, emergency department doctors—people who have been trained. Laymen are not expected to know or follow these steps. For most laymen, the most important steps are to protect the victim from further harm and call for help.

- "A" stands for "airway." Is the airway open? Can air get into the lungs? In an awake patient, you can test this by asking the person to speak; if you can talk, or if you can cough, you can move air. Our patient, Tommy, isn't really moving, and he certainly isn't speaking, so you assess the airway visually. He seems to have no serious facial trauma that would interfere with breathing. With this kind of trauma, you also want to be very careful about moving the head, but he's got to have an open airway to breathe, so if you need to move the head to open the airway, you do it.

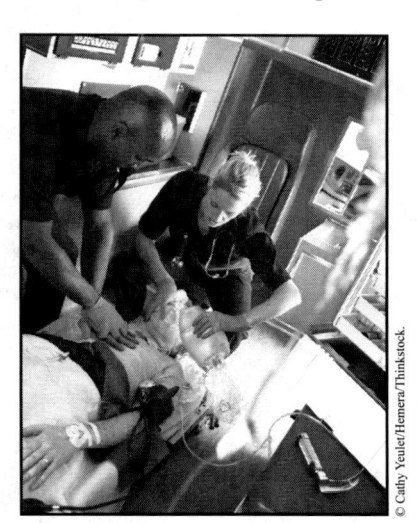

If you witness an accident, one of the most important steps is to call for emergency medical help.

- "B" stands for "breathing"—and Tommy does seem to be breathing, albeit slowly and irregularly. You look, listen, and feel: You look at the chest wall to see that it's rising and falling, at least somewhat, and you listen and feel right over the mouth to tell that at least some air is moving in and out.

- "C" is for "circulation." Is there a pulse? Is blood being circulated? Yes, there's a pulse that you can feel. It's not strong, but it is there. The assessment of circulation in this step also includes control of any serious hemorrhage. If your patient is bleeding, try to stop it with pressure and perhaps a tourniquet. If too much blood is lost, circulation will be compromised. For now, you don't see any serious bleeding.

- "D" stands for "disability," referring to your patient's neurological status. There are several scales and ways to judge overall neurological status, but one of the quickest and most widely used is the simple AVPU scale. "A" stands for "alert," meaning a normal, alert, fully awake patient. "V" stands for "voice," referring to a patient who isn't fully alert but at least responds to your voice, either by talking back or moving purposefully. "P" stands for "pain," meaning a patient who responds not to voice but only to a painful stimulus. "U" is a patient who is completely "unresponsive," who doesn't react to voice or pain at all. At this point, Tommy is a "P" on this scale.

- "E" is the last letter of the primary survey, standing for "exposure" and "environment." You need to get a look at the whole body. For practical purposes, looking at the back is done as a "log roll," with someone holding the head neutral. When Tommy is rolled, you notice that the ribs on one side of his back appear to be crushed inward. That means there is a very serious injury to his lung and that breathing may become very difficult.

At the Hospital
- Once the ambulance comes, Tommy is rushed to the hospital while you follow in your car. The philosophy of emergency medical

technicians (**EMTs**) in a serious, life-threatening situation is to spend a minimum amount of time at the scene—address only immediate threats, and only if you have the equipment and ability to address them—and then get the patient as quickly as possible to where he needs to be.

- On the way to the hospital, do as much as you can to help. One specific task, along with keeping an eye on the ABCDEs, is to try to get good IV access—get IVs started, big lines and multiple ones. EMTs would never delay transport to get those IVs in, but that access is going to be critical to give medicines, fluids, and blood products.

- The emergency department is a different sort of medical setting. In most places, as a physician, you'll make the diagnosis first, and then move logically to therapy. In the emergency department, finding a specific diagnosis is secondary. The main job is to identify the genuinely sick and get them stabilized for admission to the intensive care unit or the floor of the main hospital. It's a different sort of mindset, one where time is of the essence.

- After reassessing Tommy's ABCDEs in the trauma room, you determine that he has deteriorated across the board. In addition, he's now at U, completely unresponsive on the AVPU scale. Although many things can cause this, in a trauma situation, the big ones to think of first are those that could benefit from immediate intervention.

- First, there's direct brain injury. Tommy was going fast and then slammed into a utility pole. He was wearing a helmet, but at that speed, the collision could have done tremendous damage to Tommy's brain by directly damaging or killing cells, by shearing the connections between cells, and by damaging blood vessels necessary to deliver oxygen. This kind of damage can be difficult to assess right after an injury.

- In addition, there's brain injury from swelling, which can also decrease blood flow into the **cranium**. We'd like to get a CT scan to see what's going on in the head. Then, in the operating room, a neurosurgeon's role could be to help open up the skull and evacuate blood collections, relieving increased intracranial pressure. Monitors could also be put into the cranium to more directly measure pressure there.

- But we've got even more immediate problems to worry about. Tommy might be falling further into unconsciousness—because Tommy is in shock. That means that the body's tissues are not getting enough blood; in other words, there isn't enough perfusion. Although there may be enough oxygen in the blood, the blood isn't getting to where it's needed—so insufficient oxygen is being delivered.

- Shock can be caused by a number of different problems, but in Tommy's case, shock is being caused by what's called hypovolemia—there is just not enough circulating blood. We know that he's hemorrhaging in his chest because there's blood coming out of his **chest tubes**, and we know that he's hemorrhaging in his abdomen. We haven't been able to stop the bleeding, and as fast as we can pour blood in, it's pouring out.

- Shock can affect every organ of the body. Many problems caused by shock can pile up on one another, leading to a cascade of worsening organ failure. There are also immunological mechanisms, where damaged tissues from trauma and shock release factors into the blood that themselves lead to a massive inflammatory cascade, inflammatory overactivation, and further tissue damage and circulatory problems.

Death: Breaking the News
- Suddenly, monitors start blaring. Tommy's heart has stopped. A **defibrillator** is rushed over. You take the paddles while someone squirts clear cold goo on them to improve conduction, and you yell,

"Clear!" You shock once; nothing happens. You shock twice; a heartbeat occurs again.

- More medicines are poured into the IVs to support blood pressure and to stop arrhythmias. It has been four minutes. Moments later, a second code; the heart stops again. You shock again, with no response. Chest compressions are begun, followed by a pause for another shock. Now, the heart is quivering—not beating, just wiggling in the chest—not pumping oxygen at all. It has been eight minutes.

- One more shock leads to a few good heartbeats. A nurse reports that she feels a pulse in the neck. It's been 10 minutes. The pulse fades, softer and softer, and chest compressions are started again.

- There's an irregular recording on the heart monitor that becomes just a random squiggle. After 12 minutes, the tracing stops completely. The line becomes flat again, leading to more shocks and compressions. After 25 minutes without a strong, consistent pulse, you, the emergency department physician, look at the clock on the wall and announce the time of death while the scribe records it. Compressions stop, and the ventilator is switched off.

- You need to catch your breath and go meet the family. You're told that they're in the waiting room, and they want to come back and see Tommy right away. Families should be told this kind of news together, when possible, so that they can have each other for comfort. They also deserve to have a quiet, private area, and they need to have time with the doctor.

- You tell the family that you did everything you could, but Tommy had very serious injuries, and he couldn't survive. Some families will want more details, maybe all of the medical details, and you answer those sorts of questions as best you can. You offer your card, even as the emergency physician, for the family to call later, when more questions arise.

Important Terms

chest tube: More formally, thoracostomy tube—a tube used to drain air or fluid from the chest.

cranium: The skull, or more specifically, the part of the skull that encloses the brain.

defibrillator: A device that delivers a shock to the heart to restore a normal rhythm.

EMT: Emergency medical technician.

Suggested Reading

Nolen, *The Making of a Surgeon*.

Shem, *The House of God*.

Questions to Consider

1. What obligation should medical professionals have to stop to help people who are ill or injured?

2. How is the viewpoint of people who deal with acute injuries different—the first responders on an ambulance, versus the team in the emergency department, versus the doctors and nurses in an intensive care unit?

A Sunday Drive
Lecture 22—Transcript

Today, you're an emergency physician, but you're not yet at work. You're just driving, on the way to the hospital, heading in to do your ED shift. Drinking coffee, probably. Doesn't matter what time of day, If you're an emergency doc, you're drinking coffee.

By the way, the correct terminology is important People who work in emergency departments prefer to call it the ED. The specialty is called EM, for emergency medicine; the doctors who work in the ED are called emergency physicians. So ED is the place, EM is the specialty, EP is the specialist, and ER is a TV show.

A guy on a motorcycle passes you on the left, darting into and out of oncoming traffic. He's just flying along, probably going 60 miles an hour on a two-lane street. Up ahead of you, you see his back wheel clip the edge of a car as he darts back into your lane. The motorbike spins out of control and slams into a concrete utility pole. Today's grand rounds is going to be a little different. We know exactly what the diagnosis is; we just saw it happen. The mystery, the case that we'll see unfold, is what happens next. What happens to a human body when it's pushed to the edge of survival?

You're going to stop to help. Your foot's on the brake and you're already pulling over. In some places, laws require health care providers to stop and offer assistance, but, honestly, I don't think people stop because it's the law. You stop because you can help. First step, clear the area. You need to ensure your own safety, first, making sure no one is going to drive into you or the victim when you stop to help. You pull over, leaving your blinkers on, and leaving enough of your car in the lane to slow traffic. Then, you call for help. You're going to do what you can, but you already know that you're going to need an ambulance, and the faster they get here and get the cyclist to the hospital, the better his chance of survival. If other people have stopped to help, you could split up the jobs. Say to someone else, "you, call 911," but I wouldn't assume that somebody else has called.

407

OK, the ambulance is on the way, the area seems safe, and you approach your patient. He's lying on the ground on his back; his motorcycle helmet has been crushed and knocked off his head. You can see the word "Tommy" airbrushed across the back of the helmet. Tommy himself is lying awkwardly, his legs look broken, and one shoulder is pushed backwards unnaturally. These are the things you really can't help but notice, and afterwards, they may be the things you may remember best.

The initial care of a trauma or a critically ill patient, including any trauma patient, from any kind of trauma, from motorcycle accidents, to injuries during wartime, drowning victims, a serious fall, anything, starts with what's called the primary survey. Medical personnel go through five items, in order, and you always address the step you are on before you go on to the next step. There's a handy mnemonic to remember the five steps of the primary survey: ABCDE. The point of this primary survey is to identify and immediately deal with life-threatening problems. In the field, if there is something that is an immediate threat to life, do what you can to fix it, and if you can't fix it, continue support and get the patient transported as quickly as possible.

Now, this primary survey is for medical people, emergency medical techs and nurses, respiratory therapists, ED docs, people who have been trained. Laymen are not expected to know or follow these steps. I do recommend routinely that people take a CPR course, especially parents, or those who work with children or elderly people, so they can feel more comfortable taking the first steps in an emergency. For most laymen, the most important steps are to protect the victim from further harm, and call for help.

Today, you're an ED doctor. Let's get going on those ABCDEs. A stands for Airway. Is the airway open; can air get into the lungs? In an awake patient, you can test this by asking the person to speak. If you can talk, or if you can cough, you can move air. Our patient, Tommy, he isn't really moving, and he certainly isn't speaking. You assess the airway visually, he seems to have no serious facial trauma that would interfere with breathing, but in an unconscious patient, you know that he may not do a good job keeping his mouth open and his tongue pushed forward. You need to be very careful about moving the head; with this kind of trauma, there's a very good chance that there's a fracture in the neck, and you don't want to do something that may endanger the spinal cord. Still, he has to have an open airway to breathe, so if you need to move the head to open the airway, you do it.

B stands for breathing, and Tommy does seem to be breathing, a little bit. You look, you listen, you feel. You can look at the chest wall; it's rising and falling, at least some, and you can listen and feel right over the mouth to tell at least some air is moving in and out. But they're slow, and they're irregular, and you're hoping that the ambulance gets there soon with some equipment and people to help out.

C is circulation, is there a pulse, is blood being circulated? Yes, there's a pulse you can feel. It's not strong, but it is there. The assessment of circulation in the C step also includes control of any serious hemorrhages. If your patient is bleeding, try to stop it with pressure and perhaps a tourniquet. If too much blood is lost, circulation will be compromised. For now, you don't see any serious bleeding.

OK, help has arrived. The ambulance comes screeching up, almost simultaneously with a police car. The EMTs, those are emergency medical technicians, they jump right in. Since you're an ED doc, you know that unless you have field experience, the best thing you can do at this point is to get out of the way and let the EMTs do their job. This is highly specialized work, and it isn't really part of training for physicians. Attempts to help the ambulance team, especially in a critical situation, will usually just slow them down. They're going to start the primary survey again, from the top.

Back to A, Tommy's airway is open and more protected, now; one of the techs holds his head carefully in a neutral position, taking any load off of his spine. B,: Tommy, at this point, is barely breathing. His chest wall isn't moving well; he's maybe gasping, but he's not moving air. While one EMT keeps his head stable, another applies a mask over his mouth and nose with 100 percent oxygen and squeezes a bag to push air into his lungs. This is called bag mask ventilation, and though it can be labor intensive, it's quick to start once you have the right equipment. While bagging, you can see Tommy's chest rising and falling, so you know air is getting in and out. OK, step B is covered; that's breathing. Let's go to step C.

C, again, stands for circulation; make sure the heart is beating; make sure there are pulses; that's how you know blood getting to the body. Look for active bleeding and try to control it, usually first with direct pressure. Tommy' has reasonably good pulses, for now.

Next is D, D stands for disability, referring to your patient's neurologic status. There are several scales and ways to judge overall neurologic status, but one of the quickest and most widely used is the simple AVPU scale. A stands for Alert, meaning a normal, alert, fully awake patient. V stands for voice, referring to a patient who isn't fully alert but at least responds to your voice, either by talking back or moving purposefully. P stands for pain, meaning a patient who responds not to voice, but only to a painful stimulus. U is a patient who is completely unresponsive, who doesn't react to voice or pain at all.

The EMTs yell at Tommy. Sir, sir are you OK? He doesn't respond at all. Sir, can you open your eyes? Open your eyes! There's no response. They do a quick sternal rub; that's a quick way to give some pain, to check responsiveness, pushing on the chest with the knuckles, kind of like this. When they do this to Tommy, he kind of groans and pulls his legs up towards his chest. So at this point, Tommy is a P on the AVPU scale, he responds to pain.

E is the last step of the primary survey, standing for exposure and environment. You need to get a look at the whole body; if you don't look, you won't see. For practical purposes looking at the back is done as a log roll, with someone holding the head neutral, and in the field, this can be done in one step while rolling the patient onto a firm board to get him up in the ambulance for transport. When the team rolls Tommy, you see something not good at all. It looks like the ribs on one side of his back are crushed inwards. This means a very serious injury to his lung there, and that breathing may become very difficult.

They rush Tommy onto the ambulance; they scream away; lights and sirens blaring. You follow along in your own car to the hospital, You were heading in to work anyway, and now you know who's probably going to be your first patient.

While on the ambulance, a lot is going on. The crew reports to the ED by radio, or sometimes cell phone, and sends in data about Tommy's status and progress so the trauma team can prepare. The mantra, the philosophy of the EMTs in a serious, life-threatening situation is to spend a minimum amount of time at the scene; address only immediate threats and only if you have the equipment and ability to address them, and then get the patient as quickly as possible to where he needs to be.

On the way, en route, they do as much as they can to help. One specific task, along with keeping an eye on those ABCs, is to try to get good IV access, get IVs started, big lines, and multiple ones. EMTs would never delay transport to get those IVs in, but that access is going to be critical to give medicines and fluids and blood products.

You park your car and head into the hospital. You know the trauma team is already waiting for the patient; they're gowned and gloved, because they know something messy is coming in. IV fluid bags are hanging on poles, ready to hook up to the lines that were started on the ambulance. As soon as possible, those lines will start running in fluids called crystalloid, basically salt solutions to replace lost blood and maintain circulation.

The trauma team includes experienced nurses and techs, and a respiratory therapist. There's also an X-ray technician on hand, waiting right there shoot a CCP, that's c-spine, or cervical spine, chest, and pelvis X-ray; that's crucial in serious trauma to tell you if the neck is broken or if there's air or blood filling up the thorax. One team member is called the scribe, who stands off to the side with a clipboard, keeping track of the time and all orders and tasks that are given and carried out.

While your colleagues on the trauma team do their job, you catch your breath for a moment and shower off the blood from the field. You also need to take report from and relieve another doctor who is tired after his 12-hour shift. Tommy's going to need your attention, but there may be other patients who are critically ill who will also need your attention in the ED. And the ED, it's a different sort of medical setting. In most places, as a physician, you'll make the diagnosis first, then move logically to therapy. In the ED, finding a specific diagnosis is secondary. The main job is to identify the genuinely sick and get them stabilized for admission to the ICU or the floor of the main hospital. It's a different sort of mindset, one where time is of the essence, far more so than in other medical settings. Things happen quickly.

Speaking of which, it's time to head into the trauma room, right by the ambulance bay. Tommy's on a bed in the middle of the room so as many people can get to the patient as possible, from every direction. He's strapped to a rigid back board with a firm collar in place to prevent further spine or neck injuries. Lines are in, monitor leads are in place, blood's been sent to the lab and to the blood bank for typing. Now, you're the conductor, and this is your orchestra. Believe me, your people know what to do, often before you tell them.

You start over, at the top again. A, airway, your patient is unconscious after very serious trauma. You know you need to keep that airway open, and now you can do it the best way, with a tube, about as fat as your finger, called an endotracheal tube, or ET tube. The procedure is called intubation, and once the tube is in place, you can hook it up to either a bag to squeeze manually, or to a ventilator machine, to pump oxygenated air in an out mechanically.

Prior to placing the ET tube, medications can be given to relax the muscles and provide pain relief, though, at this point, Tommy is unresponsive and not struggling at all. You intubate Tommy, quickly, while assistants hold his neck in a safe position. Remember, he could still have a significant spinal cord injury. It's critical that the tube be placed correctly into the trachea to ventilate both lungs. You listen over both sides, and it sounds like air is going in and out. Though the sound is muffled, it's there on both sides. Other monitors and an X-ray will confirm that the tube is in place.

B, breathing, Tommy is now not making any effort, at all, to breathe. The respiratory therapist has hooked up the ET tube to a mechanical ventilator. Those muffled breath sounds you heard, that's concerning. That's what's called a pneumothorax. Air has leaked out from the lungs into the space between the lungs and the ribs, and that air is preventing the lungs from expanding. Worse, the air there is under pressure, and it's even preventing blood from getting back up into the chest and the heart.

Remember, I said, in the primary survey, you don't move to the next step until you've fixed the immediate threat. Even though the machine is pumping air in and out through the ET tube, Tommy's lungs can't inflate, so he isn't really breathing. Time for action. You open a space between Tommy's ribs, actually two spaces, one on each side, and insert what's called a chest tube, This is, again, a tube, about as fat as your finger, and when you cut into the chest to insert the tube, there is a big rush of air out. Pffft! Not just air, but blood too. You push the tubes in, and hook them up to suction to keep the space outside of the lungs clear. A lot of bright-red blood is draining into those tubes, and it keeps coming. But at least now, Tommy's chest wall is moving up and down with each breath, and listening to the chest you can hear good breath sounds on both sides. Monitors show that he's more effectively getting oxygen into his blood.

Take a few breaths yourself; it's time to move to C again, circulation. What you find isn't good. His pulses are weak, and blood pressure monitors show a very low pressure of 60/20; you'd expect a healthy young man to have a pressure of 120/80. The blood in his body isn't flowing at high enough blood pressure, strong and fast; it's barely trickling. His heart rate is rapid, 142, because his heart is desperately trying to pump as much blood as it can. But Tommy is still losing blood; he's bleeding into his chest, and that blood is pouring out of his chest tubes. Through those big IVs you start running multiple blood transfusions, as fast as you can, using devices to squeeze the bags of blood hard to push them in as fast as possible. Through other IVs, you run more fluids and medicines to support blood pressure. The blood bank has already been warned. This is going to be a long night.

While this has been going on, other staff has been exposing the patient, snipping off his clothes. Someone is working on getting in an even better line, a big, fat IV called a central line that's going into one of the big veins at the top of the thigh. You're checking pulses and looking Tommy over to see if there's any other bleeding. No open wounds are seen, but the abdomen is bruised, in the front, and now it's becoming distended, or swollen. You suspect something is bleeding in there, in his abdomen. It could be a laceration or tear of his liver or spleen, or a ruptured blood vessel, but whatever it is, it isn't good. He's bleeding inside his chest, and he's bleeding inside his abdomen as well. And that blood loss is going to make it difficult for him to maintain good circulation.

Depending on available technology, there are different ways to proceed when evaluating bleeding in the belly after trauma. If Tommy were stable, an abdominal CT scan could find the source of bleeding, but his blood pressure is very low; he's far from stable, and this is not a good time to move him to the CT scanner. A procedure called a diagnostic paracentesis can confirm that there's blood in his belly; it's simple, quick procedure. You just put a needle into the abdominal cavity to see if there's blood in there. Paracentesis won't tell you where the blood is coming from, but it can confirm active intra-abdominal bleeding, which means that your patient needs to go to the operating room quickly to stop it. In our case, we use another option, a handy quick ultrasound in the trauma room, and that confirms that there is a lot of free fluid—that's blood—in the abdomen. The surgeons have been called, and they're prepping the OR. Meanwhile, you're trying to support circulation with transfusions as best you can.

D, next, is disability, remember, at the scene of the accident, Tommy had been P on the AVPU scale, responding only to pain. Now, he's not responding at all. You do a chest rub, hard, this time, nothing. And he's not responding to the ET tube; he's not gagging or struggling; and he's not responding to IV starts or to anything at all. Pupillary reactions are another way of determining brain function. You shine a light into a pupil, and there ought to be a reflex that shrinks the pupil down. That will occur even in unconscious patients, because that reflex relies on the functioning of only the most primitive part of the brain, the brain stem, not on the big cortex part that does your conscious thinking. You shine a light, and his pupils do constrict, slowly, but they move. There is at least some brain function.

But Tommy has deteriorated. He's at U, now completely unresponsive on the AVPU scale. Though a lot of things can cause this, in a trauma situation, the big ones to think of first are those that could benefit from immediate intervention. Hypoxia, low oxygen in the blood, that's been ruled out. We have got monitors now, oxygenation, we know, is good. Hypoglycemia, very low blood sugars, that can essentially shut down the brain, but we've checked a blood sugar with the initial labs; that was OK. But there are some other causes that I think are more likely and may be more problematic to fix.

First, there's direct brain injury. Tommy was going fast, and then slammed into a utility pole. He was wearing a helmet, but at that speed, the sudden kinetic change of his brain slamming into the skull as his body suddenly decelerated from 60 to 0, that's a whole lot of energy and could have done tremendous damage to Tommy's brain by directly damaging or killing cells, or by shearing the connections between cells, and by damaging blood vessels necessary to deliver oxygen. This kind of damage can be difficult to assess right after an injury.

But there are other causes of brain injury that are even more important to look for, because they may now be causing further damage that might be preventable. The brain lives in a closed, very hard shell, the skull; that's for protection. But that can also make the brain vulnerable to damage if there is pressure or swelling inside of the skull. Increased pressure in the skull, within the cranium, can prevent blood from flowing into the skull to supply oxygen to the brain. And because there is nowhere for the swelling to go, pressure in the cranium can itself cause more brain damage as the tissue of the brain is squeezed. Tissues of the brain can be damaged from this pressure, or sometimes the brain itself can herniate, or squeeze out of the hole at the base of the brain where the spinal cord comes in. This can be catastrophic, because that area of the brain back there, it's where the control centers for breathing and blood pressure are located.

So, brain injury, directly, or from swelling, which, remember, can also decrease blood flow into the cranium, these are all interrelated, and they can all contribute to brain damage and death. We'd like to get a CT scan to see what's going on in the head. Then, in the OR, a neurosurgeon's role could be to help open up the skull and evacuate blood collections, relieving increased intracranial pressure. Monitors could also be put into the cranium to more-directly measure pressure there.

But we have even more immediate problems to worry about. We've already mentioned some important reasons for Tommy to be falling further into unconsciousness, but there's one more reason that's almost certainly contributing—Tommy is in shock. Shock means that the body's tissues are not getting enough blood. In other words, there isn't enough perfusion. Though there may be enough oxygen in the blood, the blood isn't getting to where it's needed, so insufficient oxygen is being delivered. Shock can be caused by a number of different problems. It can be cardiogenic, if the heart isn't pumping well; it can be what's called septic shock, which is caused by overwhelming infection. In Tommy's case, shock is being caused by what's called hypovolemia; there is just not enough circulating blood. We know he's hemorrhaging in his chest, remember, there's blood coming out of those chest tubes, and we know he's hemorrhaging in his abdomen. We haven't been able to stop the bleeding, and as fast as we can pour blood in, it's pouring out.

Shock can affect every organ of the body. The most noticeable, immediate, and scary symptoms relate to the brain. Shock causes listlessness, lethargy, unconsciousness, or coma. But it can also lead to damage to many vital tissues from poor oxygenation. Not enough blood to the heart muscle itself can cause a heart attack, which will not help the circulation, when the heart cannot pump well; not enough blood to the liver will cause damage to that organ, and the liver is where essential proteins to make blood clots form. Once the liver is damaged, it becomes even more difficult to control bleeding in trauma patients. Not enough blood to the tissues of the lungs will cause lung damage and resulting difficulty with breathing and gas exchange.

You can see how all of these problems can pile up, one on top of another, how shock can lead to a cascade of worsening organ failure. There are also immunologic mechanisms, where damaged tissues from trauma and shock release factors into the blood that themselves lead to a massive inflammatory cascade, inflammatory over activation, and further tissue damage and circulatory problems.

We're on the phone now with the neurosurgeon; we're on the phone with the trauma surgeon; the operating room is ready to go. Someone has reached Tommy's family. His mom and his girlfriend are headed into the hospital. Under ordinary circumstances, Tommy, or someone he's identified as a medical decision maker, would be talking with the surgeon about risks and benefits of intervention, but there really isn't time, the family isn't even here yet, and…Monitors start blaring. There's a new noise that cuts through the room, beeeeeeeeeeeeeep. Tommy's heart has stopped. This is time zero seconds of his cardiac arrest, or what's sometimes called a code blue.

You start over, ABCs. Airway and Breathing are checked quickly, the ET tube is in place, the ventilator is giving breaths, but the heart has stopped; there's no C, there's no circulation. A defibrillator is rushed over; you take the paddles; someone squirts clear, cold goo on them to improve conduction, you yell "Clear!" Shock once, nothing happens. Shock twice. There's a heartbeat, again. More medicines are poured into the IVs to support blood pressure and to stop arrhythmias. Four minutes. Moments later, a second cardiac arrest, a second code blue; the heart stops again. Shock, no response. CPR, chest compressions are begun, then a pause for another shock. Now monitors show bursts of activity from the chest leads, a shaky, squiggly line. The heart is quivering, not beating now, just wiggling in the chest, not pumping blood or delivering oxygen at all. Eight minutes.

One more shock, a few good beats, a nurse reports she feels a pulse in the neck now, 10 minutes. The pulse then fades; it gets softer and softer, and chest compressions are started again. There's a routine, in the trauma room, even at times like this, people swap in and out to do compressions to relieve the person who's starting to get tired. Now we notice an irregular, spikey looking recording on the heart monitor; then it becomes just a random squiggle. We're at 12 minutes when the tracing stops completely. Flat again. More shocks. more compressions, 14 minutes, 19 minutes. Now we're 25 minutes without a strong, consistent pulse. You, the ED physician, you look at the clock on the wall. You say the time out loud, and you say, is everyone OK with this? The team knows what you mean; it's your call, you're the doc, but you are a team, and this is a time to make sure that everyone is on the same page.

Everyone in the room nods in agreement. That's it, you say. Thanks, everyone, for the effort. The scribe records the time of death, compressions stop, the ventilator is switched off. The team did well. It was, as we say, a clean code. You need to catch your breath and go meet with the family. You're told that they're here, in the waiting room, and they want to come back and see Tommy right away.

I don't know that there's a best way to share this kind of news; this is a very personal issue, of course, both for doctors, and for families. I don't think there's a script or anything that can be used. I do think families should be told together, when possible, so they can have each other for comfort. They also deserve to have a quiet area, a private area, and they need to have time with the doctor. Sometimes, there's a doctor who's gotten to know the family as a patient slowly wound through an illness, or sometimes a nurse or therapist who also knew the patient may be there help. The hospital may have clergy or social workers available, too.

In the ER, after something sudden like this, you may be on your own. You tell the family that you did everything you could, but Tommy had very serious injuries, and he couldn't survive. Some families will want more details, maybe all of the medical details, and you answer those sorts of questions as best you can. And you offer your card, even as the emergency physician, for the family to call later, when more questions arise. Then you get back to work. You did what you could. This is the ED, where things move quickly, and there's a next patient you need to go see.

Cough, Cough, Cough
Lecture 23

For patients, when you leave the doctor's office, you should make sure that you have a clear diagnosis and that you understand what treatment you've been prescribed. Regular follow-up with your primary care doctor is essential when a problem is chronic or recurrent. Bring records of outside visits to your primary doctor, including copies of X-rays and labs, and make sure that every health provider you see knows exactly what medications have been prescribed. Doctors sometimes need to step back and look at the big picture; this can take extra time, but it can be the best way to help the patient.

Frequent Cough

- Our patient in the general medicine outpatient clinic is Margo, a 49-year-old woman who has come in with her husband with a chief complaint of "I've got this cough again." Margo says that she gets a cough frequently, a bad cough that lingers for weeks, and she keeps seeing doctors, and it gets better, and then it comes back. She thinks this time it's her allergies, because it's the fall, and she always gets this cough in the fall.

- A cough is one of the most common symptoms that drive visits to doctors. Of course, most coughs are brief, self-limited diseases that people recover from without any specific evaluation or therapy at all. Coughing is a normal protective reflex that clears the lungs of secretions and mucus and inhaled dust. But of course, too much of a cough itself is distracting and aggravating, and it can lead to impaired sleep for both the patient and family.

- Some of the most common causes of chronic, prolonged, or recurrent coughing include smoking; both active smoking and passive, secondhand smoke exposure can cause cough. Long-term smokers can develop chronic obstructive pulmonary disease with permanent destructive changes in the lungs.

- Asthma is also very common and can cause coughing as a main symptom, sometimes along with wheezing, noisy breathing, or shortness of breath. Prolonged cough can also be caused by environmental or occupational pollution. Any cause of chronic postnasal drip (including allergies or sinusitis) can cause an ongoing cough.

- Reflux—meaning gastroesophageal reflux, from stomach contents coming back up—can cause cough, as can some medications (especially ACE inhibitors, a class of blood pressure medications). Whooping cough, also called pertussis, is probably one of the most common infectious causes of prolonged coughs in adults.

- Frequent, ordinary coughs—just from common cold viruses—can kind of stack up, one after another, and seem like a chronic ongoing cough. We see this in children, sometimes, when they start day care, in young pediatricians starting training, or in teachers or day-care workers. Children or those who work around children can be victimized by very frequent viral infections.

- Less commonly, prolonged coughing can be from heart disease, chronic lung infections, or tumors or cysts in the lungs or bronchial tubes. Problems outside of the chest have to be considered, too—such as something in the larynx or throat, or neurological conditions that lead to excessive secretions or an impaired ability to keep the airways clear.

- Also, any sort of immune-compromising condition can lead to recurring or persistent coughing. Occasionally, we see what's called a psychogenic cough, sometimes related to stress.

- We can ask about the quality of the cough, to try to nail down exactly what it sounds like. There are a few specific coughs that do have very characteristic sounds. Croup is an illness of children—young children and babies mostly—with a cough that sounds like the bark of a seal or a dog. But croup is very uncommon in adults.

- Another characteristic cough is the cough of pertussis, or whooping cough. Classically, this is a staccato, one-after-another cough that goes on for a minute or more, followed by one big inspiration—a whoop. But many people with whooping cough don't actually sound like that and don't make that whoop.

- There's also a distinction that can be made between a wet and dry cough. A dry cough is likely related to irritation, or some condition without a lot of excess phlegm; a wet, phlegmy cough is likely related to infection or inflammation, perhaps caused by sinus disease or allergies.

- But there's a lot of overlap. Pneumonia can sound to some people wet or dry, and so can asthma. And two people listening to the same cough often disagree on whether it's wet or dry. Cough descriptions are not very reliable or helpful, and they certainly shouldn't be something that leads you to narrow down the diagnosis without corroborating information.

- The physical exam reveals that Margo is a healthy woman, overall, but she has an annoying, severe, recurring cough. She also wheezes, at least sometimes, on the physical exam. A wheeze is an almost musical whistling noise that is classically caused by narrowing of the airways in the chest. That can be from a one-time illness—such as pneumonia, where mucus in the airways causes narrowing—or by some kind of tumor or mass that's pressing on one or more airways.

- From Margo's history, this is a recurrent, come-and-go cough that is associated with a wheeze that comes and goes. That's very suggestive of one single, common diagnosis: asthma. In fact, many of the medications Margo's been using on and off for years are actually asthma medications, so doctors have been thinking about asthma before. But apparently this has never been communicated clearly to Margo.

- A first test that's part of the evaluation of any chronic or recurrent cough is a chest X-ray. It's simple and cheap and allows us to can see the heart and lungs and the larger tubes of the airways. Margo's chest X-ray looks fairly normal, but the lungs are hyperinflated—it looks like Margo is taking extra-deep breaths—and there are little areas of slightly denser lungs, suggesting a little bit of fluid in those areas.

- You look back at some older films that have been taken over the last few years, and there is often that hyperinflation, and sometimes there are those little consolidated areas in different places. It's the pattern—what's seen in the series of X-rays, along with the findings of repeated physical exams revealing a wheeze that comes and goes—that is suggestive of asthma.

- One other confirmatory test is done: By using a device to measure Margo's breathing, called a **spirometer**, we see that Margo's airways are clamped down small, especially during exhalation. Then, we give her a medicine called a bronchodilator—a very common asthma medication used to relax and open her breathing tubes—and afterward, her spirometry testing normalizes. We've documented a breathing obstruction that responds quickly to bronchodilators, confirming the diagnosis of asthma.

Asthma

- Asthma is very common. It affects about 25 million people in the United States, including 7 million children. It causes symptoms by two interrelated mechanisms in the lungs: Part one is inflammation—swelling and mucus accumulation in the airways. Part two is what's called

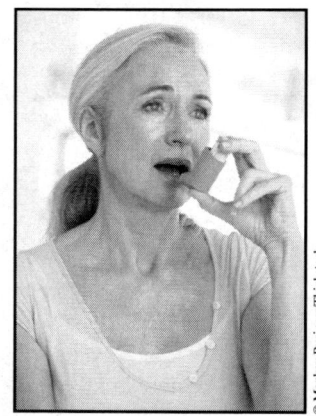

Asthma, which makes it difficult for a person to breathe, can be controlled with inhalers.

bronchoconstriction, where muscles that wrap around the airways constrict, causing narrowing.

- The main symptoms of asthma, when it's flaring up, are coughing, shortness of breath, and a feeling of chest tightness. Sometimes there can be chest or, more rarely, abdominal pain as well. Symptoms can range from mild to quite severe or even life threatening, and they very characteristically wax and wane, getting better or worse depending on triggers.

- However, many people with asthma have at least some amount of chronic inflammation and symptoms as a baseline, though they may not complain about daily problems.

- People with asthma can have triggers that lead to a flare-up of symptoms, sometimes called an asthma attack. Common triggers can be exercise, cold air, respiratory infections (including common cold viruses), tobacco smoke, or allergies.

- These triggers lead to cough even in people without asthma, which can be a source of diagnostic confusion. For example, allergies themselves cause cough, but usually, there are other symptoms of allergies, such as a runny or congested nose or itchy eyes—or a common cold. Everyone gets some cough with their colds, but when someone's colds often lead to a prolonged, severe cough, that also suggests the possibility of underlying asthma.

Preventing and Controlling Symptoms
- Although there is no cure for asthma, there are important steps to prevent and control symptoms—steps that may also help prevent the overall progression of asthma to a more life-threatening disease. Nonmedical steps can include avoiding tobacco, including secondhand exposure, and avoiding other identified triggers when possible.

- Also, control of allergic symptoms with allergy medications, environmental measures, or immunotherapy can help control asthma, at least in people with allergic triggers.

- Beyond that, medications can very effectively improve the health of people with asthma—when they're used correctly. There are both quick-relief medications, such as bronchodilators, which are taken quickly at the onset of asthma symptoms for quick relief. These are sometimes called "rescue" meds, and they can also be used as a pretreatment right before exposure to an individual's known trigger, such as exercise or visiting a family with a cat.

- However, there is a dark side to these rapid rescue medications: Overuse of them, overly frequent use, makes the body less responsive to their effects. Over-relying on these quick medicines may mean that when there's a more severe attack, these important medicines will not work. In fact, overuse of rescue meds is a risk factor for death from asthma.

- The most important steps in prevention are making the right diagnosis and teaching the family about asthma, including avoiding triggers, controlling symptoms, and using medications correctly, both as preventives and as rescue therapy when there are symptoms. People with asthma need an action plan for when their symptoms occur, and they need to know when to head to the hospital when symptoms are severe or not improving.

- Some things to look for, both for patients and their family, that mean an attack is potentially severe include needing to use rescue medications over and over—that is, taking more puffs than typically needed to control a flare-up. Also, look for unremitting cough, gasping, trouble speaking complete sentences, or any patient who is becoming upset, agitated, confused, or lethargic. These kinds of symptoms warrant immediate communication with a doctor or a quick trip to the nearest emergency department.

- For anyone with chronic symptoms, or symptoms that are intermittent but common or severe, a daily "controller" type of medication is needed. Controllers are underused in the treatment of asthma and are sometimes used incorrectly. They're meant for daily use, or at least daily use for long stretches of time—for example, through all of allergy season. They do not work quickly, so they're not the first thing to grab when there is an asthma attack. But regular use prevents flare-ups and controls daily symptoms.

- Many of the medicines used for both rapid relief and long-term control of asthma are given in inhalers, small canisters that create a puff of medication to breathe in. They're great because they put the medicine where it's supposed to go, in the lungs, without many side effects. But they're often used incorrectly. It turns out that proper technique is difficult to master, and it takes repeated teaching and practice. In almost all cases, a plastic spacer device can improve effectiveness when prescribed alongside these inhalers, though they're underused.

Important Term

spirometry: Tests of lung functioning.

Suggested Reading

Adams, *The Asthma Sourcebook*.

Questions to Consider

1. What are the advantages and disadvantages of medical care at a primary care office versus an urgent care center?

2. How do you know whether a cough should be treated with antibiotics?

Cough, Cough, Cough
Lecture 23—Transcript

Hello again. Today we're back in general medicine, the outpatient clinic, and we have a very old and very common disease to diagnose. It was named by Hippocrates, about 400 years before the common era, using the Greek word for wind or to blow. Physicians both in ancient India and the Roman Empire found herbs that were probably effective treatments. Those herbs, which are still in use, contain chemical compounds similar to what are used in modern pharmaceutical products today. Pliny the Elder of Rome, in addition to herbs, also suggested, specifically for this illness, drinking the blood of wild horses and eating millipedes soaked in honey. Those ideas, probably, didn't help quite as much.

Our patient is Margo, a 49-year-old woman, who's come in with her husband with a chief complaint of, "I've got this cough again." Margo says she gets a cough frequently, a bad cough that lingers for weeks, and she keeps seeing doctors. It gets better, and then it comes back. She thinks this time it's her allergies, because it's the fall, and she always gets this cough in the fall. Her husband chimes in. Yup, she's always coughing."

You speak up, to clarify the history. "Margo, do you mean you always cough, every day, for a long time? Or do you mean you have a cough that comes and goes, that there are times when the cough is completely gone?" Margo says, "Oh, it comes and goes. I have it bad now," she says, "but it goes away, and it always comes back." Margo's husband, his name is Randall, he says, "I don't know about that. You're always coughing, you know." He says this directly to Margo. "When do I cough?" She asks. "You cough all the time," says Randall. "You always cough at night, and when you go outside, and especially in the morning, and…" Well, that's what happens sometimes, when you try to take a medical history. Sometimes you ask what you'd think is a simple question, and it kind of gets away from you. Margo and Randall are arguing now, so you try to settle things down, trying to redirect the conversation. "Margo," you say, "let's focus on this cough, now. What's it like, how long have you had it, what other symptoms are there?"

Margo says she's had this cough for two weeks. Randall's back there; he's shaking his head, but we're trying to ignore him for now. She says it's worse in the morning, and it's wet. Now, Randall interrupts, he says it's a bronchitis cough. Margo kind of shushes him, and says, none of her cough medicines are working this time, so she knew she had to come see the doctor.

What medicines? You ask. Randall says, "Look at this, doctor," as Margo upends her purse, dumping out bottles and inhalers and sprays all over the exam table. You kind of rake through it. You're seeing inhalers for asthma, and allergy medicines, steroid pills, antibiotics, all sorts of bottles, all sorts of dates, from all sorts of different doctors. Many places, urgent cares, ERs, it looks like every bottle has a different doctor's name.

"You've got all the records, you know," Margo says, and sure enough, you can see scanned into your electronic health record copies of multiple visits to clinics and urgent care centers across several years. There are also scattered X-ray reports, some letters from specialists, an allergist, an ENT; there's of papers scanned in there. "You should go look through those," Randall says.

Now, this is a style thing, coming up. I've been stressing how important a good history can be. I think it would be reasonable to step outside of the room to reduce distractions and try to go through these old medical records, maybe not line by line, but at least to get a feel for these visits. But personally, I've always found that a story from the patient is more useful, at least at first, than looking at other doctor's records.

So, we want more history. But time for a pause, let's think in broad terms about coughing. A cough is one of the most common symptoms that drive visits to doctors. Of course, most coughs are brief, self-limited diseases that people recover from without any specific evaluation or therapy at all. Coughing is a normal, protective reflex that clears the lungs of secretions and mucus and inhaled dust. But of course, too much of a cough itself is distracting and aggravating, and can lead to impaired sleep for both the patient and the family, as Randall has been quick to point out.

Some of the most common causes of chronic, prolonged, or recurrent coughing include smoking, both active smoking, and passive, second hand, smoke exposure; those can both cause cough. Long-term smokers can develop COPD, or chronic obstructive pulmonary disease, with permanent destructive changes in the lungs. Asthma is also very common and can cause coughing as a main symptom, sometimes along with wheezing, noisy breathing, or shortness of breath.

Prolonged cough can also be caused by environmental or occupational pollution. Any cause of chronic post-nasal drip, including allergies or sinusitis, can cause an ongoing cough. Reflux, meaning gastroesophageal reflux, from stomach contents coming back up, that can cause cough, as can some medications, especially ACE inhibitors, a class of blood pressure medications. Whooping cough, also called pertussis, is probably one of the most common infectious causes of prolonged coughs in adults.

It's also worth mentioning that frequent, ordinary coughs, just from common cold viruses, can kind of stack up, one after another, and seem like a chronic, ongoing cough. We see this in children, sometimes, when they start day care, or in young pediatricians starting training, or in school teachers or day care workers. Children or those who work around children can be victimized by very frequent viral infections.

Less commonly, prolonged coughing can be from heart disease, chronic lung infections, or tumors or cysts in the lungs or bronchial tubes. Problems outside of the chest have to be considered, too, like perhaps something in the larynx or throat, or neurologic conditions that lead to excessive secretions or an impaired ability to keep the airways clear. Also, any sort of immune compromising condition can lead to recurring or persistent coughing. Occasionally, we can see what's called a psychogenic cough, sometimes related to stress. So, a pretty long differential, but I think with some history clues we can narrow things down.

More history, we can ask about the quality of the cough, to try to nail down exactly what it sounds like. There are a few specific coughs that do have very characteristic sounds. Croup is an illness of children, young children and babies mostly, with a cough that sounds like the bark of a seal or a dog. And it really does sound like that. But croup is very uncommon in adults. Another characteristic cough is the cough of pertussis, or whooping cough.

Classically, this is a staccato, one-after-another cough—cough, cough, cough, cough, cough that goes on for a minute or more, followed by one big inspiration, a whoop. But many people with whooping cough don't actually sound like that and don't make that whoop.

There's also a distinction that can be made between a wet and a dry cough. We think of a dry cough as being caused by irritation, or some condition without a lot of excessive phlegm; versus a wet, phlegmy sort of cough, likely related to infection or inflammation, perhaps caused by sinus disease or allergies. But there's a lot of overlap. Pneumonia can sound to some people wet or dry, and so can asthma. And two people listening to the same cough often disagree on whether it's wet or dry. Bottom line, I don't think cough descriptions are very reliable and helpful, and they certainly shouldn't be something that leads you to narrow down the diagnosis without corroborating information.

In any case, Margo and Randall are still arguing about what the cough sounds like, so we're not going to get a straight answer on that today. Let's get some answers to some more specific questions. Margo doesn't smoke, and isn't around smokers; she doesn't take any ACE inhibitors or other medicines that trigger cough. That already takes out some of the categories we've reviewed. She's also had no chronic or recurrent fevers and no weight loss, and really, no other symptoms, like chronic diarrhea or skin problems. Together, all of that makes immune problems unlikely. Margo works from the home, doing telephone marketing, so she's not exposed to a whole lot of children or their infections.

What about allergies? Though cough can be caused by chronic post-nasal drip from nasal allergies, we'd expect to have a report of other allergic symptoms. Margo denies frequent sneezing or runny noses or nasal congestion, so allergy really is unlikely. In fact, Margo denies now that she has any congestion or runny nose at all, so I don't think her cough could be caused by post nasal drip from an upper respiratory infection or sinusitis.

How about reflux? Margo denies classic heartburn symptoms, and also denies more-subtle possible symptoms of reflux, like a tickling or something-stuck feeling in her throat. She also doesn't really think her cough is worse after meals or when she's lying down, though Randall does chime in that she coughs a lot at night, when she's sleeping.

Now, some red flag questions for cough, a few questions to make sure we're not missing something scary. We had already asked about fevers and weight loss, if those were present, especially chronic or recurrent fevers. If those were present, especially chronic or recurrent fevers, we'd have to think about tuberculosis, or cancer. Another red flag for both of those diagnoses would be coughing up blood. Now, anyone with a severe cough can occasionally cough up just a bit of blood from broken vessels in the throat, but coughing up significant blood makes us worry. Margo hasn't had any of that. She also denies shortness of breath, which could have been a sign of heart disease, COPD, or rare but serious diseases of the lungs that could have caused scarring and fibrosis.

One other point, and I think it would be best to try to get a clearer answer. Is this a recurrent cough that keeps getting better and worse or a chronic cough? Margo and Randall kind of disagreed on that question. We flip though the prior records, and we see chief complaints and histories that include "cough for three weeks" or "cough for 20 days" or "coughing has come back," So, at least, the impression for now looks like this is more of a recurrent than persistent cough. That's an important distinction. Lung cancer or tuberculosis or some kind of mass pressing on the lung really should cause more of a persistent cough, one that's always there, or one that's gradually getting worse and worse. We'll want to keep an open mind, but for now, the history suggests that Margo has some kind of intermittent problem, or a diagnosis that causes symptoms that come and go.

While we're looking at those old records from other physicians, there are some diagnoses that keep popping up—bronchitis, and sinusitis, and upper respiratory infection, sometimes allergies, and occasionally wheezing or walking pneumonia or reflux. All of these different diagnoses span over several years, but they're all associated with the same chief complaint; it's always coughing. No wonder Margo and Randall are frustrated. It's all cough, and she keeps being told different things, and the cough keeps coming back, anyway.

You're still kind of pawing through the pile of medications. "Do any of these work," you ask? "Sure, says Margo." "Nah, says Randall." You say, "I think I can tell which of you is the glass half full one." Everyone starts laughing, and that starts Margo coughing. It's quite a cough, loud, and strong. "That's the cough," says Randall. "See? it's bronchitis." Margo's just kind of waving him away, sort of catching her breath.

OK, let's do our exam. Margo is Caucasian, and when she stops coughing, she looks like she's in good shape and feeling well. Vital signs are done, including a respiratory rate and a quick pulse-ox. They're all normal. HEENT is normal; Margo isn't congested; the lining of her nose isn't swollen; and she's not sniffling at all. Her heart exam is normal. When you listen to her lungs, they sound clear; when you ask her to take a deep breath, she starts coughing again, so you try a few more times, and finally, you get to hear some nice, deep breaths, and you can hear a bit of a wheezy sound through the stethoscope when Margo breathes out from low down on one side of her chest.

"That's it, then," says Randall. "That's bronchitis. They always say it's bronchitis when they hear that." That wheeze you heard, what does that mean? A wheeze is a noise from an airway that's constricted, a tight noise, typically heard in expiration when a patient breathes out. It sounds like [wheezing]. Lung sounds can sometimes fool the examiner. A wheeze that sounds like it's a noise from the lung, down here, can actually be a noise transmitted from up here. Still, from what we hear, the exam suggests there's something going on in the lung itself.

And, Randall's offhanded comment, "when they hear that, it's bronchitis," that tells us something; that tells us that Margo has had wheezing before, but maybe not every single time she gets a cough. Aha! Clues are stacking up now; they're subtle, but they're there. So, what do we have? A healthy woman, overall, but with an annoying, severe, recurring cough. And wheezing, at least sometimes, on the physical exam.

A wheeze is a noise, and sometimes the word wheezing is used by people to describe any kind of noisy breathing. But to a physician with a stethoscope, a wheeze is more specific. That specific, almost musical whistling noise is classically caused by narrowing of the airways in the chest. That can be from a one-time illness, like pneumonia, where mucus in the airways causes narrowing, or by some kind of tumor or mass that's pressing on one or more airways. But from Margo's history, this is a recurrent, come and go cough, associated, we think, with a wheeze that comes and goes. And that's very suggestive of one single, common diagnosis—asthma. In fact, many of the medications Margo's been using on and off for years are actually asthma medications, so doctors have been thinking about asthma before. But apparently, this has never been communicated this clearly to Margo.

Margo says, "I don't have asthma," and Randall chimes in "They said you had that, remember, bronchial asthma, that one doctor said…," and Margo cuts him off. She says, that was asthmatic bronchitis; that's different, and the two of them, they're arguing again. Margo starts coughing again, too. We need confirmation. Though I think it might be entirely appropriate to diagnose asthma based on the information we have so far, this has been going on for a long time, and it would be best to confirm the diagnosis so we know exactly what kind of plan to suggest.

A first test that's part of the evaluation of any chronic or recurrent cough is a chest X-ray. It's simple test; it's cheap, and it allows us to see the heart and lungs and the larger tubes of the airways. A chest film can not only tell us what the lungs look like today, but can also can be compared to prior films to see if anything spotted in the lungs is persistent, suggesting perhaps an anatomic problem or a tumor. Today's chest X-ray looks fairly normal, but there are subtle findings we can see. The lungs are hyper-inflated. It looks like Margo is taking extra-deep breaths. And there are little areas of slightly denser lungs, suggesting a little bit of fluid here and there. You look back at some older films that have been taken over the last few years, and there is often that hyperinflation, and sometimes there are those little consolidated areas in different places.

These subtle lung findings can be a source of confusion and misdirection. They can be seen with pneumonia, especially mild pneumonias that are sometimes called walking pneumonia. But when they come and go like in Margo's case, these areas are called atelectasis, referring to small parts of underinflated lung tissue. Atelectasis that shifts around like this is very characteristic of asthma, though it can't be documented by one single chest X-ray. Again, it's the pattern, what's seen in the series of X-rays, along with the findings of repeated physical exams revealing a wheeze that comes and goes, that's what is suggestive of asthma.

So asthma is not a one-time diagnosis. The first cough or the first wheeze, that's not something that's appropriate to diagnose as asthma. But neither is it appropriate to wait through years and years of frequent coughing and wheezing to make the diagnosis.

One other confirmatory test is done. We use a device to measure Margo's breathing, called a spirometer, and with that, we see that Margo's airways are clamped down small, especially during exhalation. Then we give a medicine called a bronchodilator, that's a very common asthma medication used to relax and open her breathing tubes. And afterwards, her spirometry testing normalizes. We've documented a breathing obstruction that responds quickly to bronchodilators, That confirms the diagnosis of asthma.

Asthma is very common; it affects about 25 million people in the United States, including seven million children. It causes symptoms by two interrelated mechanisms in the lungs. Part one is inflammation, swelling and mucus accumulation in the airways. Part two is what's called bronchoconstriction, where muscles that wrap around the airways constrict, causing narrowing. The main symptoms of asthma, when it's flaring up, are coughing, shortness of breath, and a feeling of chest tightness. Sometimes there can be chest, or more rarely, abdominal pain. Symptoms can range from mild to quite severe, or even life-threatening, and they very characteristically wax and wane, getting better or worse, depending on triggers. However, many people with asthma have at least some amount of chronic inflammation and symptoms as a baseline, though they may not complain about daily symptoms.

As we talked with Margo and her husband, it became clear that she did have chronic symptoms. Her cough was sometimes better, and sometimes worse, but as is characteristic of asthma, it sounds like there had always been some coughing, especially at night. She had also stopped exercising many, many years ago, because she found that after exercise she'd cough and cough, and it was embarrassing in the locker room. Again, that's characteristic of asthma, though it's only become clear, now, in retrospect.

Back to triggers, people with asthma can have triggers that lead to a flare-up of symptoms, sometimes called an asthma attack. Common triggers can be exercise, cold air, respiratory infections, including common cold viruses, tobacco smoke, or allergies. These triggers lead to cough, even in people without asthma, which can be a source of diagnostic confusion. For instance, allergies themselves cause cough, but usually, there are other symptoms of allergies, like a runny nose or congestion or itchy eyes. Or a common cold, everyone gets some cough with their colds, but someone whose colds lead to a prolonged, severe cough, that also suggests the possibility of underlying asthma.

When we talked with Margo about this, that cold viruses can trigger a prolonged asthma flare, she and Randall finally found something to agree about. Yes, whenever a cold went through the family, Randall would be sick for a week or so; he wouldn't even see the doctor, but when Margo got the same cold, she'd be sick for weeks, and she'd end up with a bunch of prescriptions.

Although there is no cure for asthma, there are important steps to prevent and control symptoms, steps that may also help prevent the overall progression of asthma to a more life-threatening disease. Non-medical steps can include avoiding tobacco, including second-hand exposure, and avoiding other identified triggers when possible. Also, control of allergic symptoms with allergy medications, environmental measures, or immunotherapy can help control asthma, at least in people with allergic triggers.

Beyond that, medications can very effectively improve the health of people with asthma—when they're used correctly. There are both quick-relief medications—those are those bronchodilators I mentioned earlier, They're taken quickly at the onset of asthma symptoms for quick relief. These are sometimes called rescue meds, and they can also be used as a pre-treatment right before exposure to an individual's trigger, like exercise or visiting a family with a cat. However, there is a dark side to these rapid-rescue medications; overuse of them, overly frequent use, makes the body less responsive to their effects. Over relying on these quick medicines may mean that when there's a more severe attack, these important medicines will not work. In fact, overuse of rescue meds is a risk factor for death from asthma.

And people do die from asthma, about nine a day in the United States, or over 3,000 a year. There is a risk of death, even among people with less severe disease, like Margo. The most important steps in prevention are, number one, making the right diagnosis, and number two, teaching the family about asthma. That's avoiding triggers, controlling symptoms, and using medications correctly both as preventives and as rescue therapy when there are symptoms. People with asthma need an action plan for when their symptoms occur and need to know when to head to the hospital when symptoms are severe or not improving.

Some things to look for, both for patients and their family, that mean an attack is potentially severe. Needing to use rescue medications over and over, that is, taking more puffs than typically needed to control a flare up. Also, look for unremitting cough, gasping, trouble speaking complete sentences, or any patient who's becoming upset, agitated, confused, or lethargic. These kinds of symptoms warrant immediate communication with a doctor, or a quick trip to the nearest emergency department.

For anyone with persistent asthma symptoms, or symptoms that are intermittent but common or severe, a daily controller type of medication is needed. Controllers are underused in the treatment of asthma and are sometimes used incorrectly. They're meant for daily use, or at least, daily use for long stretches of time, say, through all of allergy season. They do not work quickly, so they're not the first thing to grab when there is an asthma attack. But regular use prevents flare-ups and controls daily symptoms. For instance, Margo's night cough, that's a chronic symptom she's kind of gotten used to, and at least at first, she didn't even think it was a problem. But it certainly disrupted her sleep, and once we got it under control, she and her husband both started sleeping better.

Many of the medicines used for both rapid relief and long term control of asthma are given in inhalers. These are little canisters that create a puff of medication that's breathed in. They're great, because they put the medicine exactly where it's supposed to go, in the lungs, without many side effects. But they're often used incorrectly. It turns out, the proper technique with these things is difficult to master, and it takes repeated teaching and practice. A plastic spacer device improves effectiveness and should always be prescribed to use with asthma inhalers.

So we went through Margo's collection of medications, clarifying which to use now, which are meant to treat active wheezing, and which are meant to be her every day controllers. We also treated this acute attack with an oral steroid, prednisone, not something we want to do repeatedly, but an important step in establishing good control. We'll also make sure that Margo's had a chance to learn about asthma, preventing triggers, and using her medications the best way. She will stay on her controller medicine and add in her rescue medicine at the first sign of cough. We'll have regular follow up to ensure that she stays in good control, with no cough and feeling well, and we'll try to get her lungs in good shape so she can resume exercising, too.

Looking back, why did it take Margo so long to get the right diagnosis and a good, long-term management plan? The fundamental problem was in communication. There was fractionated care, with Margo visiting a number of urgent cares, a variety of places that treated each illness separately, rather than looking at the big picture. And Margo had never understood exactly what the prescribed medicines were or how to use them.

Our own doctor language probably made matters worse. Some doctors had referred to "asthmatic bronchitis," which is kind of a euphemism for asthma, without clearly explaining their thoughts. Perhaps everyone was relying on the primary care doc to pull the threads together, but the primary care doc, until now, wasn't seeing the patient regularly.

So, for patients, when you leave the doctor's office, every doctor's office, or ED, or urgent care, you ought to make sure you have a clear diagnosis and that you understand what treatment you've been prescribed. Regular follow up with your primary care doctor is essential when a problem is chronic or recurrent. Bring records of outside visits to your primary, including copies of X-rays and labs, and make sure every health provider you see knows exactly what medications have been prescribed. And for those of us who are doctors, or planning to be one, we sometimes need to step back and look at the big picture, not just the reason the patient came in today. That can take extra time, but it can be the best way to really help your patient.

We have one more case in our grand rounds series, one more medical mystery to work through. The clues, I promise, will be there waiting for you, as long as you listen and look. See you next time.

A Confused Father
Lecture 24

The case presented in this lecture illustrates the risks of side effects of medications and, especially, of what's sometimes called **polypharmacy**—taking multiple medications. It is important that elderly patients have an advocate to help them at appointments and make sure the correct history is available. Once a patient is sick, he or she might not be in the best condition to communicate with the doctor and follow through on plans. That goes for mental health and cognitive concerns, but even for almost any general medical concern. In addition, a single doctor who has known a patient well for years can be a strong ally.

Dementia, Delirium, and Depression

- In the general medicine clinic, our patient is a 90-year-old gentleman named Isaac. He is brought in by his son. You've known Isaac for many years, though he's a snowbird who you see for routine care only about six months out of the year. It's April, and he's come back to town from his usual winter stay in Boca Raton, Florida.

- His son says that he's just not right—that he hasn't been right since he came back. The doctors in Florida said that he has Alzheimer's disease, but Isaac doesn't seem to agree.

- You last saw Isaac about six months ago, and at least then, he was in pretty good shape. His wife had died about a year ago, and you had been worried then about him continuing to live alone. After the funeral, Isaac's son moved back to town into an apartment he could share with his father. That turbulence, his wife's death and moving, had seemed to cause some confusion and a little forgetfulness, maybe not unexpected at Isaac's age.

- At the time, you had him see a neurologist and then a psychiatrist, who had prescribed medication for depression. Isaac seemed to improve and settled into a new routine. Now, it seems—just from a first impression—that Isaac has had a big step backward in function and cognition.

- Isaac's son reports that Isaac has some good days and bad days—some days when he seems confused. Most days, he doesn't talk, and he can't really dress himself anymore. His son adds that most of the time, he just looks confused.

- Dementia is a progressive decline in memory and at least one other cognitive area. It is very strongly related to age. Dementia is rare under age 50, but it affects 8 percent of those at age 65. By age 90, almost 40 percent of people have at least some dementia.

- The common causes of dementia are almost all related to chronic and progressive brain damage, occurring most often from age-related diseases like strokes or Alzheimer's or Parkinson's disease. Damage can also be related to chronic infections like HIV or from toxins like alcoholism.

- Most causes of dementia cannot be reversed, but in at least some, the progression can be slowed with therapy. Rarely, symptoms of dementia can be caused by thyroid disease, vitamin deficiencies, or a brain tumor.

- The way that different people show symptoms of dementia can vary, but there is always some degree of memory loss. There will also be other evidence of problems with cognition, such as difficulty with language and communication or problems carrying out learned and purposeful movements.

- Sometimes there can be a decline in the ability to recognize objects or tell what they're for. Some people will also have changes in personality and perhaps a loss of social inhibition in their actions or speech.

- One specific cause of dementia that's been mentioned is depression. This is sometimes called pseudodementia in the elderly, because depression can contribute to the symptoms of dementia, and dementia itself can present with symptoms similar to depression. In addition to a sad mood, elderly patients with depression can have symptoms affecting sleep, energy, appetite, and motivation.

- In contrast to dementia, which is slow and progressive, **delirium** is an acute disorder of cognition that is treatable and often reversible. It has a quicker onset, often on the scale of hours or days, and it may be accompanied by excessive drowsiness. The symptoms of delirium fluctuate and are often dominated by easy distractibility, inattention, and disorganized thinking.

- Some of the causes of delirium in elderly patients include infections or illness of almost any organ—pneumonia, urinary tract infections, or kidney disease, for example. Injuries, pain, or stress can all cause or exacerbate delirium, especially stays in the hospital or the intensive care unit.

- Many prescription or nonprescription drugs can contribute, as can low blood sugar or dehydration. Any big changes in life—moving, for example, or the loss of a loved one—can trigger or worsen delirium in elderly people at risk.

- Complicating all of this is that elderly patients with dementia can also have delirium—basically, an acute and treatable decline in function on top of a chronic, slow process. There is a lot of overlap in the causes and presentation, but it's important to try to think of these two processes separately because delirium, once diagnosed, can often be reversed. Depression can also coexist with both delirium and dementia, further muddying the diagnostic waters.

- Based on the first impression, it is possible that Isaac could have all three of these: dementia, delirium, and depression. His decline was more rapid than typical dementia, though sometimes the early signs of dementia could have been subtle and overlooked, especially if they were occurring right after his wife's death. Some degree of delirium could certainly be going on—and depression as well.

- The physical exam, overall, shows neurological problems across multiple areas of cognitive functioning. Isaac has memory problems, plus an inability to do simple arithmetic, and he can't seem to do ordinary motor tasks. There is at least some element of dementia.

- The neurological exam does not show any specific areas of motor weakness or sensory loss, what we would call focal neurological findings, making a specific, isolated brain lesion from a tumor or stroke unlikely. Whatever is going on, it must be a diffuse process throughout the cortex of the brain.

Taking Multiple Medications

- Isaac's list of medications is not a huge list—for a 90-year-old man. He has a medicine for irritable bowel syndrome, an older medicine that's called an antispasmodic that slows gut contractions. He had been using that for years, and it was meant to be used as needed. Isaac's well-meaning son has been giving that medicine every day, thinking that it would improve his dad's appetite.

- Isaac is also taking an antidepressant; he's been on that for about a year or so. The dose, though, was increased a few months ago.

- In addition, Isaac went to the hospital for a urinary tract infection (UTI) four months ago in Florida. A UTI is definitely a cause of delirium in elderly patients, and older men are at risk for them because of urinary retention sometimes caused by an enlarged prostate. Because his doctors suspected some

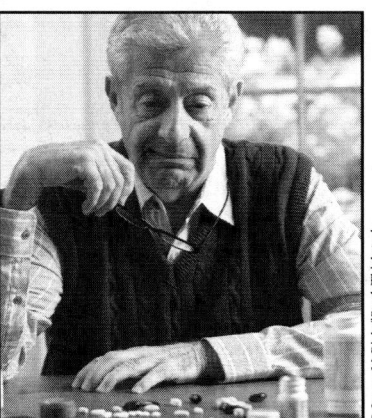

Elderly people who seem to have dementia could instead be experiencing cognitive problems as a result of being on multiple medications.

retention, he was prescribed a medication to prevent urinary retention, a common medication that's usually very well tolerated.

- However, all three of these medications have, in part, a similar pharmacological action. They all affect receptors of a neurotransmitter called acetylcholine, so they're all called anticholinergics. And there is an additive effect of using three anticholinergic medications with the same patient: You're much more likely to see anticholinergic side effects. Those can include a lot of different manifestations, including dry mouth, increased heart rate, and constipation, but—more importantly for Isaac—impaired concentration, memory, and attention.

- Isaac and his son are told to stop all three medications and make a follow-up appointment in one week. We also make arrangements for him to see a psychiatrist with expertise working with geriatric patients, and we contact a social worker to visit the home to help make sure that there are reasonable accommodations to prevent falls.

- One week later, Isaac is a different man. He walks in to the appointment, and he shakes your hand with strength and confidence. Tests of memory are still not at par with those of a young man; Isaac has some trouble repeating back reversed digits, but his **apraxia**, his inability to perform tasks, has disappeared.

- When asked about his wife, Isaac becomes tearful and sad. He talks about being lonely and about not wanting to be a burden to his son. So, there still may be an element of depression, and social support will still be essential.

- Isaac may have a mild degree of dementia as well. But addressing the medical cause of delirium—in this case, the medications he had been prescribed—was a huge step in improving Isaac's life and the life of his family.

Drug-Induced Cognitive Impairment
- Drug-induced cognitive impairment occurs in about 12 percent of elderly patients with suspected dementia. Almost any class of medications can do this, including commonly used blood pressure medications, psychiatric medications, pain medicines (including ordinary nonsteroidal pain medicines like aspirin and ibuprofen), medications for allergy or GI conditions or diabetes, and even many over-the-counter medicines.

- Some of these medicines cause their mischief directly, as a side effect. Or, some medications affect the metabolism of other medications, so it might be the combination, or interactions between the medications, especially when combined with other health issues, that lead to cognitive problems.

- The more medications taken, the higher the quantity of different pills, the more likely any side effect will be, including cognitive problems. The risk of delirium on three medications is about three times the risk on one; if taking five medications, the risk increases ninefold.

- The exact risk depends on what medicines are taken in what combination and at what doses, and on other health factors, so it's impossible to know the exact risk for any one patient. But the risk is substantial, and it gets higher and higher as the number of medications increases.

- The single most important step to reduce the risk of drug-induced cognitive impairment is to minimize the number of medications taken. The minimal effective doses should always be used, and medicines should be taken for the shortest possible length of time. The highest risk medications, especially sedatives and combinations of anticholinergic medications, should be avoided when possible.

- It's also crucial that every prescribing physician have a complete and accurate list of all medications taken and doses, including all over-the-counter meds and supplements. Patients can help by keeping a single, printed, up-to-date list or by bringing every single one of their medicine bottles to every single doctor's appointment.

- Caution is especially important when new medications are prescribed or doses changed, and of course, it's important that medicines be used correctly. If there is any concern about cognitive impairment, a family member or other responsible individual may be needed to take charge of medications to make sure they're used as intended.

- Medications certainly have their role. Medical problems like diabetes and arthritis need to be treated. Pain, especially, needs to be recognized and addressed, though that doesn't necessarily mean that pain has to be treated with medication.

- Drug withdrawal, too, can lead to delirium, so patients shouldn't stop taking medications on their own. Tapering down a long list of medications should be done under a doctor's supervision and advice and may need to be done in a stepwise, gradual fashion.

Important Terms

apraxia: Inability to perform purposeful actions.

delirium: An acute deterioration in brain function, typically occurring from intoxication, infection, or other specific disorders.

polypharmacy: An informal term referring to a condition where many medications are taken at once, often leading to adverse reactions.

Suggested Reading

Goldacre, *Bad Pharma.*

Mace, *The 26-Hour Day.*

Questions to Consider

1. How can you tell the normal forgetfulness that accompanies aging from dementia?

2. Of all the tools that doctors use to evaluate patients, what is the most useful? Most cost effective? Most reliable?

A Confused Father
Lecture 24—Transcript

Welcome, everyone, to our final grand rounds! Today we'll meet our last patient, and then we'll sum up some of the lessons we've learned, both about being a good doctor and about being a good patient.

The ancients knew that with age comes cognitive decline. Pythagoras, the Greek mathematician and physician of the 6th century B.C.E., divided the life cycle into five stages, the last of which, he said, began at age 81. He named this last stage the senium, and thought of it as an inevitable period of decline and regression. From the word senium comes senile, implying that age and senility are linked, and perhaps, inevitable. A Greek judge, Solon, about 50 years earlier, had incorporated this unavoidable decline into laws regarding inheritance. Men could direct their inheritance to any heir they wished, "providing judgment was not impaired by pain, violence, drugs, old age, or the persuasions of a woman."

We're in clinic today, general medicine clinic, and our patient is an 82-year-old gentleman named Isaac. He's brought in today by his son. You've known Isaac for many years, though he's a snowbird who you see for routine care only about six months out of the year. It's April, and he's come back in town from his usual winter stay in Boca Raton. You extend your hand to shake his, and you say hello. You say, "What can I do for you?" Isaac, hesitantly, he takes your hand for a brief squeeze. "He's just not right, doc," says his son. "He hasn't been right since he came back." The docs in Florida say he has Alzheimer's, but I wanted you to check him out.

You're shocked, really. You last saw Isaac about six months ago, and at least then, he was in pretty good shape. His wife had died about a year ago, and you had been worried then about him continuing to live alone. After the funeral, Isaac's son had moved back to town into an apartment he could share with his father. That turbulence, his wife's death and moving, had seemed to cause some confusion and a little forgetfulness, maybe not unexpected at Isaac's age. You had had him see a neurologist, and then a psychiatrist who had prescribed medication for depression. Isaac had seemed to improve and kind of settle into a new routine. Now it looks like, just from a first impression, Isaac has had a big step backwards in function and cognition.

Let's get more of the story from Isaac's son. He says they had been doing pretty well, he thinks, six months ago, when they made their usual winter move down south. And when they got there, his dad still seemed OK. His son works in consulting, mostly just using a computer and Skype from home with clients, so he had already decided to just stay with his dad in Florida. But after a few months, he thought dad was getting more withdrawn. They had met a new doctor in Florida and went to see him, and that doctor thought the depression was getting worse, so they adjusted his antidepressant medication.

Over the next few weeks, he noticed that Isaac was having trouble using the computer to read emails and would have occasional periods of irritability or crying, and would sometimes seem to be confused about how to dress himself. At one point, he had a particularly bad day and almost seemed like he had forgotten how to walk. That day he was taken to the ED and was diagnosed with a urinary tract infection. Treatment of that infection did help; he was able to walk, and his mind seemed to be clearer afterwards. His doctor had started another medicine to relax his bladder to prevent further infections.

Still, Isaac seemed to continue to have some good days and some bad days, some days when he seemed kind of out of it or confused, and he was referred to a neurologist who diagnosed him with Alzheimer's disease. Now, most days now, he doesn't talk, and he can't really dress himself anymore, and his son says, mostly, he just looks confused.

At this point, Isaac looks up at you, and you almost see a familiar sparkle in his eyes. He squints a little, and he looks at you, and he says, "I know you, doctor. How are you? How are your children?" He reaches over to shake hands again, though kind of turns his palm downwards, more like a hold than a shake. Still, you're happy to hear his voice, and you take his hand. "I'm doing fine, Isaac, thanks for asking. How about yourself?" Isaac says, "They say I have Alzheimer's. I don't know about that." His son looks shocked. It's easy to assume that someone who's not talking isn't listening, or that someone who seems out of it is unlikely to follow a conversation.

OK, we need a brief differential diagnosis to go forward, taking our traditional moment to organize our thoughts so we remember to ask the right questions. What's the cause of Isaac's cognitive decline? Let's start very broadly. Let's look at two big categories—dementia and delirium. Dementia is a progressive decline in memory and at least one other cognitive area. It is very strongly related to age. Dementia is rare under age 50, though it affects eight percent of those age 65. By 90, almost 40 percent of people have at least some dementia. The common causes of dementia are almost all related to chronic and progressive brain damage, occurring most often from age-related diseases, like strokes or Alzheimer's or Parkinson's disease. Damage can also be related to chronic infections, like HIV, or from toxins, like alcoholism. Most causes of dementia cannot be reversed, but at least, in some of the cases, progression can be slowed with therapy. Rarely, symptoms of dementia can be caused by thyroid disease, vitamin deficiencies, or a brain tumor.

The way that different people show symptoms of dementia can vary, but there was always some degree of memory loss. There will also be other evidence of problems with cognition, such as difficulty with language and communication, or problems with carrying out learned and purposeful movements. People with dementia, for instance, they may not be able to carry out the steps needed to comb hair or to use a coffee maker. Sometimes there can be a decline in the ability to recognize objects, or tell what they're for. Some people will also have changes in their personalities, and perhaps a loss of social inhibition in their actions or their speech.

One specific cause of dementia that's been mentioned is depression; this is sometimes called pseudo-dementia in the elderly, because depression can contribute to the symptoms of dementia, and dementia itself can present with symptoms similar to depression. In addition to a sad mood, elderly patients with depression can have symptoms including sleep problems, low energy, decreased appetite, and poor motivation.

Now, in contrast to dementia, which is slow and progressive, delirium is an acute disorder of cognition that is treatable and often reversible. It has a quicker onset, often on the scale of hours or days, and it may be accompanied by excessive drowsiness. The symptoms of delirium fluctuate, and are often dominated by easy distractibility, inattention, and disorganized thinking. Some of the causes of delirium in elderly patients include infections or illness of almost any organ—pneumonia, urinary tract infections, or kidney disease, for example. Injuries, pain, or stress can all cause or exacerbate delirium, especially stays in the hospital or the ICU. Many prescription or non-prescription drugs can contribute, as can low blood sugar or dehydration. Any big changes in life, moving, for instance, or the loss of a loved one, can trigger or worsen delirium in elderly people at risk.

Complicating all of this is that elderly patients with dementia can also have delirium, basically, an acute and treatable decline in function on top of a chronic, slow process. There is a lot of overlap in the causes and presentation, but it's important to try to think of these two processes separately, because delirium, once diagnosed, can often be reversed. Depression can also co-exist with both delirium and dementia, further muddying the diagnostic waters.

So what do you think, based on the first impression? Does Isaac have dementia or delirium or depression? From what we know, I think he could have all three. His decline was more rapid than typical dementia, though sometimes the early signs of dementia could have been subtle and overlooked, especially if they were occurring right after his wife's death. Some degree of delirium could certainly be going on, and depression as well. Let's see if we can clear this up with some additional history.

Isaac's appetite has been up and down, sometimes, some days better than others. He does have a history of irritable bowel syndrome, so his son thinks sometimes abdominal upset has caused some skipped meals; he has been giving Isaac an older medication that's been used for years to help with those belly symptoms. There has been no vomiting and no headaches, and that goes against a brain tumor. There's also been no history of weakness of a limb or slurred speech that would suggest a stroke or other damage to a small, specific area of brain.

By this point of the history, Isaac is answering some questions and he's participating himself. Isaac denies any symptoms at all, no aches or pains, no cough or fever, no urinary symptoms. When asked about that, his son adds that he's still taking that medication to help with his bladder. Isaac has had no trouble with sleeping, and overall, Isaac says, he feels pretty good.

You look back through the medical record, and overall, Isaac has been in great shape. He's been taking an antidepressant since shortly after his wife's death, and you see that about four months ago the dose was increased. Other than the history of occasional stomach upset caused by irritable bowel syndrome, he's really had no other health concerns. He's had the usual screening tests for his age, including cholesterol and EKGs and a stress test, and you have some labs that were done while he was out of town, including normal thyroid tests, tests of vitamin levels, and other routine blood work. All of that looks fine. You also have a copy of a CT scan that was done a few months ago. And that does show just some shrinking of the brain to a small degree; that's not unexpected for Isaac's age, and it really isn't really diagnostic. Still, the CT is further confirmation that there isn't a tumor or a bleeding vessel in the brain.

On to our physical exam. Isaac is now sitting up. He looks more alert. He's a tall man, kind of wispy white hair; he looks well-groomed and dressed and not at all neglected. His temperature and other vital signs are normal, and the remainder of the general medical exam is unrevealing. Focusing on the neurologic exam, we find that his strength and reflexes are normal, and he has normal sensations in all of his extremities. There are some simple tests we use to confirm this, using the pointy end of a broken tongue depressor to test if he can feel a sharp pinprick, and bottom of a tuning fork to see if he can feel vibrations.

We ask Isaac a few questions about what's called his orientation; he knows his own name and the city you're in, but not the year. You'd say he's alert and oriented to name and place but not time. You ask him to remember three common objects, say a car and an orange and a hat. Isaac can immediately repeat those three back to you, but five minutes later he cannot remember any of them. Isaac can't repeat a series of numbers backwards, and can't perform a simple calculation like 100 minus 7. He finds it difficult to follow multistep commands, and is unable to pantomime pouring a cup of coffee; that last finding is a test for what's called apraxia, or motor planning. You can ask anything that's culturally appropriate and something that your patient ought to be able to do, like taking money out of a wallet or opening a can of tuna. Isaac seems to understand the questions, but can't seem to get his body to act out the actions.

That physical exam, overall, is showing neurologic problems across multiple areas of cognitive functioning. Isaac has memory problems, plus an inability to do simple arithmetic; he can't seem to do ordinary motor tasks, either. There is at least some element of dementia here. The neurologic exam does not show any specific areas of motor weakness or sensory loss, what we would have called focal neurologic findings, making a specific, isolated brain lesion from a tumor or stroke unlikely. Whatever's going on, it must be a diffuse process throughout the cortex of the brain.

But is this just dementia? You shouldn't be so sure. You're still struck by your recollection of your last visit. How did Isaac decline so rapidly? That's part of the value of seeing patients for years, that gut feeling that you know people, and know what they're like. In this case, you're just not satisfied that this is only a case of age-related dementia.

I want to go back the quote I used at the start of this lecture, from the Greek judge Solon, whose law in about 600 B.C.E. allowed for people to make their own decisions about inheritance. Men could make their own decisions, "providing judgment was not impaired by pain, violence, drugs, old age, or the persuasions of a woman." Solon here was making a declaration about mental competence and listing things that even 2,500 years ago were known to interfere with thinking.

First, Solon said pain, which remains a well known and often unrecognized cause of delirium, especially in the elderly. Although the mechanisms of how pain leads to impaired thinking aren't clearly understood, it's well known that older people in pain from urinary tract infections or arthritis or GI conditions, like diverticulitis, they can have dramatic declines in their cognitive ability, both from the pain itself and sometimes from the medications used to treat the pain. Pain, I think, can refer both to physical pain from illness or injury, but also the mental pain of depression and isolation and loneliness that so many older people experience. Both of these kinds of pains, by the way, are transmitted and processed by the same pathways in the brain.

Solon's list also includes violence, which could certainly cause brain injury. Elder abuse is a real phenomenon now, too, and can present as depression, withdrawal, and cognitive decline. The last item on Solon's list, the "persuasions of a woman," I'm not going to go into much more detail there, but I suppose a modern parallel would be anyone who takes advantage of the fear and isolation that older people may feel. One more item from Solon's list, and that's the one I want to focus on the most—drugs; 2500 years ago, and the Greeks even then knew that their drugs could interfere with clear thinking. And we've got far more drugs now, that are far more powerful and more widely used.

Isaac's medicines, let's review. It's not a huge list for an 82-year-old man. He has a medicine for irritable bowel syndrome, an older medicine that's called an antispasmodic that slows gut contractions. He had been using that for years, and it was meant to be used as needed. By the way, for those of you still getting used to doctor lingo and writing prescriptions, Latin for "as the need arises" is *pro re nata*, so drugs prescribed to be used as needed are abbreviated PRN. Now, Isaac's well-meaning son had been giving that medicine every day, thinking it would improve his dad's appetite.

Isaac is also taking an antidepressant; he's been on that a year or so. Though the dose, remember, had been increased a few months ago. And, he went to the hospital for a urinary tract infection four months ago in Florida. A urinary tract infection, we usually abbreviate that UTI, is definitely a cause of delirium in elderly patients, and older men are at risk for them because of urinary retention sometimes caused by an enlarged prostate. Because his doctors suspected some urinary retention, he was prescribed a medicine to prevent urinary retention, a common medicine that's usually very well tolerated.

But, all three of these medications have, in part, a similar pharmacologic action. They all, all three of them, affect receptors of a neurotransmitter called acetylcholine, so they're all called anticholinergics. And there is an additive effect of using three anticholinergic medications in the same patient; you're much more likely to see anticholinergic side effects. Those can include a lot of different manifestations, including dry mouth, increased heart rate, and constipation, but more importantly for Isaac, impaired concentration, memory, and attention.

Isaac and his son are told to stop these medications, just stop all of them, and make a follow-up appointment in one week. We also make arrangements for him to see a psychiatrist with expertise working with geriatric patients and contact a social worker to visit the home to help make sure that there are reasonable accommodations to keep Isaac safe and prevent falls.

And one week later, Isaac is a different man. He walks in to the appointment; he shakes your hand with strength and with confidence. Tests of memory are still not at par with those of a young man; Isaac has some trouble repeating back reversed digits, but his apraxia, his inability to perform tasks, that has disappeared. When asked about his wife, Isaac becomes tearful and sad, and talks about being lonely, and talks about not wanting to be a burden to his son. So, I think there may be an element of depression, still, here, and social support will still be essential.

Isaac may have a mild degree of dementia as well. We'll want to get him involved, perhaps, in a day program or other activities to engage his mind, which can prevent or slow the progression of age-related dementia. Here's another quote from Solon, the Greek judge who had listed so many of the causes of cognitive decline. "I grow old learning something new every day." Continuing to learn may be one of the best ways to keep an aging mind sharp.

But addressing the medical cause of delirium, in this case, the medications that had been prescribed, was the biggest and most important step in improving Isaac's life and that of his family. Drug-induced cognitive impairment occurs in about 12 percent of elderly patients with suspected dementia. Almost any class of medications can do this, including commonly used blood pressure medications; psychiatric medications; pain medicines, even including ordinary, non-steroidal pain medicines, like aspirin or ibuprofen; medicines for allergy; or GI conditions; or diabetes; and even many over-the-counter medicines. Some of these medicines cause their mischief directly, as a side effect. Or, some medications affect the metabolism of other medications. So it might be a combination, or interactions between the medications, that lead to cognitive problems.

One principle, though, is that the more medications taken, the higher the quantity of different pills, the more likely any side effect will be, including cognitive problems. The risk of delirium on three medications is about three times the risk on one. If taking five medications, the risk increases nine-fold. The exact risk depends on what medicines are taken, in what combinations, and on what doses, other health factors as well, so it's impossible to know the exact risk for any one patient. But the risk is substantial, and it gets higher and higher as the number of medications increases.

So the single, most important step to reduce the risk of drug-induced cognitive impairment is to minimize the number of medications taken. The minimal effective doses should always be used, and medicines should be taken for the shortest possible length of time. The highest risk medications, especially sedatives and combinations of anti-cholinergics, should be avoided when possible. It's also crucial that every prescribing physician have a complete and accurate list of all medicines taken and doses, including all over-the-counter meds and supplements. Patients can help by keeping a single, printed, up-to-date list, or just by bringing every single one of their medicine bottles to every single doctor's appointment.

Caution is especially important when new medications are prescribed or doses are changed, and of course, it's important that medicines be used correctly. If there is any concern about cognitive impairment, a family member or other responsible individual may be needed to take charge of medications to make sure they're used as intended.

That being said, medications certainly have their role. Medical problems, like diabetes and arthritis, need to be treated. Pain, especially, needs to be recognized and addressed, though that doesn't necessarily mean that pain has to be treated with medication. Drug withdrawal, too, it can lead to delirium, so I don't mean to imply that patients should stop taking medications on their own. Tapering down a long list of medications should be done under a doctor's supervision and advice, and may need to be done in a stepwise, gradual fashion.

Today's case, of course, illustrated the risks of side effects of medications, and especially of what's sometimes called polypharmacy—taking multiple medications. We also saw how important it was that our patient had his own advocate, in this case, his son, to help him at appointments and to make sure the correct history was available. Once a patient is sick, he or she might not be in the best condition to communicate with the doctor and follow through on plans. That goes for mental health and cognitive problems, of course, but even for any general medical condition that's distracting and worrying, really, almost any concern.

We also saw that a single doctor who's known a patient well for years can be a strong ally. ERs and urgent cares have their place, but when care is fractionated, with different people focusing on individual problems, doctors are more likely to overlook the big picture, and patients are less likely to get the care they need.

And that's what this course really has been about—how to give and get the best medical care for yourself and your family. We've been through some interesting cases, and you've learned, I hope, some solid medical information and some doctor lingo. But what's more important than knowing about individual diseases is knowing how doctors think and how patients can use that information to get better health care.

For instance, we've seen again and again that doctors rely on the patient's narrative to reach a diagnosis. That may have seemed like a surprising thing to say at the beginning of this series, but now you know that even in this day of lab tests and CT scans and all sorts of equipment and technology, most diagnoses rely on the history, the story of the illness, or the story that the patient brings to the doctor. This is what happened, this is what happened next. Doctors need to take the time to listen to their patients, after all, it's the patient's story; it's not the doctor's. A few directed questions can help focus on what's going on, but the story needs to unfold. Sometimes, the whole story isn't complete at the first encounter; it may take multiple visits to figure out what's going on. That doesn't necessarily mean that the doctor missed something or made a mistake.

The physical exam is a great tool, starting with the vitals, and including both a good overview and specific observations to look into concerns raised by the history. There is no such thing as an absolutely complete physical exam.

I guess one could be done, but it would take a few hours, but the most critical organ systems need to be evaluated, along with a more in-depth exam of the most concerning areas. Like the history, the first exam might not supply all of the answers, and sometimes physical exams have to be repeated to reveal the clues that are needed.

Tests and labs, these really are an essential part of medicine, but as we've seen, maybe not in the way people think. Labs and tests confirm diagnoses to rule out things that are very serious and critical. But labs and tests can also, themselves, be misleading. There's no way to "test for everything," and tests have to be interpreted with caution and that eye on the big picture.

We've seen a few times the idea of a therapeutic trial, coming up with what is called a working diagnosis, then seeing what happens when that's treated. A response to a treatment, or a non-response to treatment, that itself is a valid test and can help confirm or refute the working diagnosis. That the first idea didn't work doesn't mean it was a mistake, but sticking with the wrong plan, not making changes in the diagnosis or treatment when a plan isn't working, that is a mistake.

A physician's most important skill doesn't involve a little hammer, or a stethoscope, or a lab slip or prescription pad. It is, actually, listening. Paying attention to what's said, listening for clues, sometimes asking the right questions to get the story you need. Doctors need to keep an open mind, stay curious, and keep reading and learning. There is always more to learn, and we need to be humble about what we don't know.

So, what can patients do to help their doctors and help get themselves the best possible care? Be honest. Be ready to tell your story, maybe even again and again. Keep in mind that it may take multiple visits and repeated encounters to get to the bottom of a diagnosis. Sometimes, even with the best doctors, you won't get a clear answer at first. In fact, not all problems even have a clear answer, but that doesn't mean they can't be addressed. Sometimes care has to be coordinated between specialists or between different medical facilities. Help that process along by making sure copies of labs and reports get to everyone involved, especially your primary physician. Keep your follow-up appointments, and make sure you get the results of tests and labs and understand them. No news isn't necessarily good news—if it was important to do a test, it's important for the patient to get the results.

There are some simple questions that a patient should always feel comfortable asking. Simple things, like, "What are you thinking, doctor?" or, "What do you think the problem might be? Are there other diagnoses that we still need to worry about?" Ask the doctor, "What are the next steps for tests or treatments?" Or, simply, "What, exactly, do you want me to do?"

And, perhaps, the most important questions of all, "When should I expect to feel better, and what should I do if I'm not feeling better then?" Those last questions are crucial, not only because they focus on information patients need to know, but also because they reinforce the collaboration between the doctor and patient. In other words, they bring the conversation away from the disease and the tests and the medicine, and back directly to the patient.

If you're a patient wanting to understand how doctors think, from this grand rounds series you've learned some valuable information that will help you become a more effective part of the doctor-patient team. And if you're planning to become a physician yourself, watch for those clues that your patients bring you. The most effective encounters, the ones that really help keep patients healthy, are the ones when patients and doctors help each other solve the mysteries.

Glossary

adhesion: Surfaces stuck together, typically referring to organs and tissues within the abdomen.

AED: Automated external defibrillator.

agonal: Occurring just before death.

ANA: Antinuclear antibodies, a common blood test used in the evaluation of autoimmune and rheumatologic disease.

anemia: Low red blood cell count.

angina: Literally, "pain"—most often referring to angina pectoris, a kind of chest pain associated with decreased oxygen delivery to the heart muscle.

anorexia: Lack of appetite or disinterest in eating.

antibodies: Serum immunoglobulins that are part of the immune system.

aphasia: Inability to understand or express speech.

apnea: Cessation of breathing.

apraxia: Inability to perform purposeful actions.

arrhythmia: An irregularity in the heart rhythm. Although this term is used commonly, a more exact term that is preferred is "dysrhythmia."

arterial blood gas: A blood test that measures pH and gases, including oxygen and carbon dioxide.

arthralgia: Joint pain without evidence of inflammation.

arthritis: Joint inflammation, typically manifested by stiffness and pain accompanied by swelling.

ascites: Abdominal swelling caused by accumulated fluid in the abdominal cavity.

atelectasis: Partially collapsed areas of lung, typically observed on a chest X-ray.

autoclave: A container that can be heated under pressure, typically used to sterilize medical equipment.

bacteria: A unicellular microorganism lacking a nucleus.

bariatric surgery: Surgery intended to assist weight loss.

bilious vomiting: Vomiting stained by bile, typically green or yellow; often an indication of abdominal obstruction.

blanching: To become white or colorless when squeezed or pressed.

board certified: Maintaining requirements by a medical specialty board, typically including passing examinations and fulfilling educational and practice requirements.

bone scan: A nuclear study that identifies areas of active bone turnover, typically from infection, trauma, or tumor.

bruit: A noise caused by turbulent flow in a blood vessel.

candida: A common species of yeast.

cardiorespiratory monitor (often abbreviated "CR monitor" or just "monitor"): An electronic device that measures and displays vital signs and often heart and breathing rhythms in real time.

catarrh: Excessive mucus in the nose or throat.

catheter lab (often abbreviated "cath lab"): Referring to an area of a hospital or clinic where procedures involving catheterization of blood vessels are undertaken. These include studies and interventions of the heart, brain, and other vasculature.

cerebrovascular accident: Stroke—brain damage caused by insufficient blood flow.

chest tube: More formally, thoracostomy tube—a tube used to drain air or fluid from the chest.

chief complaint (often abbreviated "CC"; "chief concern" is also used): A traditional part of a medical encounter that is typically recorded in the patient's own words, expressing the main reason that the patient sought care.

complete blood count (CBC): A common laboratory test that quantifies the different types of cells in the blood.

concussion: Brain trauma leading to symptoms of brain dysfunction.

confluent: Running together or atop one another, often referring to a rash characterized by individual spots that coalesce and touch each other, appearing as one larger area.

congestive heart failure: Insufficient output of blood from the heart, leading to fluid accumulation.

computed tomography scan (CT scan): A study that uses a series of X-rays to construct two-dimensional images of internal structures.

crackles (also called "rales"): A physical exam finding of the lungs, crackles sound very much like the "snap, crackle, and pop" of milk poured over breakfast cereal.

cranium: The skull, or more specifically, the part of the skull that encloses the brain.

C-reactive protein (CRP): A blood protein that can be measured in the laboratory. An elevated CRP is an indication of inflammation.

defibrillator: A device that delivers a shock to the heart to restore a normal rhythm.

delirium: An acute deterioration in brain function, typically occurring from intoxication, infection, or other specific disorders.

dementia: A chronic disorder of brain functioning, most typically marked by memory problems in addition to other manifestations.

deny: In medical lingo, "deny" means that the patient says the symptom in question did not occur. It does not imply that the patient is being untruthful.

differential diagnosis: A list of candidate diagnoses to explain a medical problem.

diplopia: Double vision.

dyschezia: Painful defecation.

edema: Swelling, typically of an extremity.

EKG: Electrocardiogram—sometimes abbreviated ECG.

EMR: Electronic medical record—sometimes abbreviated EHR for "electronic health record."

EMT: Emergency medical technician.

encephalitis: Inflammation of the brain, most typically caused by infection.

encephalopathy: Dysfunction of the brain from any cause.

endocrine: Relating to glands that secrete hormones into the blood.

ENT: A surgical specialty standing for "ear, nose, and throat"—sometimes referred to as otorhinolaryngology.

epilepsy: A neurologic disorder characterized by recurrent seizures.

erythrocyte sedimentation rate (often abbreviated "sed rate" or "ESR"): A blood test of inflammation.

family practice: A board-certified medical specialty that provides primary care to patients of all ages, often including obstetric care and minor surgery.

fever: An elevated body temperature.

functional illness: Symptoms that cannot be ascribed to any abnormality on an objective test, such as an X-ray or a blood test.

general practitioner: A physician who treats general conditions; this title does not require a residency or board certification.

generic: Referring to medications, "generic" means manufactured by a company that does not own the patent.

genetic: Relating to the genes, or the sequences of DNA encoded in cells that direct their functioning.

glucosuria: Glucose in the urine.

grand rounds: Medical education sessions typically presented to physicians and students, usually surrounding a single case presentation.

HEENT: "Head, ears, eyes, nose, and throat"—referring to these areas of the physical examination.

hematochezia: Visible blood in the stool.

hematocrit: A measure of the volume of blood that is taken up by red blood cells, expressed as a percentage.

hemoglobin: The molecule in red blood cells that binds oxygen. "Hemoglobin" often refers to a quantitative lab measurement of the concentration of this molecule in a blood sample.

hernia: A condition where an organ protrudes through the wall of the area surrounding it.

history of present illness (HPI): A chronologic account of a patient's symptoms.

homeostasis: Physiologic equilibrium, as maintained by mechanisms that control vital processes.

hormone: A substance secreted into the blood that controls functions at a distant site—for example, insulin.

hypoglycemia: Low blood sugar concentration. Contrast with hyperglycemia (high blood sugar) or euglycemia (normal blood sugar.)

hypoventilation: Insufficient breathing, resulting specifically in increased carbon dioxide in the blood.

idiopathic: Of unknown cause.

IgE: Immunoglobulin E, a specific subtype of antibody that's often associated with allergic disease.

IgG: Immunoglobulin G, the most common subtype of antibody circulating in blood.

ileus: A cessation of the normal movements of the gut wall.

immune globulin: Proteins that assist immunity, often called "antibodies."

incidentaloma: An informal word referring to something found on a test or radiology study that is unrelated to the problem being investigated.

inflammation: A physiologic reaction to infection or stress that can include redness, swelling, pain, and warmth.

intellectual disability (MR): Impaired cognitive or intellectual functioning. Often used synonymously with or as a preferred term for "mental retardation."

intern: A graduate of medical school training in the first year after graduation.

internal medicine: A medical specialty that concentrates on the diagnosis and management of nonsurgical problems in adults.

internist: A physician practicing internal medicine.

intravenous (IV): Within a vein.

intubation: Placing a tube within a hollow organ, most commonly referring to an endotracheal (breathing) tube placed in the trachea (airway).

jaundice: A yellow color to the eyes and skin caused by excessive bilirubin in the blood.

laparoscopy: A surgical procedure using optical instruments inserted through the abdominal wall to view the inside.

laparotomy: A surgical procedure including an incision into the abdominal cavity.

lesion: A region of an organ or tissue that has been damaged.

liver function tests (LFTs): More properly, "transaminases"—a collection of blood tests that indirectly measures the health of liver cells.

lumbar puncture (LP): Sometimes called a "spinal tap"—inserting a needle between the vertebrae to collect cerebrospinal fluid or instill medication.

magnetic resonance imaging (MRI): Using a strong magnetic field and radio waves to get detailed images of internal organs.

metabolic: Related to chemical processes that sustain life.

metastatic: Cancer appearing at a site distant to the original cancer, caused by migrating and then proliferating cells.

murmur: A noise heard over the chest with a stethoscope caused by turbulent blood flow through the heart.

myositis: Inflammation of muscle.

narcotic: A class of pain relievers derived from opium or morphine.

nausea: A feeling of queasiness, or that one is about to vomit.

negative: In medical use, "negative" means that the inquired symptom or finding is absent. It does not imply that this is good or bad.

neuropathy: Damage or malfunction of nerves.

nystagmus: A rapid, flicking movement of the eyes.

opioid: An opium-like compound, informally synonymous with "narcotic."

organic illness: An illness that includes objective abnormalities on a blood test or radiologic study that correlates with symptoms.

palpate: To feel, as in part of the physical exam.

paracentesis: Inserting a needle into the abdominal cavity to obtain fluid.

pathology: Diseased tissue, or the collective features of a disease—or the branch of medicine that studies diseased tissues.

peritonitis: Inflammation in the lining of the abdomen.

petechiae: A physical finding of the skin, appearing as small broken blood vessels or red-purple, non-blanching spots.

plasmapheresis: A medical procedure that separates out the plasma from the whole blood and then filters out certain elements, typically proteins, before returning the blood to the body.

platelets: A kind of blood cell involved in clotting.

polycythemia: Excessively high red blood cell count.

polypharmacy: An informal term referring to a condition where many medications are taken at once, often leading to adverse reactions.

positive: In medical lingo, "positive" is used to denote a finding that is present. It does not imply whether this finding is good or bad.

primary: A problem or finding that isn't caused by something else. For example, a primary headache isn't caused by some other medical condition.

pro re nata (PRN): Literally, "as the thing is born" or "as the need arises"—refers to a medication that's ordered to be given only as needed.

pulse oximeter (often abbreviated "pulse ox" or "POX"): A device that measures the pulse and oxygen saturation in blood.

pulse rate: A count of heartbeats per unit time, such as beats per minute.

purpura: Coalescing petechiae, or a large area of skin with bruising and broken blood vessels, leading to bleeding within or under the skin.

red blood cells: The cells in the blood that carry oxygen.

referred pain: Pain that is perceived in a different location than where the tissue damage is occurring.

review of systems (ROS): Part of the medical interview, with a series of questions organized by organ system to see if specific symptoms have been present.

scintillation camera: A camera that detects radiation, used in nuclear medicine studies.

secondary: A symptom or problem caused by some other medical problem. For example, a secondary headache may be caused by a sinus infection, concussion, or brain tumor.

seizure: A sudden disruption in the normal electrical activity of the brain, accompanied by altered consciousness, movements, or other neurologic manifestations.

sepsis: A whole-body inflammatory condition, triggered by serious infection.

seroconversion: When blood tests show that a person has been exposed to an infectious agent by demonstrating the presence of specific antibodies against that infection.

shock: A life-threatening state of insufficient blood flow to multiple organs.

spirometry: Tests of lung functioning.

stenting: Using a hollow tube to hold open a hollow organ, typically a blood vessel.

stricture: A narrowing of a hollow organ, such as the esophagus or a blood vessel.

superinfection: An infection that occurs on top of a first infection.

syncope: Synonymous with "faint"—a brief loss of consciousness caused by insufficient cerebral blood flow.

syndrome: A group of symptoms that occur together with a specific condition.

tachycardia: Fast heart rate.

tenderness: Pain that is increased with palpation.

vertigo: A spinning sensation, or feeling that one's environment is spinning around.

vestibular: Related to the sense of balance and position sense.

virus: A small infectious agent that does not contain its own cells or organelles.

vital signs: Collectively, clinical measurements of pulse rate, blood pressure, respiratory rate, and temperature.

vitamin: One of a group of compounds that are essential to be ingested in small quantities to maintain health and life.

wheezing: A physical exam finding of the lungs, heard best with a stethoscope. Wheezing sounds like air rushing through small tubes and is most typically heard in expiration.

white blood cells: The cells in the blood that are part of the immune system.

Bibliography

Adams, Francis. *The Asthma Sourcebook*. New York: McGraw-Hill, 2006. Written by a physician specializing in pulmonary medicine, this book for patients is comprehensive and well organized. Includes information on asthma prevention and treatment, along with a directory of resources, further information, and support groups.

Barkley, Russell A. *Taking Charge of ADHD: The Complete, Authoritative Guide for Parents*. New York: The Guilford Press, 2000. A great guide for parents about day-to-day management, homework, discipline, and living together in peace—while helping your child gain the skills he or she needs to succeed.

Barry, John. *The Great Influenza: The Story of the Deadliest Pandemic in History*. London: Penguin Books, 2005. Biology plus politics led to up to 100 million deaths in one year, 1918—the worst flu pandemic in history. Could it happen again?

Brazelton, T. Berry. *Touchpoints: Birth to Three*. Cambridge, MA: Da Capo Press, 2006. Written with love and humor for parents and anyone else who wants to understand what babies and young children do and think. This is the classic guide to infant development.

Buchholz, David. *Heal Your Headache*. New York: Workman Publishing Company, 2002. Getting a little out of date—especially regarding current medications—but still a great resource for understanding, preventing, and treating migraine headaches.

Burns, David. *Feeling Good: The New Mood Therapy*. New York: Harper, 2008. A self-help book for depression that relies on techniques of cognitive-behavioral therapy to teach people how to recognize and change problematic patterns of thought. A few small clinical trials have shown that this book can help people with major depression.

Carpenter, Kenneth. *Beriberi, White Rice, and Vitamin B: A Disease, a Cause, and a Cure.* Berkeley, CA: University of California Press, 2000. A thought-provoking tale that starts with a simple observation—that chickens fed only white rice die—and then traces the work of dozens of scientists to elucidate and cure what was once a common disease.

Chokroverty, Sudhansu. *Questions and Answers about Sleep Apnea.* Burlington, MA: Jones and Bartlett, 2008. Authoritative, practical insight for doctors, patients, and families.

De Kruif, Paul. *Microbe Hunters.* Boston, MA: Mariner Books, 2002. Heroes and stories make the history of microbiology come alive in this entertaining and informative book, first published in 1926.

Dickens, Charles. *The Pickwick Papers.* Knoxville, TN: Wordsworth Classics, 1998. Dickens's first novel is a classic of comic writing, featuring a host of memorable characters—including one with a prescient presentation of a modern scourge.

Fletcher, Anne. *Inside Rehab: The Surprising Truth about Addiction Treatment and How to Get Help That Works.* New York: Viking Adult, 2013. Addiction may be incurable, but it is certainly treatable—and this book explores the best treatment options available and how to find them.

Garrett, Laurie. *The Coming Plague: Newly Emerging Diseases in a World out of Balance.* London: Penguin Books, 1995. Where's the next disease coming from—and are our environmental and political policies causing it? Provocative, and perhaps not always 100 percent accurate in its predictions, but Garrett's book will give you a lot to think about.

Gawande, Atul. *Complications: A Surgeon's Notes on an Imperfect Science.* New York: Picador, 2003. Doctors are far from infallible, as illustrated in these entertaining case histories.

Giudice, Linda, ed. *Endometriosis: Science and Practice.* Hoboken, NJ: Wiley-Blackwell, 2012. Written for physicians, this textbook is a compilation of chapters from the world's experts. May be a bit heavy for a casual reader—but if you want solid science, this is it.

Goldacre, Ben. *Bad Pharma: How Drug Companies Mislead Doctors and Harm Patients*. London: Faber & Faber, 2013. Pulling no punches, a comprehensive account of how the pharmaceutical industry can game the system for profits—even while providing life-saving medications we all depend on.

Gratzer, Walter. *Terrors of the Table: The Curious History of Nutrition*. New York: Oxford University Press, 2005. An entertaining history of food and nutrition, written for laypeople, though with considerable science and an entertaining take on the characters and quackery that have colored the journey. Includes fascinating accounts of the history of nutritional disease, including scurvy, rickets, beriberi, and pellagra.

Green, Peter, and Rory Jones. *Celiac Disease: A Hidden Epidemic*. New York: William Morrow, 2010. Despite the provocative title, a well-balanced and informative view of this common disease, including up-to-date information on pathophysiology and testing.

Groopman, Jerome. *How Doctors Think*. Boston, MA: Mariner Books, 2008. Entertaining and enlightening insights into the mind of a physician and the art of medicine.

Hillman, Robert, et al, eds. *Hematology in Clinical Practice*. New York: McGraw-Hill Professional, 2010. Cutting edge and at times almost too detailed—but if you want to understand blood and its diseases, this textbook covers it.

Hochberg, Z. *Vitamin D and Rickets*. Basel, Switzerland: S Karger, 2003. From its fascinating history through its modern presentation, this comprehensive book covers just about anything anyone could want to know about what was once called the "English disease."

Jelinek, George. *Overcoming Multiple Sclerosis: An Evidence-Based Guide to Recovery*. Sydney, Australia: Allen & Unwin, 2010. Written by a physician with MS, this book starts out focusing on his personal story, but also contains a wealth of information about practical ways to cope, diet and exercise, and modern medical therapies.

Kapit, Wynn. *The Physiology Coloring Book*. San Francisco: Benjamin Cummings, 1999. Don't let the title fool you—this is a serious book that teaches real physiology at a medical school level. And you don't really have to color it.

Klein, Grady, and Alan Dabney. *The Cartoon Introduction to Statistics*. New York: Hill and Wang, 2013. Before you try to read the medical literature, you need to understand how science and statistics work. This is a great place to start.

Lindley, Richard. *Stroke: The Facts*. New York: Oxford University Press, 2008. A guide for families and patients struggling with stroke risks, therapy, and rehabilitation. It's illustrated and friendly, but nonetheless provides solid information.

Link, John. *The Breast Cancer Survival Manual*. New York: Holt Paperbacks, 2012. A wonderful and comprehensive guide to breast cancer and how to fight it—based on the best available evidence.

Mace, Nancy. *The 26-Hour Day: A Family Guide to Caring for People with Alzheimer's Disease, Other Dementias, and Memory Loss in Later Life*. New York: Grand Central Life & Style, 2012. The practical guide to helping families deal with dementia with kindness and love.

Mayo Clinic. *Mayo Clinic Healthy Heart for Life*. Birmingham, AL: Oxmoor House, 2012. Practical, up-to-date, and actionable advice that you can use to get your heart healthy and keep your heart healthy.

Meniere Man. *The Self Help Book for Meniere's Disease*. Page Addie Press, 2012. Funny, personal, yet practical, this Australian author and Ménière's disease sufferer has decided that it's up to you to improve your own health.

Montgomery, Kathryn. *How Doctors Think: Clinical Judgment and the Practice of Medicine*. New York: Oxford University Press, 2005. Several years before Groopman's popular book, Montgomery wrote this overlooked gem about the application of clinical judgment—the art of medicine.

Mukherjee, Siddhartha. *The Emperor of All Maladies: A Biography of Cancer*. New York: Scribner, 2010. A Pulitzer Prize–winning history of cancer research, filled with personal tales from a gifted writer and practicing oncologist.

Nolen, William. *The Making of a Surgeon*. Nashville, TN: Mid List Press, 1999. The classic memoir of a surgeon's transformative life.

Offit, Paul. *Autism's False Prophets: Bad Science, Risky Medicine, and the Search for a Cure*. New York: Colombia University Press, 2010. A provocative story about how the autism community was fooled into a false idea—and how that misdirection is costing lives.

———. *Deadly Choices: How the Anti-Vaccine Movement Threatens Us All*. New York: Basic Books, 2010. Do you think that anti-vaccine propaganda isn't going to hurt you or your family? Think again. A gripping story of how a small number of zealots has created a controversy that's causing a public health debacle.

Plotkin, Stanley, et al, eds. *Vaccines: Expert Consult*. Saunders, 2012. Hefty, well referenced, and authoritative—if you want solid, unbiased, comprehensive vaccine information, you'll find it here.

Pollan, Michael. *Food Rules: An Eater's Manual*. London: Penguin Books, 2009. Short, easy, simple, and livable rules for improved health and a longer life.

Reynolds, Richard, and John Stone, eds. *On Doctoring*. New York: Simon and Schuster, 2010. A collection of stories and poems about medicine and doctors—appealing, at times hysterical, at times heartbreaking. If you want to understand what it feels like to be a doctor, this is a good place to start.

Rogozov, Vladislav, and Neil Bermel. "Auto-Appendectomy in the Antarctic." *BMJ: British Medical Journal* 339, no. 7735 (2009): 1420–1422. The most detailed account of the most celebrated case of self-surgery every reported, written by the surgeon's son. Quite graphic photographs provide all the proof you'll need.

Sacks, Oliver. *The Man Who Mistook His Wife for a Hat: And Other Clinical Tales*. New York: Touchstone, 1998. The mysteries of the human brain explored by a practicing neurologist in a series of fascinating cases.

Sheff, David. *Beautiful Boy: A Father's Journey through His Son's Addiction*. Boston, MA: Mariner Books, 2009. This book is intense and emotional, and the author makes you feel as though you're living though his nightmare of his son's crystal meth addiction.

Shem, Samuel. *The House of God*. New York: Berkley Trade, 2010. Every medical student reads this—a fictional but realistic view of what happens in a hospital, or at least what your doctors probably don't want you to know. Profane, hilarious, blistering, and not for everyone.

Shilts, Randy. *And the Band Played On: Politics, People, and the AIDS Epidemic*. London: St. Martin's Griffin, 2007. Reads like a thriller, or even a horror story—written by an early victim of AIDS (though before he knew he was infected), this book is a legacy of the human tragedy of AIDS.

Solomon, Andrew. *The Noonday Demon: An Atlas of Depression*. New York: Scribner, 2002. A personal story interwoven with information about many aspects of depression: history, symptoms, and treatment. A rare book that's well written, moving, and informative.

Spence, David, and Henry J. M. Barnett, eds. *Stroke Prevention, Treatment, and Rehabilitation*. New York: McGraw-Hill, 2012. Written for medical professionals, this multiauthored book covers the most reliable information about strokes for patients and physicians alike.

Stern, Scott, Adam Cifu, and Diane Altkorn. *Symptom to Diagnosis: An Evidence-Based Guide*. New York: McGraw-Hill Medical, 2009. Written for medical students, doctors, and other health care providers, this book starts with the symptom and explains the appropriate evaluations, in case-study format. Appropriate and accessible even to those without formal medical training.

Thomas, Lewis. *The Youngest Science*. London: Penguin Books, 1995. Looking back at a lifetime in clinical medicine, a physician's essays illustrate what we've learned, what we've lost, and what we have yet to accomplish.

Wanderer, Alan A. *Hives: The Road to Diagnosis and Treatment of Urticaria*. Bozeman, MT: AnsonPublishing, LLC, 2003. Getting a little out of date, but nonetheless, the basic science and information in this book is still dependable.

Weinberg, Robert. *The Biology of Cancer*. New York: Garland Science, 2013. Detailed and very up-to-date information about the cellular, biochemical, and genetic basis of cancer, written at a college to medical school level.

Wen, Laura, and Joshua Kosowsky. *When Doctors Don't Listen: How to Avoid Misdiagnoses and Unnecessary Tests*. New York: Thomas Dunne Books, 2013. Real-life case presentations reveal how doctors can make mistakes—and how patients can help prevent them.

Internet Resources

AIDS.gov. http://aids.gov/. Government-sponsored site that includes links to news, comprehensive background information, and resources to help families and patients with HIV and AIDS.

American Cancer Society. http://www.cancer.org/. Solid information and resources from the American Cancer Society about cancer prevention and treatment.

American Diabetes Association. http://www.diabetes.org/. The American Diabetes Association site features in-depth and practical information about preventing and fighting diabetes.

American Heart Association. http://www.heart.org. The American Heart Association's website is a truly encyclopedic site of solid information on heart health and modern treatments for heart disease.

Centers for Disease Control (CDC). http://cdc.gov/. The authoritative site for health information on epidemic disease, vaccinations, and traveler's health.

———. http://www.cdc.gov/flu/. The CDC's guide to influenza prevention and treatment, including links to maps showing flu activity in your area.

———. http://www.cdc.gov/measles/pubs-mmwr.html. A compilation of articles about measles from the CDC.

———. http://www.cdc.gov/ncbddd/sicklecell/index.html. Information from the CDC that is organized into topics such as general information about sickle-cell disease, living with sickle-cell disease, and links to ongoing research.

Endometriosis.org. http://endometriosis.org/. News, links to support groups, solid information—just about anything anyone needs to know and the resources people need to get healthy.

Medscape. http://emedicine.medscape.com/. Written for physicians but open to the public, this site includes monographs on almost any disease you'd want to learn about—the symptoms, the cause, the treatment.

MS Soft Serve. http://mssoftserve.org/. A unique and wonderful nonprofit site that provides great information for learning about multiple sclerosis at your own pace.

Pediatrics. http://pediatrics.aappublications.org/content/122/5/1142.full. From the American Academy of Pediatrics, a well-referenced and authoritative guideline to the prevention of vitamin D deficiency in infants, children, and adolescents.

Vestibular Disorders Association. http://vestibular.org/. Detailed and informative site about Ménière's disease and other vestibular disorders, with plenty of links to solid information and resources.

WebMD. http://www.webmd.com/depression/. For people who think they might be depressed, for their families, or for those recently diagnosed, this site offers solid information on resources and management.

Notes